Aphasia

Aphasia

· · · · · · · · · · ·

A Clinical Perspective

D. FRANK BENSON

ALFREDO ARDILA

New York   Oxford

OXFORD UNIVERSITY PRESS

1996

Oxford University Press

Oxford   New York
Athens   Auckland   Bangkok   Bombay
Calcutta   Cape Town   Dar es Salaam   Delhi
Florence   Hong Kong   Istanbul   Karachi
Kuala Lumpur   Madras   Madrid   Melbourne
Mexico City   Nairobi   Paris   Singapore
Taipei   Tokyo   Toronto

and associated companies in
Berlin   Ibadan

Copyright © 1996 by Oxford University Press, Inc.

Published by Oxford University Press, Inc.,
198 Madison Avenue, New York, New York 10016

Oxford is a registered trademark of Oxford University Press

Library of Congress Cataloging-in-Publication Data
Benson, D. Frank (David Frank), 1928–
Aphasia : a clinical perspective /
D. Frank Benson, Alfredo Ardila.
p. cm. Includes bibliographical references and index.
ISBN 0-19-508934-0
1. Aphasia.
I. Ardila, Alfredo.   II. Title.
[DNLM: 1. Aphasia.   WL 340.5 B474ab 1996]
RC425.B457   1996   616.85'52—dc20
DNLM/DLC   for Library of Congress   95-31243

9 8 7 6 5 4 3

Printed in the United States of America
on acid-free paper

Preface

In 1979 one of us (D.F.B.) published a monograph called *Aphasia, Alexia, and Agraphia* that stressed the clinical-neuroanatomical approach developed at the Boston Veterans Administration (VA) Hospital in the 1960s and early 1970s. Although the book was limited to the neurologist's view of acquired language disorder, it proved to be of value for many disciplines and has been consistently used as a text.

Some years ago Alfredo Ardila suggested that a second edition of the 1979 monograph was needed as the original had become dated. But second editions, while demanding a great deal of work, are intellectually confining. Instead, we decided to write a new book on aphasia based on our combined experiences and attempting to incorporate many of the advances made in the understanding of aphasia over the last fifteen years. We have retained the clinical approach of the original monograph but covered many of the new approaches to the various facets of language impairment.

The senior author (D.F.B.) spent fifteen years as a member of the team of aphasia specialists that worked at the Boston VA Hospital Aphasia Research Center (sometimes referred to as the "Boston School of Aphasia"). As a fellow under the direction of such eminent figures as Norman Geschwind, Harold Goodglass, Edith Kaplan, Robert Sparks, and Frederick Quadfasel and later as a co-investigator, D.F.B. worked with the many neurology fellows who trained in aphasia and neurobehavior at the Boston VA Hospital. Many of these former colleagues have attained eminent positions in the field of aphasia and related disorders. In addition, a number of accomplished young psychologists, linguists, and speech pathologists also trained or worked at the Aphasia Research Center of the Boston VA Hospital during this period. From this combined experience, a multidisciplinary approach to acquired language disorder was developed. The neurologic aspects of this team approach were featured in the original monograph.

The co-author (A.A.) of this book had a different background. After initial training in psychology in Bogota, Colombia, A.A. attended Moscow State University where he received a doctorate degree in neuropsychology under the renowned neuropsychologist Aleksandr R. Luria. In his four years in Moscow, he not only mastered the Russian language but also became familiar with Luria's approach to the psychological functions of the brain, including language function. The Luria approach, while basically psychological, was developed from a vast experience in the clinical evaluation of brain-injured subjects; it also has a strong clinical orientation. After returning to his native Colombia, A.A. actively pursued a career in research and teaching covering a variety of neuropsychological subjects but maintained a special interest in aphasia and related disorders.

In this book we have tried to combine the clinical and neuropsychological approaches of these two major schools of thought on aphasia developed in the second half of the twentieth century. We have also reviewed some of the other approaches to the investigation of aphasia taken in the past few decades. Both the Boston and the Russian schools view aphasia as a clinical problem, not an academic exercise, however; thus the main focus of this book is on the clinical aspects of aphasia and related disorders.

The relatively recent advent of neuroimaging, the advances in the assessment of language disorders, and to a lesser degree the modeling efforts of neurolinguists have enhanced our ability to localize and characterize aphasia-producing brain lesions. These developments have had considerable importance in aphasia research and have provided valuable insights for the clinician. As much as possible, material from all three fields has been incorporated into this volume.

The authors would like to thank their many colleagues who have offered them inspiration, constructive criticism, and a breadth of experience and knowledge. In many ways, we have acted largely as conduits, using this volume to express ideas that have been gathered from many sources. Much of the material demands interpretation, however, and most of the interpretations in this book are our own.

Finally, we wish to give sincere thanks to Ms. Bonita Porch whose expertise provided not only effective secretarial supervision but also invaluable editorial assistance and constructive criticism during the entire production of the manuscript. Her efforts, particularly in the final excruciating months, were instrumental in the completion of the volume. And both authors wish to express our appreciation for the patience and loyal support provided by our wives, Donna Benson and Monica Rosselli-Ardila. The dedication, support, and selfless efforts of these three individuals made this volume possible.

Los Angeles, Calif.   D. F. B.

March 1995   A. A.

Contents

I Basic Considerations

II Syndromology

III Related Disorders

IV Rehabilitation

I

BASIC
CONSIDERATIONS

. . . .

1

What Is Aphasia?

· ·

Aphasia is the loss or impairment of language function caused by brain damage.

Despite considerable variation in wording reflecting attempts at greater precision, this basic definition is accepted by virtually all clinicians and investigators dealing with aphasia. The appearance of fundamental agreement is illusory, however. Aphasia was born of controversy, has a history of ongoing disagreements about appropriate approaches and remains a contentious topic. Rather than cooly discussed, viewpoints on aphasia are often hotly argued and the debate has sometimes become downright acrimonious. In recent years, investigators appear increasingly willing to accept and utilize distinctly different approaches; a tendency remains, however, for viewpoints on aphasia to be both diverse and contested.

Much of the longstanding controversy can be traced directly to the definition of aphasia—not what aphasia is, but what it represents. All aphasiologists agree that aphasia is an impairment of language function and almost all accept that it is a result of brain damage. The controversy stems largely from differing interpretations of the word *language*, a knotty problem that must be faced before a meaningful discussion of aphasia can be presented.

Language refers to a system of communication, but over the years the term has accumulated a number of additional, divergent connotations, many of which are not germane to a discussion of aphasia. In most instances, the nonuniform uses of the word are the products of specialized academic disciplines. Merely listing some of the scholarly uses of *language* will highlight the problem and provide a background to develop a working definition of aphasia for this book.

The interpretation of literature, the comparison of national tongues and dialects and the analysis of linguistic structures are well-established, respected scholarly disciplines. All three are acknowledged to be studies of language, but they use the term in distinctly different ways. Some scholars in these disciplines have utilized aphasia as a resource for their studies. As it is a problem of language, for instance, it has been argued, emphatically and reasonably, that aphasia falls within the province of linguistics (Jakobson, 1964). Numerous models of the mechanisms of language formulation have been devised in recent years; when appropriate, the features of aphasia have been used to support or refute the models. Increasingly, language attributes highlighted by the study of aphasia (e.g., disordered grammar) are built into the proposed linguistic models.

Language is also a cognitive function, however, and falls within the province of psychology. Any number of psychological subspecialties have developed particular interests in communication, verbal symbolism, language development and other language-oriented topics. With increasing frequency, abnormal language (aphasia) is used for investigative work by branches of psychology. Students of developmental psychology have carefully charted the development of language and utilized the delayed acquisition or actual loss of language in childhood to derive and support theories of language development. Both experimental psychologists and learning-theory specialists have utilized observations on aphasia to investigate aspects of their own disciplines. On the basis of their models, they offer explanations of language disorder. Most of these investigators use secondhand information, observations and/or theories culled from the aphasia literature and carefully selected to bolster the preferred theory of language function.

The most directly involved of the psychological subdisciplines is the comparatively new discipline of neuropsychology which stands between neurology and psychology. Much current neuropsychological research deals with the residual cognitive capabilities of persons with damaged brains, and aphasia has always ranked among the most important areas for neuropsychological investigation. Psycholinguistics, a robust relation of neuropsychology, investigates variations in the use of language based on multiple factors, including brain damage (Goodglass, 1993).

In addition to the direct concerns of the linguist and the psychologist, other academic specialists have serious if somewhat more tangential interests in language and aphasia. Based on the observation that language and thought are intimately intertwined, philosophers have long expressed interest in language and, to a limited degree, its impairments. Philosophical speculations concerning the relationship of language and thought go back for centuries and are still being developed (Arendt, 1978; Corballis, 1991; Dennett, 1986; Fodor, 1983; Popper and Eccles, 1977). Language as an attribute of mind remains a contemporary theme that clearly influences the definition of language.

Both speech and language are functions of the brain; neuroanatomists, neurophysiologists, neuropathologists, neurochemists and other neuroscientists include language in their studies of brain function and at times utilize pathologically derived language breakdown as a research tool. Most neuroscientists deal with more basic nervous system operations but one recently established discipline—neurolinguistics—is devoted to study of the organization of brain mechanisms that are active in verbal functions. Using current linguistic theories, neurolinguists investigate the neurophysiological mechanisms underlying language manipulations (perception and production), verbal memory, hemispheric lateralization of language involvement and similar problems. Many of the theories of language function proposed by neurolinguists derive directly or indirectly from observations of aphasic subjects.

Aphasia interferes with verbal output, impinging upon the function usually called speech, and aphasia has become a concern of the specialty known as speech pathology. Most formal therapy for aphasia is provided by individuals trained in speech (language) therapy. Although interest in aphasia therapy developed relatively recently, speech (language) pathology has become a strong specialty. Speech pathologists have also produced several theories of language, consistent with their approach to verbal function. Speech pathology was originally taught in schools of education; in addition to the obvious educational aspects of retraining an aphasic subject to communicate, this drew educators into aphasia therapy, producing a particularly rich source for theories that link language and learning.

Aphasia produces disorders in behavior and may eventually result in serious adjustment problems; both psychiatrists and clinical psychologists have become involved with aphasic patients. These specialists also contribute to discussions of aphasia. Both psychiatric influences on the meaning of language and the psychological consequences of language impairment are of significance in characterizing aphasia.

Finally, aphasia is a product of brain damage and thus falls within the scope of neurologists. Aphasia was an early and decidedly important influence on the development of neurology as a medical specialty and remains the most firmly established example of neurologically based behavior disorder. By correlating language-processing disorders with focal brain lesions, the anatomically oriented neurologist brings yet another approach to the study of language.

Each group mentioned above has legitimate reasons to study aspects of aphasia. Fascinating but widely diverse characterizations of language coexist and each has significance within the chosen sphere. It is easy to see, however, that an operational definition of language used in one discipline may disagree or even compete with that held by other groups. Thus, disagreement over definition prevails. The various consequences of the breakdown of language in aphasia can be used to support or refute theories of language function that are based on diverse approaches. Since its inception, aphasia has been a malleable pawn in attempts to understand one of the brain's most important attributes—language. The controversies involve the clinical characteristics of aphasia far less than the theories of language function. Because aphasia is an important disorder, a purely clinical approach is meaningful for its own sake. Unfortunately, aphasia is difficult to discuss without reference to some theory of language function and most clinical studies of aphasia postulate some mechanism of language organization. The clinical studies generate their own quota of theoretical disagreement.

Definitions

Based on the varied approaches to aphasia it can be anticipated that individual investigators will define the basic terms surrounding language and language defects idiosyncratically. To counteract this problem, a number of key terms will be discussed here. Although they are also idiosyncratic, these definitions will at least provide a degree of consistency in this book.

Aphasia

There is comparatively little disagreement over the definition of *aphasia* itself. Many different investigators (Adams and Victor, 1977; Benson and Geschwind, 1971; Darley, 1975; Goodglass, 1993; Luria, 1966; Nielsen, 1936) give almost identical definitions that are paraphrases of the first sentence of this chapter: *aphasia is the loss or impairment of language function caused by brain damage.* Among the more detailed definitions, Darley, Aronson, and Brown (1975) describe aphasia as "a multi-modality reduction in the capacity to decode (interpret) and encode (formulate) meaningful linguistic elements. It is manifested in difficulties in listening, reading, speaking and writing." Kertesz (1985) defined aphasia as "an acquired loss of language due to cerebral damage, characterized by errors in speech (paraphasias), impaired comprehension, and word-finding difficulties (anomia)." For virtually all investigators, the basic meaning remains similar; the controversy centers on the meaning of language, not the meaning of aphasia. In fact, the level of disagreement is sufficiently low that many discussants accept that the reader is fully cognizant of the term's meaning and offer neither definition nor characterization.

Speech, Language, and Thought

The terms *speech, language,* and *thought* have gathered many meanings, most differing only slightly. Yet a meaning useful for one discipline may have limited relevance for others. Differences in the definitions of these terms are detected only by careful scrutiny, but they can engender obscurity. To obviate this problem here, we will introduce operational definitions for these terms and the three functions will be further separated on the basis of disorders that involve only one of the functions.

Speech can be defined as the mechanical aspect of communication; oral speech demands the combination of appropriate neuromuscular activity to produce phonation and articulation. Purely oral speech disorders, usually termed *dysarthrias*, are based on defects in the neuromuscular activities (respiration, phonation, articulation) needed to produce oral speech. Both writing and gesture can be considered forms of speech and many neuromuscular defects (both central and peripheral) can interfere with their function in language. In most discussions, however, only the oral-communication aspect is implied by the term *speech*.

Patients with speech disorders but no disturbance of either language or thought are common in clinical practice. Laryngitis is the most frequent cause of "pure" speech disorder but an entirely neurological example is bulbar paralysis due to poliomyelitis or amyotrophic lateral sclerosis that can produce dysarthria, hypophonia, and even mutism. Although the impairment of mechanical speech may be extreme, language remains intact. If a substitute means of communication can be established, the patient demonstrates full and appropriate language capability. Advanced parkinsonism may affect the motor competency of the verbal output mechanism so seriously that no output occurs; again, no language problem need be present. Many other examples of speech loss not associated with either language or thought disorder are recognized (Metter, 1985).

Language can be separated from the purely mechanical aspects of speech, but, as already noted, a simple operational description of language is difficult. If language is defined as the communication of meaningful symbols, language disturbance would incorporate difficulties in comprehending (decoding) and/or programming (encoding) communication symbols. Aphasia is the clinical expression of language disturbance and although it is frequently combined with either speech or thought disorder (or both), it can occur as a pure abnormality of symbolic communication.

Because aphasia is a language disorder, some fundamental linguistic terms deserve definition. These will be discussed in detail in Chapter 4. Four basic subdivisions of language—gesture, prosody, semantics, and syntax—deserve recognition. *Gesture* refers to nonverbalized motor acts that convey meaning (e.g., shaking the fist). *Prosody* refers to a number of physical characteristics of vocal output including rhythm, melody, and intonation (e.g., an angry or sad intonation). *Semantics* represents the system of meanings conveyed by language (e.g., the use of a word or symbol for an object or action). *Syntax* reflects the method used to combine words into a meaningful relationship (e.g., the difference between "mother's brother" and "brother's mother"). Impairment in any of the four subdivisions of language can disturb communication. In medical practice, however, disturbances of prosody or gesture without problems in the syntactic or semantic aspects of language are usually not classed as aphasic language impairments. In this book, *language* will refer only to phonology (study of vocal sounds), morphology (study of the forms and structures of verbalization), semantics, and syntax, unless modified (e.g., gestural language).

Thought, the third term, is the most resistant to description. Many philosophers insist that language and thought cannot be separated (Arendt, 1978; Merleau-Ponty, 1964; Watson, 1930). A number of clinical observations indicate that a significant distinction exists between language and thought. Just as relatively pure speech and pure language disorders can occur in patients, certain disease states represent relatively pure "thought" disorders. For instance, schizophrenia can produce a characteristically abnormal verbal output with neither speech nor language defect. Thus, the psychotic schizophrenic who manifests severe disorder of rational thought can express the irrational thoughts through competent use of language. Word selection and grammar are not only intact in such patients but may be remarkably apt (Benson, 1973). Similarly, severely depressed patients may have disordered ideation but little or no problem verbally expressing their morbid thoughts. In some stages of dementia, significant deficiencies in thought processing can be demonstrated in patients whose language is relatively intact; as dementia progresses, however, most such individuals develop serious problems in speech or language. It is not unusual for a patient with early Alzheimer's disease symptomatology to show an adequate vocabulary and fully normal syntactic competence but deficient cognitive abilities.

Disturbances in communication via writing (agraphia) and gesture (disordered body language) are common in clinical practice. They may be based entirely on peripheral motor problems such as muscular dystrophy, but both language disturbances and abnormal ideation can also produce abnormalities of writing and gesture.

In the evaluation of aphasic patients, when disorder of one function (speech, language, or thought) is present, at least some symptoms relating to the others are almost always present. Pure states are relatively rare and most aphasic patients have problems in two or even all three categories. Nonetheless, speech, language or thought can be involved separately and each has independent significance. Aphasia should be considered a disturbance of language and kept separate from disturbances of thought or speech (Benson, 1975). Disorder of either thought or speech in an aphasic individual is a nonlanguage complication. In the common situation where a language disturbance is coupled with either speech or thought disturbance, the individual disorders must be recognized; etiology, prognosis, and therapy will vary depending on the mix of problems, and theories of language function can be seriously compromised if the distinction is not recognized.

Summary

This book is designed to provide clinical information concerning aphasia for the use of practicing neurologists, neuropsychologists, and speech (language) pathologists. It will present as much useful clinical information as possible and will unabashedly utilize a classic localizationist approach to aphasia. The information presented here is intended neither to confirm nor to refute any present or past theory of language. Rather, it represents a collection of clinical observations from the authors' experiences and from the world literature.

Most aphasia literature is couched in terms that presuppose a single theory of language function. Individually, most such presentations are understandable; the literature as a whole, however, contains so many conflicting theories that coherence is lost. Writings on aphasia are notorious for their inexact use of terminology and confusing theories. As far as possible, theoretical aspects will be avoided in this volume, but aphasia is a multidisciplinary subject and valuable information concerning language function is available from many sources. When pertinent, nonclinical data of potential value to the clinician will be included.

The goal of this book is to aid the practicing clinician in understanding and caring for patients with aphasia. Some of the clinical observations discussed in this volume may prove useful for scientific investigation of language but the picture of aphasia described here remains incomplete. Additional observations are constantly being added to this already huge corpus, and both better care for the aphasic patient and improved theories of language function can be anticipated in the future.

2

Historical Background

······································

Writings on the history of aphasia naturally tend to be slanted toward the views of their authors. Some reveal a strong national prejudice, some emphasize the contributions of specific investigators and others have a particular theoretical bias. Especially recommended reviews are those of Freud (1891/1953), Head (1926), Weisenburg and McBride (1935/1964), Benton and Joynt (1960), Brain (1961), Quadfasel (1968), Hécaen and Albert (1978), Benson (1979a), Arbib, Caplan, and Marshall (1982), Lecours and colleagues (1983), and Goodglass (1993).

The modern conception of aphasia can be said to have commenced with the 1861 presentation by Broca of a case of aphasia associated with a focal brain lesion. Acquired language loss following brain injury had been reported far earlier, however, and a critically important historical prodrome preceded the 1861 presentation. The surveys of pre-Broca reports by Benton and Joynt (1960), Benton (1964), Boller (1977), and others showed that acquired language disorders had been noted for many centuries. Benton and Joynt (1960) asserted that "almost all the clinical forms of aphasia—complete motor aphasia, paraphasia, jargon aphasia, agraphia and alexia—had been described before 1800." In most instances, however, these reports detailed individual cases only crudely describing the language disorder along with many other effects of brain injury. Most of the pre-Broca reports made no attempt to correlate the observation of language disorder with either the site of brain damage or the characteristic language process disturbed. Although acquired language impairment has been recognized since antiquity, it was not separated from other manifestations of brain damage.

Prodrome: From Gall to Broca

Among the first to attempt or even to suggest the correlation of individual psychological functions with discrete areas of the brain was Franz Joseph Gall (Gall and Spurzheim, 1810–1819) (Figure 2.1). Gall contended that the apparently uniform mass of tissue that makes up the brain contained separate organs (areas) and that each organ subserved a specific intellectual or moral faculty. Based on considerable dissection of human and animal brains (Gall easily ranks among the foremost neuroanatomists of his day) and his knowledge of the psychophilosophical tenets of the day, Gall categorized human brain function into three major subdivisions: (1) vital force; (2) inclinations of the soul; (3) intellectual qualities of the mind. He localized the vital force to the brainstem and considered the soul to be a function of the basal ganglia. The intellectual qualities of the human mind were located in various but consistent regions of the cerebral cortex (Young, 1970/1990).

Gall distinguished six varieties of memory—(1) verbal memory—the sense of words and names; (2) grammatical memory—the talent for languages and philosophy; (3) memory of the relation of numbers; (4) memories of locality; (5) memories of colors; and (6) memories of the tonic harmony of music. In Gall's vision of brain function, each major psychological function could be localized to an organ situated in the convolutions of the brain. Based on a general rostral-caudal division of functions and abetted by a limited number of clinical observations, Gall localized the faculty of speech, a product of verbal and grammatical memories, to the most anterior parts of the cortex—the frontal lobes (Young, 1970/1990).

Gall's views were revolutionary, sufficiently divergent from the scholastic dogma of the era to be declared heretical. Gall was forced to vacate his post in Vienna, eventually settling in Paris with a student-collaborator, J. C. Spurzheim. Gall and Spurzheim produced a multivolume opus on human and animal neuroanatomy (1810–1819) that included some of the localization philosophy propounded by Gall. Not long after this, Gall and Spurzheim separated. Spurzheim focused his efforts on delineation of human psychological qualities through measurement of the variability of skull size and shape (craniology), an approach that eventually became the "science" of phrenology that was practiced widely in the nineteenth century. Spurzheim and his followers proposed many additional mental faculties (up to forty) and provided psychological counseling based on presumed differences in these faculties as indicated by the individual's skull configuration. Phrenology was originally devised as a serious endeavor to understand brain function, but it eventually became tainted by distortion and outright fraud and has now come to epitomize mental chicanery.

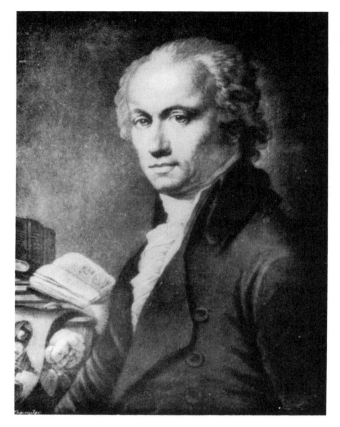

Figure 2.1. Franz Joseph Gall (1758–1828). (From Hedderly, 1970).

Unfortunately, Gall's name and reputation have been stigmatized by the aura of deceit that surrounds phrenology. Gall maintained his belief in the correlation of brain anatomy with psychological functions but was unable to advance beyond his original premises. A unitary, spiritually guided conception of mind prevailed; most of Gall's contemporaries violently opposed the idea that mental functions could be separated, much less localized within parts of the brain. In particular, Pierre Flourens (1846), an accomplished experimentalist who pioneered ablation techniques for the study of brain function, vehemently criticized phrenology and discredited Gall's attempts to localize mental functions within the separate areas of the brain. Flourens (1846) maintained that the qualities of feeling, willing, and perceiving represented a single, essentially unitary, faculty residing in a single biological organ—the brain. This view predominated through the first half of the nineteenth century and contained the basic premises promoted by later holistic approaches such as those of K. S. Lashley, the Gestalt psychologists and others. Very few scholars of influence supported Gall and his premise of localization of function within the brain.

There were exceptions, however. The most prominent proponent of Gall's thesis was Jean-Baptiste Bouillaud (1825), a powerful and influential academic physician in early nineteenth-century France. Based on over forty case observations, Bouillaud, in 1825, published a paper entitled "Clinical Research Able to Show That the Loss of Speech Corresponds to a Lesion of the Anterior Lobules to the Brain and to Confirm Mr. Gall's Opinion on the Seat of Articulated Language." Throughout his life Bouillaud continued to champion the views of Gall but met with strong opposition and little support. The unitary theories of Flourens and the scholastics prevailed.

Debate on whether the brain was unitary in function waxed and waned during these years, with the controversy becoming particularly strong during meetings of a Parisian anthropological society in 1861. Pierre Gratiolet, an embryologist who had previously demonstrated a primitive skull with a relatively small brain volume (1854), opened a discussion on whether brain size alone determined the cultural level of the subject. Indirectly, the deliberations also pondered whether the brain functioned as a whole or was composed of multiple organs or centers. Engaged in the ensuing discussion were a physician, Ernst Auburtin (Bouillaud's son-in-law), and Paul Broca, a surgeon. Auburtin firmly supported the theory of localization of mental functions within discrete brain areas and in a report to the anthropological society he emphasized the importance of pathological studies including some that provided evidence suggesting frontal lobe localization of the faculty of speech. The cogency of this premise impressed Broca who invited Auburtin to examine one of his patients who had lost the faculty of speech. Shortly after this examination the patient expired, the brain was removed and Broca demonstrated it the following day at the April 1861 meeting of the anthropological society. The incident received relatively little attention, but four months later Broca (1861a) presented a more extensive neuroanatomical report that stressed the frontal locus of brain damage in combination with the loss of the faculty of speech. Three months later, Broca (1861b) reported postmortem findings of a second patient with longstanding loss of verbal function (see Figure 2.2). These communications produced considerable excitement in the medical world and the first epoch in the history of aphasia commenced.

Epoch I: From Broca to Marie

The clinical observations and subsequent correlations with postmortem material presented by Broca were widely discussed and the technique of clinical-

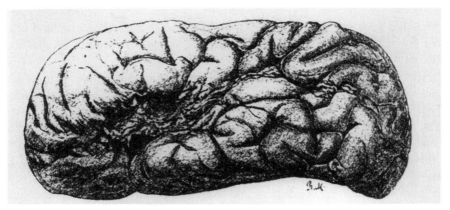

Figure 2.2. Drawing of the fixed specimen of the brain of Broca's second patient. Note posterior-inferior frontal location of old cortical scar. (From Brain, 1961).

anatomical correlation was immediately reported, but other reports observed disturbed language function in patients whose lesion did not involve the frontal lobes. A striking example (observed by Broca) was of a patient, demonstrated by Charcot, who had suffered a loss of speech for many years but at postmortem had no obvious frontal lobe damage (Head, 1926). The patient's lesion involved the first and second temporal gyri, the greater part of the insula, and much of the corpus striatum. By this time Broca was aware that the left hemisphere was involved more than the right. In 1863 Broca reported eight cases in which language output (speech) was abnormal and in which the left frontal lobe was damaged at postmortem. One additional case in that report had right frontal damage but no speech disturbance. Broca stated: "Here are 8 cases where the lesion is situated in the posterior portion of the third frontal convolution . . . and a most remarkable thing, in all of these patients the lesion is on the left side. I do not dare make a conclusion and I await new findings." Additional cases were reported and in 1865 Broca bluntly stated, "We speak with the left hemisphere." It has been suggested that Broca leaped to this conclusion because of the discovery of an earlier report by Dax (1836) noting that right hemiplegia was far more common than left hemiplegia in patients with an acquired speech disturbance (Benton and Joynt, 1960; Dax, 1865). Dax's early report had never been published, and Broca is rightly credited with the formal declaration of hemispheric specialization for language.

In 1868 Broca presented an invited lecture on the "Physiology of Speech" at the annual meeting of the British Association for the Advancement of Science (Head, 1926). He not only presented evidence favoring the left hemisphere as the site of speech but divided acquired language disturbances into two major categories, *"aphemie"* and *"amnesie verbale."* According to Broca, aphemie was a disorder in which verbal output was limited, whereas amnesie verbale was a disorder in which the patient pronounced words adequately but lost the ability to associate ideas with words. Broca considered the latter to be a memory disorder affecting spoken and written words.

Although Broca clearly outlined major differences in aphasia, he was not prepared to localize any faculty of language except that of articulate speech. Other investigators, however, recognized the potential for a series of functional components within language and their possible neuroanatomical correlation. The seminal presentation on language and brain was a dissertation by a young neuroanatomist/neuropsychiatrist, Carl Wernicke (1874), who presented descriptions of two distinct types of aphasia—motor and sensory—as well as anatomical-pathological demonstrations to support this division (Geschwind, 1967c; Wernicke, 1874). Wernicke also postulated a third language disorder (presently called conduction aphasia) based on his bimodal sensory-motor scheme of brain function. Wernicke's original proposal was modified, expanded, and clarified over the next few years to become the cornerstone of clinical-anatomical correlation studies.

A paper, "On Aphasia," published in *Brain* (Lichtheim, 1885) presented a simple diagrammatic illustration of Wernicke's anatomical-psychological model of language function (see Figure 2.3). Lichtheim's scheme, supported by selected case reports, provided a powerful presentation of the anatomical basis of selected language functions, and the Wernicke-Lichtheim model remains the basic structure of most brain-language correlations.

Many other works purporting to show neuroanatomical localization of spe-

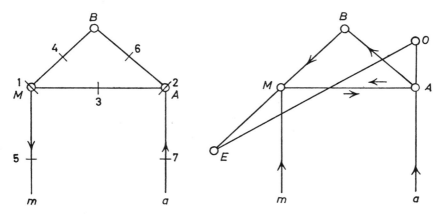

Figure 2.3. Diagrams of the Wernicke-Lichtheim (1885) model of the neural basis of language: *(A)* auditory; *(M)* motor; *(B)* ideation. In the right-sided diagram, *E* = motivation. The numbers in the left-sided diagram indicate areas in which disconnection would produce distinct language and/or cognition disorder. (From Lichtheim, 1885).

cific language functions have proposed to augment the basic Wernicke-Lichtheim scheme. Charcot (1877, 1889), Bastian (1898), Exner (1881), Kussmaul (1877), Dejerine (1914), Henschen (1922), Nielsen (1936), and others produced variations on this classic postulation. The various schemes were not always in agreement and, altogether too often, the proposed anatomical correlation of a variation of language impairment was based on a single case. Most reports were observations of language function made during the life of the patient and ascribed to a neuroan-atomical locus of pathology demonstrated at postmortem. The psychological find-ings were expressed in the jargon of the day, and with few exceptions the anatomi-cal description involved the cortical surface only. Selected cortical areas were proposed as "centers," essential for a specific language function (although some investigators were aware of and even described networks). Proposed centers in-cluded such entities as a gleidokinetic center, a writing center, an auditory-verbal image center, a center for symbols, a center for object images, and numerous others. Discussion and debate concerning the neuroanatomical loci of various psy-chological functions became popular; a phrenology of language was developed. During the late nineteenth century many cases of aphasia, correlated with post-mortem data, were reported in detail, along with postulations of functional activi-ties carried out by various brain centers. Much of this early correlative material was collected by Solomon Henschen, who published a report on 1,337 cases of aphasia with sufficient neuroanatomical localization information to allow clinical-pathological correlation (Henschen, 1922). Henschen's monumental work was published too late, however, to exert any influence on the early development of aphasia investigations and remains virtually unknown.

Epoch II: From Marie to Geschwind

During the period in which the clinical-pathological correlations prevailed, a group of scholars steadfastly adhered to another, quite different view of language disturbance—one that stressed overall brain function. An early and eventually influential proponent of this more unitary psychological approach was John Hughlings Jackson (1864, 1915, 1932), an English neurologist who carefully stud-ied patients with aphasia from a dynamic, psychological viewpoint rather than from the static, neuroanatomical basis favored on the continent. Jackson was aware of and influenced by Broca, and vice versa (Arbib, Caplan, and Marshall, 1982). Unfortunately, Jackson's writings were difficult to understand and his opinions were neither recognized nor accepted for many years. In 1891 Sigmund Freud published a monograph, obviously influenced by Jackson, that proposed a holistic approach to aphasia and roundly criticized the contemporary "diagram-makers." Freud's monograph received scant attention (it sold only 257 copies in ten years). Not until the dramatic and easily comprehendable presentations of Pierre Marie (1906a,b,c) did the holistic point of view influence a wide audience.

Marie (Figure 2.4) presented a series of papers provocatively entitled "The Third Frontal Convolution Does Not Play Any Special Role in the Function of Language," reopening the Gall-Flourens arguments. Marie's statement did not go unchallenged; opposing articles were published and another debate, similar to that of 1861, took place in 1908 (Lecours et al., 1992). Jules Dejerine, a proponent of the localizationist approach opposed Marie's broader, more holistic viewpoint. Based on reexamination of the brains of Broca's first two patients, Marie claimed that the frontal-lobe pathology reported by many investigators was not the cause of the disordered language activities (Brais, 1992; Cole, 1968). Marie

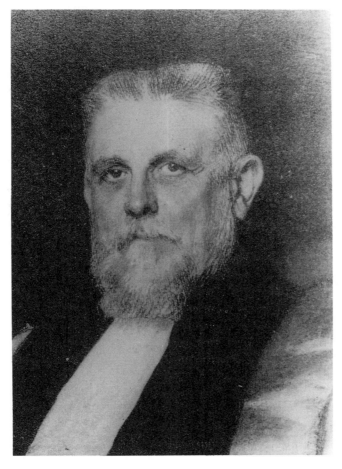

Figure 2.4. Pierre Marie (1853–1940). (From Haymaker and Schiller, 1953).

asserted that every aphasic patient suffered some degree of intellectual dysfunction, but he accepted only the disturbance originally described by Wernicke as a true aphasia. The Dejerine-Marie debate was, typically, unresolved, but the influence of the holistic approach on aphasia steadily increased from that point and garnered many significant advocates over the early part of the twentieth century (Head, 1926; Wilson, 1926; Pick, 1931/1973; Isserlin, 1929, 1931, 1932; Weisenburg and McBride, 1935/1964; Wepman, 1951; Bay, 1964; Schuell, Jenkins, and Jimenez-Pabon, 1964; Critchley, 1970b).

During this epoch a number of students of aphasia (including Marie [Marie and Foix, 1917]) recognized that damage to certain neuroanatomical locations consistently produced specific clusters of clinical symptoms but their approach to language deficits emphasized the psychologic and linguistic residuals rather than the neurologic or anatomical defects. One influential investigator, Henry Head, observed and tested a series of aphasic subjects and from the data collected, proposed a linguistic categorization of aphasia (1926) with four distinct types—verbal aphasia (defective articulatory and auditory functions), nominal aphasia (disconnection of the sign from its meaning), syntactical aphasia (defective grammatical arrangements), and semantic aphasia (defective intellectual, including nonverbal, function). Head's classification satisfied academic and intellectual needs and was cited frequently for almost a half century but did not prove useful in clinical practice (Brain, 1961; Humphrey, 1951; Weisenburg and McBride, 1935/1964). Following Head's lead, subsequent investigators utilized various linguistic-psychological approaches to the study of aphasia. One result, the introduction of linguistic terminology to the aphasia literature, further compounded an already unmanageable terminology problem. Head (1926) had described the era of the diagram makers as "chaos," and then added a bewildering new complication.

Some brain scientists, not otherwise psychologically oriented, were also unwilling to accept the direct correlation of focal brain lesions with specific language impairments. Constantin von Monakow (1914, 1928) stated that there was no aphasia, only aphasic patients; he postulated that all cerebral pathology was accompanied by variable areas of malfunction including involvement of some regions distant from the primary site, a function he termed "diaschisis." The widespread scattering of anatomic dysfunction produced the variability in clinical impairment that characterized individual aphasic patients. While Monakow accepted that damage to the language area of the brain was the immediate source of language impairment, he recognized only motor and sensory variations and believed that enough distant dysfunction existed to invalidate localization of more specific language malfunctions in a given patient. Arnold Pick, a psychiatrist, studied aphasia from an almost purely psychological perspective and stressed two "moments"—psychological (the structuring of thought), and linguistic (the formulation of articulated language) (Pick, 1913, 1931/1973). Pick viewed aphasia as a disturbance of the mental activities connecting thought formation with its expression through language. Gestalt psychology (Koffka, 1935), best exemplified in aphasia by the work of Goldstein (1948) and Conrad (1954), promoted a strongly holistic approach to language impairment. In this formulation, damage to brain structure interfered with the basic function *(Gestalten)* of language by disturbing the global reactivity of the brain; aphasic symptomatology was derived from a combination of injury-produced sensory-motor and psychological functions of the brain. Under the Gestalt approach, psychological concepts could augment or even be substituted for the neuroanatomically based theories. Scientific support for the holistic approach came from the animal experiments of Lashley (1929), who interpreted his early investigations as demonstrations that cerebral functions were not the product of specific neuroanatomical structures but, rather, were based on integrated participation of masses of cerebral tissues. Lashley and his followers introduced rigid measurements and careful observations to their psychological studies, but in the end their investigations reaffirmed the importance of specific cerebral structures for selected psychological functions including language (Chapman and Wolfe, 1959; Gardner, 1985; Lashley, 1929).

Although it is accurate to divide the approaches to aphasia into two distinctly different camps (anatomically based localizationists and psychologically based holists), almost all investigators of impaired language utilize ideas from both approaches. Identical case material can be described in such different manners as to support totally diverse postulations for the language defect. Several influential aphasiologists have been linked with one theoretical approach but have produced meaningful work in the other. As an example, Kurt Goldstein (1948), recognized as a staunch proponent of the holistic (organismic) approach to aphasia, published some of the most clearly defined case descriptions of aphasia available in contemporary literature, often including excellent neuropathological correlation. The Russian neuropsychologist Aleksandr Luria (1947/1970, 1966) (Figure 2.5) expressed strong antilocalizationist views but provided excellent descriptions of aphasic syndromes and their anatomical correlations.

Interest in aphasia waned considerably during the first half of the twentieth century. It was revived when the care of brain-injured World War II servicemen led to the introduction of aphasia therapy, a new academic specialty that fostered increased interest in language impairment. Early aphasia therapy approaches remained holistic, and the unitary, brain-as-a-whole approach prevailed until the 1960s.

The first important publication in the postwar period was *Traumatic Aphasia* (1947), Luria's book based on the systematic observation of hundreds of war-wounded patients. Luria (Figure 2.5) took a midway stance between the localizationist and holistic approaches. He considered language to be a complex functional system, requiring many different steps in both comprehension and pro-

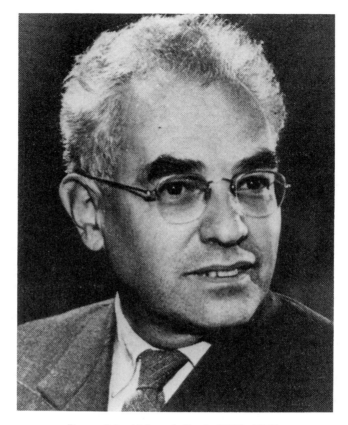

Figure 2.5. Aleksandr Luria (1902–1977).

duction; simultaneous participation of multiple cortical areas would be required for language processing. Although each cortical area performs a specific process, it also participates in different functional systems. Thus, the first temporal gyrus participates in phoneme discrimination, and its damage causes difficulty in all functional systems requiring phoneme discrimination (e.g., understanding spoken language, writing). Luria (1963) proposed a classification of aphasic disturbances based on the language features impaired. He also proposed a method for assessment of aphasic disorders based on error-analysis: the pass/fail criterion is not as important as the characteristics of the language errors produced and the associated errors in other cognitive abilities (syndrome analysis approach). Luria's approach to aphasia led to techniques for aphasia rehabilitation.

In the United States during the early 1950s, Hildred Schuell, a speech pathologist, studied the errors made by aphasic patients and promoted selected rehabilitation procedures. Her Minnesota Test for the Differential Diagnosis of Aphasia (Schuell, 1955) was used extensively for several decades. She proposed a typology of aphasic disorders based on severity rather than features and considered that a single general language factor could account for most of the deficits in the aphasic patient.

During the mid-1950s, the work of Roman Jakobson attracted a number of linguists to the aphasia arena. Jakobson observed that linguistics is the study of language, that aphasia is a language phenomenon, and that aphasia, therefore, lies in the domain of linguistics (Jakobson and Halle, 1956). Jakobson proposed a classification of aphasic disorders (Jakobson, 1964) based on linguistic concepts and influenced by the clinical reports and interpretations of aphasic disorders presented by Luria. Jakobson's linguistic analysis of aphasia phenomenology influenced, in return, the later publications of Luria (1976 a,b).

The American psychologist Joseph Wepman (1961) developed an aphasia examination based on the proposition that language operations could be defined as combinations of sensory input and motor output and that these functions could be sampled. He further proposed that there were five types of aphasia (syntactic, semantic, pragmatic, jargon, and global) (Wepman and Jones, 1964). Wepman's aphasia assessment has been widely used and portions have been incorporated into some current neuropsychological assessment battery tests.

Epoch III: Geschwind and the Return of Localization

The 1960s witnessed a remarkable increase in the interest in aphasia that coincided with the arrival of a vigorous new investigator, Norman Geschwind (1962, 1965a, b, 1967c) (Figure 2.6). Based on a few carefully studied cases—alexia without agraphia (Geschwind and Fusillo, 1966), anterior callosal disconnection (Geschwind and Kaplan (1962), and conduction aphasia (Geschwind, 1965)—and an extensive review of German, French, English, and American aphasiology literature, Geschwind proposed (actually reintroduced) a relatively novel concept, cortical disconnection, to explain many of the language and psychological impairments of aphasia. A brain lesion could affect either discrete cortical areas (the "centers" discussed in earlier literature) or the fibers connecting several of these areas (as suggested by some early investigators) or both. The differences in symptom clusters would then be based on the specific locus of the lesion, a return to anatomical-psychological correlation theory. In a series of papers published in *Brain* in 1965, Geschwind (1965a,b) presented the concept of disconnection and directly challenged the then dominant holistic theory. While not excluding considerable validity for the holistic concept, Geschwind warned that failure to consider the anatomical basis of language was actively misleading. His combination of pertinent clinical observations, superb scholarship, and vigorous presentation of a rational scientific-philosophic approach won the day. Localization theories

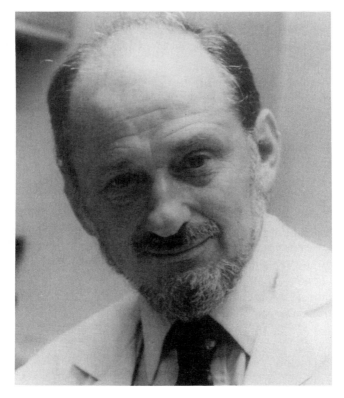

Figure 2.6. Norman Geschwind (1926–1984). (From Benson, 1983).

returned to a position of importance in the investigation of acquired language impairment.

Although he was rapidly promoted and eventually honored with a chair of neurology at Harvard, Geschwind's major investigative efforts in aphasia were centered at the Boston Veterans Administration (VA) Hospital where a number of specialists in related fields focused their interest on aphasia. While far from exclusive, the main focus of the Boston VA aphasia group was on the neuroanatomical localization of aphasia-producing lesions, a clinical-anatomical correlation that stressed the role of the neurologist. A number of young North American neurologists came to Boston for training in aphasia. M. Albert, M. Alexander, F. Benson, J. Brown, J. Cummings, M. Denckla, M. Freedman, S. Greenblatt, V. Henderson, A. Kertesz, A. Rubens, and R. Strub all were fellows at the Boston VA Aphasia Research Center. In addition, a number of foreign neurologists— F. Boller, A. Damasio, F. Denes, T. Landis, J. Meadows, T. von Stockert, A. Yamadori—had some of their training at the Boston VA facility. Following Geschwind's appointment to Harvard, a number of neurologists who trained under him at Boston City Hospital spent some time at the Boston VA Aphasia Research Center; these included A. Galaburda, K. Heilman, M.-M. Mesulam and E. Ross. These physicians became proficient in the clinical-anatomical correlation techniques introduced by Geschwind and most combined this competency with expertise in newly developed techniques in neuroanatomy, neurophysiology, neuropsychology, psycholinguistics and neurolinguistics, brain imaging, and/or language therapy. The neurologists trained at the Boston VA Aphasia Research Center provided a rich and continuing influence on the understanding of aphasia.

During the 1960s and 1970s, in addition to the training program in aphasia, the Aphasia Research Center included an active psychology/psycholinguistic research unit under the direction of Harold Goodglass and Edith Kaplan and an active, innovative language therapy program under Robert Sparks and later Nancy Helm-Estabrooks. Both programs produced a number of individual investigators who became prominent in their fields and have significantly advanced understanding of both aphasia and language.

Not all aphasia-oriented research activity was centered in Boston in those years. Many other neurologists, psychiatrists, and psychologists around the world became active in aphasia research. Major contributors included De Renzi and Vignolo in Italy; Hécaen, Lecours, and Lhermitte in France; Leichsner and Poeck in Germany; Gloning and Gloning in Austria; Luria in Russia; Maruszewski in Poland; Avila, Azcoaga, Caceres, and Medilaharsu in Latin America; and Sasanuma in Japan. The diversity of investigators and approaches that evolved during this period produced multiple directions for aphasia research. The correlation of focal neuroanatomical functions with psychological activities, particularly language, was in active ferment.

Following closely upon the renewed academic interest in language pathology, technical advances allowed the production of images of brain lesions in the living human; information from the new neuroimaging techniques provided a revolutionary new capability for more precise demonstration of the anatomical substrate of language dysfunction and a strong confirmation of the nineteenth-century anatomical-psychological observations. Both the psychological and the neuroimaging correlation studies of aphasia continue to the present and have provided robust support for the localization approaches. Geschwind energized a rebirth of the nineteenth-century brain-language correlation studies which have been strongly abetted by advances in technology.

Epoch IV: Language Modeling

Activity in the investigation of language and its impairment during the past three decades stemmed from many disciplines in addition to neurology. Important advances, both theoretical and pragmatic, were made in other disciplines.

Originally independent but increasingly interlocked with the developing localization approaches was a revolution in linguistics that utilized and influenced
aphasia. The prime influence behind this activity was Noam Chomsky, who in a
series of publications starting the late 1950s (but first reaching wide attention in
the mid-1960s) greatly altered the approach to structural linguistics and created a
model-building process for the study of language (Chomsky, 1957, 1972, 1980).
With this approach, a model of linguistic function could be formulated, appropriate experimentation devised, and the model proved or refuted by observation.
In the original formulations (as practiced by Chomsky and his immediate followers), the anatomical basis of language was ignored. Many subsequent investigators, however, found that aphasic subjects could be used as experimental material
to validate aspects of the models; these investigators were, of necessity, forced
to use portions of the terminology and classification of aphasia. Three loosely
interconnected areas of language study that have been developed in these years
deserve discussion—psycholinguistics, neurolinguistics, and, almost totally independent, speech pathology; all three disciplines utilize models of language function. While these disciplines often stand aloof from the traditional neurologic
models of language function, whenever brain correlations are conjectured, observations of aphasic subjects are utilized to provide hard data.

Psycholinguistics

Stemming from a combination of formal linguistics and psychology, a number of
important advances in the description and analysis of language have been made.
Based on multiple approaches to language including aphasia, Jakobson suggested
three dichotomies of language: (1) encoding/decoding, (2) limitation/disintegra-
tion, and (3) contiguity/simultaneity (Jakobson, 1964) (see Figure 2.7). While perhaps not fully satisfactory, these three dichotomies provided a solid structure on
which to develop psycholinguistic theory. Luria, who was equally critical of both
the early anatomical and the subsequent holistic approaches, utilized his own clinical experience and his background in developmental psychology to devise an
approach to aphasia based on linguistic properties loosely correlated with neuroanatomy. Luria's linguistic classification (1966, 1976a,b), unlike Head's (1926),
was eminently practical and has been used by many students of language disturbance (particularly psychologists).

A major figure in the early development of psycholinguistics was Harold
Goodglass (Figure 2.8), a psychologist working at the Boston VA Aphasia Research Center whose growing knowledge of linguistics led to major studies of
agrammatism, semantic fields, phrase length, and naming characteristics in aphasic patients. Of greater importance, Goodglass's laboratory devised and perfected
psychologically precise testing techniques for use in aphasia evaluation (Goodglass
and Kaplan, 1972, 1983).

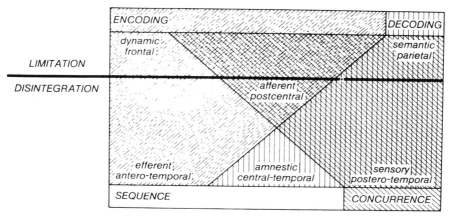

Figure 2.7. The three dichotomies of language proposed by Jakobson. (From Jakobson, 1964).

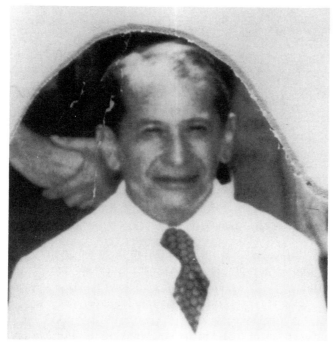

Figure 2.8. Harold Goodglass, leading American expert in the psycholinguistics of aphasia. (From personal files of DFB).

Advanced psycholinguistic studies have been carried on in many academic centers throughout the world. Investigators who have carefully studied aspects of aphasia with psycholinguistic techniques include Avila (1976), Buckingham (1981 a,b, 1989), De Renzi and Vignolo (1962), Gardner (1973), Hécaen and Angelergues (1965), Lecours et al. (1983), Poeck (1972), and others. Although their interests have been broad, many of the investigations reported by psycholinguists have been based on study of aphasic subjects.

Neurolinguistics

Neurolinguistics, a field related to but functionally distinct from psycholinguistics, developed directly from formal linguistics; psychological influences were considerably decreased but are still influential. Neurolinguistics attempts to correlate the principles of linguistics with the neural functions of the brain. Again, Jakobson's linguistic analysis of aphasia provided a major influence; his theories were expanded and altered by formal linguists such as Chomsky (1968), Fodor (1975), Katz (1972), Miller, Galanter, and Pribram (1960), and others. The production of language by a normal subject was the investigative focus for the neurolinguist. Models of language functions were devised, tested, debated, and validated (or refuted). Chomsky's models—generative grammar, transformational grammar, and universal grammar—remain topics of debate but each exerted a strong influence on subsequent studies of language. A number of neurolinguists have evaluated aphasic subjects in attempts to investigate individual language functions. Influential individuals in this field include Blumstein (1973), Zurif (1972), Caramazza (1986), Berndt (1988a,b), Lecours (Lecours, Lhermitte and Bryans 1983), Marshall and Newcombe (1973), and Caplan (1992). The sharply focused, neurolinguistic approach to language function has produced many provocative and appealing theories over the past few decades.

Although not specifically related to discrete brain regions or to neurological parameters, the psycholinguistic and neurolinguistic models of language processing provide dynamic new approaches to concepts of brain function.

Speech (Language) Pathology

Although its primary goal is to improve communication in aphasic patients, language therapy demands rigid assessment techniques and practical working theories of brain function. This combination of demands has led to an independent (nonlinguistic, nonanatomical) model of human language activity.

No formal field of language therapy existed until World War II. Many relatively healthy survivors of that war had suffered brain injuries that caused aphasia. Language therapy was initiated, simultaneously, in a number of countries.

Luria (1947/1970) outlined therapeutic techniques and provided some advice for rehabilitation. Wepman (1951) developed both assessment and therapeutic methods. As the field of language therapy developed, it was embraced in formal, university-based speech programs and a new discipline—speech (language) pathology—was created. A group of speech pathologists dedicated to aphasia therapy appeared, led by practitioners such as Eisenson (1954), Darley (1975), Schuell (1955), Sarno (1969), Holland (1980), Sparks (Sparks, Helm and Albert, 1974), Basso (1989), Brookshire (1983), Helm-Estabrooks (Helm-Estabrooks, Fitzpatrick, and Barresi, 1982), and Whurr (1974).

The assessment techniques devised by aphasia therapists have become powerful tools for the evaluation of aphasic subjects. The assessment techniques have improved in both sensitivity and specificity and many of the techniques have become standard for language evaluation. These will be described in Chapter 6.

A number of the approaches to language therapy developed by speech pathologists have been innovative. Starting with the standard techniques of education (e.g., rote practice), aphasia therapists have utilized material from the programmed learning efforts that began in the 1950s and more recently have borrowed ideas from psychology, neurology, and education to create novel rehabilitation techniques. Some of the most creative approaches to aphasia in recent years have risen from the efforts of the speech pathologists.

As much as the linguists and more than the psychologists or neurologists, the speech pathologists have tended to follow their own directions. As a group, speech pathologists have maintained a more holistic approach to language function. Most of the influential early therapists (Darley, Schuell, Wepman) took a unitary, holistic approach. A second generation of language therapists (Sarno, Holland, Basso, Helm-Estabrooks, Tsvetkova) adopted anatomically based classification schemes to a greater degree but focused on the residual brain function, not the anatomically based impairment, as the basis for language therapy. The holistic approach to aphasia has a practical appeal for the therapist attempting to develop the best possible communication capability in a patient from the totality of residual functions.

Rehabilitation after brain damage in general, and rehabilitation of language disorders in particular, continue to attract considerable interest. A new, more inclusive approach, known as cognitive rehabilitation, has emerged. This embraces attempts to deal not only with language disturbances but with associated cognitive disturbances (memory, perceptual, attentional, etc.) that result from brain damage. The efforts of speech pathologists have been considerably reinforced by techniques developed for cognitive rehabilitation. The aphasic subject is now approached in a considerably broader manner. Although still technically immature, cognitive rehabilitation promises continued improvement in the treatment of aphasia.

Summary

Starting from a rather limited focus, the study of aphasia has diversified and passed through a number of different stages. An original clinical-anatomical localization approach led to a reaction that brought holistic views to prominence. This was followed by a resurgent localizationist approach that utilized modern brain-imaging techniques. Aphasiology has now evolved into a diversified subspeciality that combines neurological, psychological, linguistic, and rehabilitation approaches. To a greater or lesser degree, each approach is interdependent with the others.

3

Variations within Aphasia

· ·

Any attempt to investigate a case of aphasia demands recognition of a number of crucial variables. First is an obvious but easily overlooked factor: no two individuals have identical backgrounds (social, spiritual, material) for thought or language (Benson, 1992; James, 1890/1983). Individual variation in mental content is extreme and this naturally influences language production. Second, brains are not identical anatomically or physiologically. The causes and effects of these variations are obscure, but they defeat any attempt to look upon the brain as a fixed "printed-circuit". A third point concerns the language(s) used by the individual. Not only the lexicon but also the rules of grammar differ between languages, and these variations between languages and even within a single language are crucial to the investigation of aphasia (Segalowitz and Bryden, 1983). Many other factors influence the comprehension and production of language, and a few will be discussed below.

Hemispheric Specialization

With the demonstration by Broca (1865) and his contemporaries that aphasia was almost invariably associated with left-hemisphere damage and that a similarly located lesion in the right hemisphere produced little or no overt language disturbance, the localization of a specific brain function to a single hemisphere (hemispheric specialization) became an established fact (Milner, 1974). Lateralization of language function is now so universally accepted that the unnatural state that it represents routinely goes unnoted. Asymmetry of function in a relatively symmetrical biological organ is an anomaly that, with only minor, almost debatable exceptions, occurs only in the human brain. The human body contains many paired organs (e.g., kidneys, lungs, eyes, reproductive glands) in which the functions of right and left members are identical. Damage to one of the pair alters function in degree only. Human cerebral hemispheric specialization for language is almost unique in biology.

Many hypotheses about the specialization of mental activities within one cerebral hemisphere or the other have been proposed (Bradshaw and Nettleton, 1981). Based on observations following section of the human corpus callosum, Sperry (1985), Bogen and Bogen (1969), Lishman (1969), Gazzaniga (1970), Levy (1974), and many others have suggested that each hemisphere is capable of separate mental activity. It has been argued that the human brain contains two "minds" (Wigan, 1844; Orenstein, 1972), that each hemisphere processes information in a different way (logical/analytic; propositional/apositional, etc.) (Bogen, 1969; Semmes, 1968; TenHouten, 1985). Hemispheric differences have been described for music (Gates and Bradshaw, 1977; Bever and Chiarello, 1974), visuospatial functions (Cummings, 1985a), psychiatric disorders (Flor-Henry, 1969; Robinson and Price, 1982; Ross, 1981), education (Wittrock, 1985; Goldberg and Costa, 1981) as well as more basic cerebral functions such as attention (Heilman et al., 1985a,b,c; Mesulam, 1981), emotion (Ross and Mesulam, 1979; Benson, 1984), language (Fromkin, 1985; Zaidel, 1978; Gazzaniga and Sperry, 1967), computations (Hécaen, 1962; Spiers, 1987) and for many other high-level "cortical" functions.

Following the initial period of exuberant and often rather fanciful postulations concerning specialized activities of the two hemispheres, a period of retraction was inevitable (Smyth and Sugar, 1975). Disclaimers have been voiced, possibly most ardently and effectively by Efron (1990) who denied, but only partially disproved, the existence of hemispheric specialization. Although many of the hypotheses put forward over the past two decades remain controversial, a strong consensus affirms that at least some high-level psychological functions are performed better (or in a different manner) by one or the other hemisphere.

Lateralization of Language Function

Approximately 99% of all right-handed individuals are said to have language function in the left hemisphere (Carter, Satz, and Hohenegger, 1984; Kertesz, 1985). With a lesion in a particular left-hemisphere location, most humans who prefer the right hand for unimanual activities will become aphasic whereas damage to the corresponding anatomical area in the right hemisphere will not significantly disrupt language. Called *dominance*, hemispheric specialization for language was solidly established following Broca's declaration that "we speak with the left hemisphere" (1865); considerable support for this observation was gathered by his contemporaries. Two rules of cerebral hemispheric dominance for language were originally formulated in the nineteenth century (Benson, 1985b) and can be paraphrased as follows:

1. The left hemisphere is crucial (dominant) for language in the right-handed individual.
2. The right hemisphere has a similarly dominant position for language in the left-handed individual.

The dictum of left-hemisphere dominance for language became so strong that dichotomies such as dominant/nondominant and major/minor were used to distinguish the functions of the two hemispheres. It was even assumed that the right hemisphere was a "spare" that could take over some crucial functions if trouble developed in the "major hemisphere." The correlation of handedness and language function became a matter of serious study (Bryden, 1988). Cases were collected, the literature reviewed, the data collated, and many studies published (Table 3.1 summarizes one report of lateralization of language).

In general, these early studies of the correlation between handedness and language dominance demonstrated that when right-handed individuals suffered left-hemisphere damage approximately two-thirds became aphasic; in contrast, only about one-third of individuals who claimed to be left-handed became aphasic after left-hemisphere damage (Luria, 1947/1970). Very few right-handed individuals who suffered right-hemisphere damage became aphasic (usually 1 to 2%) whereas about 25% of left-handers developed aphasia following a right-hemisphere lesion (Gloning, 1977). Investigators came to realize that for the ma-

Table 3.1. Lateralization for Language in a Sample of 262 Subjects, Obtained by Means of the Sodium Amytal Test

Handedness	Number of Cases	LANGUAGE REPRESENTATION (%)		
		Left	*Bilateral*	*Right*
Right	140	96	0	4
Left	122	70	15	15

Adapted from Rasmussen and Milner, 1977.

jority of individuals (right-handed or left-handed), aphasia was associated with left-hemisphere lesions. The left hemisphere was dominant for language not only in right-handers but also in left-handers.

Dominance for handedness, however, is not a simple dichotomy. Depending on the task requested or the question asked of the subject, the number who favor the right or left hand varies widely (Annett, 1970; Bryden, 1982) (see Table 3.2 for an example of such studies). Furthermore, the percentage of left-handers found in different groups can differ, depending on cultural influences, age, education, and/or genetic factors (Ardila et al., 1989a; Bryden, 1982; Gilbert and Wysocki, 1992; Harris, 1990). Healey, Liederman, and Geschwind (1986) presented a fifty-five-item handedness questionnaire to 290 adult subjects. Using a Varimax Factor Analysis they observed four factors that accounted for about 80% of the variance: (1) distal fine motor movements requiring continual modification of a motor program (e.g., writing); (2) activities governed by a program requiring little modification once initiated (e.g., to press the button of a phone); (3) proximal/axial coordination (e.g., holding a baseball bat); (4) ballistic movements of the proximal and/or axial musculature (e.g., throwing a dart). Handedness proved to be multidimensional; different aspects of hand preference can be delineated.

Table 3.2. Percentages of "Left," "Either," or "Right"
Responses to Different Handedness Questions,
in a Sample of 2,321 Subjects

	HANDEDNESS		
TASKS	Left	Either	Right
Dealing cards	17.02	3.32	79.66
Unscrewing jar	16.50	17.49	66.01
Shoveling	13.53	11.89	74.58
Sweeping	13.49	16.89	69.62
Threading needle	13.10	9.74	77.16
Writing	10.60	0.34	89.06
Striking match	9.95	8.74	81.31
Throwing ball	9.44	1.29	89.47
Hammering	9.22	2.54	88.24
Using toothbrush	9.18	8.49	82.33
Using racquet	8.10	2.59	89.31
Using scissors	6.20	6.81	86.99

Adapted from Annett, 1970.

A new pair of rules, based on observations like those above, became prevalent in the 1970s:

1. The left hemisphere is crucial (dominant) for language in the right-handed individual.
2. Non-right-handers (the newly promoted euphemism [Annet, 1970] that includes those who are left-handed or ambidextrous) show much less definite hemispheric lateralization of language; some may have language dominance in the right hemisphere, some in the left hemisphere (Subirana, 1958) and some have mixed hemispheric dominance.

Additional observations confirmed that language function is considerably less lateralized in non-right-handed individuals, suggesting that they have bilateral language function (Luria, 1947/1970; Gloning, 1977; Goodglass and Quadfasel, 1954). Gloning and colleagues (1969) noted that aphasia following brain injury in non-right-handers occurred with greater frequency than in right-handers, and Luria (1947/1970) reported a better recovery rate from aphasia in non-right-handers. It seems probable that some degree of bilaterality of language function is also present in most of the right-handed population (Benson, 1985b; Castro-Caldas and Confraria, 1984), but the presence of severe language disturbance (aphasia) following left-hemisphere damage, compared to a relatively minimal disturbance in language function following right-hemisphere damage, in the individual who prefers his right hand for most activities indicates that the hemispheric lateralization of language function is strong in the majority of humans.

Language lateralization may depend, to a degree, on the specific language used by the individual. Every language has idiosyncrasies with regard to phonology, syntax, and semantics, and writing systems vary widely among different languages. Any of these factors may be relevant for language lateralization. Thus, the percentage of crossed aphasia in right-handers (aphasia associated with a right-hemisphere lesion) appears to be higher in many Indo-European languages (from less than 1% to 3.5%, but generally from 1 to 2%) (Joanette, 1989; Sweet, Panis, and Levine, 1984) than it is among Spanish-speaking populations (below 1%).

Aphasia has been less widely studied in non-Indo-European languages. Gao and Benson (1990) reported a 2.9% incidence of crossed aphasia in Chinese aphasics, while Yu-Huan, Ying-Guan, and Gui-Qing (1990) found an even higher percentage in their Chinese subjects. In a sample of eighty-one Mandarin Chinese–speaking stroke patients, Gao and Benson (1990), found aphasia patterns similar to those observed in Indo-European languages: almost all aphasic right-handers and about 80% of left-handed aphasics had damage located in the left hemisphere. Yu-Huan, Ying-Guan, and Gui-Qing (1990), on the other hand, reported a higher percentage of motor aphasia in Chinese who spoke a different dialect.

It seems likely that a basic universality in the organization of language in the brain, as proposed by Chomsky (1957, 1968), does exist. Minor differences may be present, however, depending on specific language idiosyncracies.

Language Area

Following the observations of Broca and Wernicke, it became clear that two different left-hemisphere zones were involved in language (Broca's area and Wernicke's area). Later, Dejerine (1891, 1892) developed the concept of alexia with damage to the occipital lobe (alexia without agraphia) or the parietal lobe (alexia with agraphia) and proposed a language zone in the left hemisphere that includes three areas.

1. Anterior, including the posterior part of the foot of F3, the frontal operculum, and the immediate surrounding zone, including the foot of F2, and probably extending to the anterior insula
2. Inferior or temporal, encompassing the posterior first and second temporal gyri
3. Posterior, the angular gyrus ("center of the visual images of the words").

Luria (1966, 1947/1970) proposed different levels of language recognition and production, depending on the integrated activity of language-dedicated areas in the left temporal, parietal, and frontal lobes. In his view each of these brain areas is specialized for a particular aspect of language processing such as phoneme discrimination or verbal memory.

Luria (1947/1970) superimposed on brain templates the loci of lesions that produced specific language disorders to determine which areas are critical for language. From these data he drew an outline of the "speech" area of the human left hemisphere. Figure 3.1 presents a crude outline of Luria's proposed language area and compares it with five previously published outlines of the areas of the left cortex most often associated with language impairment.

The Boston group (Albert et al., 1981; Benson, 1979a; Benson and Geschwind, 1971, 1985; Geschwind, 1965; Goodglass and Kaplan, 1972) asserted that the central perisylvian area was crucial for language and that focal damage within this area could produce three different language disorders: frontal (Broca aphasia), parietal (conduction aphasia), and temporal (Wernicke aphasia). In their view damage to dominant-hemisphere tissues surrounding the central perisylvian language area was associated with transcortical (or border zone) aphasias.

The language areas described by Dejerine, Luria, and the Boston group are similar to those suggested by many other investigators. Marie and Foix (1917),

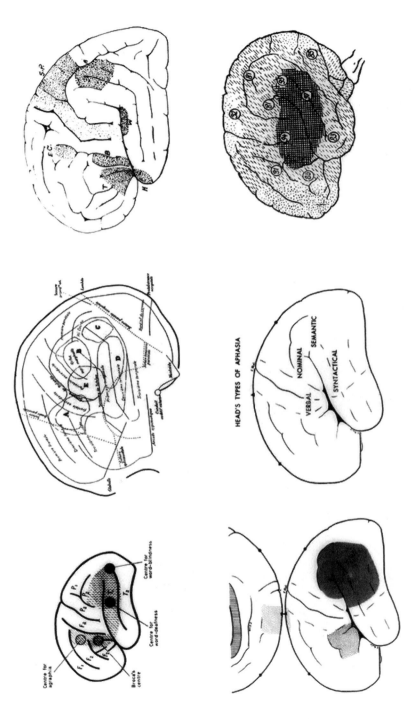

Figure 3.1. Six representations of "the language area." Clockwise from upper left: Froment (as reproduced by Brain, 1961); Marie and Foix (as reproduced by Penfield and Roberts, 1959); Nielsen (1962); Luria (1947/1970); Head (1920) (as reproduced by Penfield and Roberts, 1959); Penfield and Roberts (1959).

Penfield and Roberts (1959), Nielsen (1936), and others have produced basically similar demonstrations of the brain areas crucial to language. All of the areas suggested as the site of language function lie within the vascular territory of the left-middle cerebral artery. Figure 3.2 represents a composite outline of the left-hemisphere language area as demonstrated by clinical data collected over the past century.

Childhood Language Disorders

The study of abnormalities of language in childhood has a long, confused history, and the term *childhood aphasia* remains controversial. Language abnormality is a relatively common problem of childhood but the language symptoms produced by brain abnormalities in children are complicated by developmental variability (Carter, Satz, and Hohenegger, 1982). The language disorders of childhood often fail to fit the classical syndromes of aphasia in adults and often represent very different clinical problems. Two major divisions of childhood language abnormality are recognized: (1) *developmental language disorder*, and (2) *acquired aphasia of childhood* (Alajouanine and Lhermitte, 1965; Guttman, 1942; Woods, 1985b).

By definition, children with developmental language disorder fall outside the accepted definition of aphasia since they have never developed normal language that can be lost or impaired. Not all language retardation is complete, however; when partial language develops, it poses a complex diagnostic problem. Inasmuch as the language symptoms are based on failure of anatomical and psychological

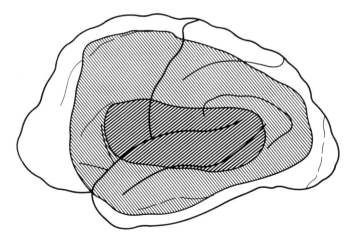

Figure 3.2. Language area. Central area indicates perisylvian language area. Surrounding area represents extrasylvian language area. (From Benson, 1979a).

functions to develop normally rather than on focal cerebral damage, neither the clinical features nor the anatomical correlations of adult aphasia are necessarily present in childhood developmental language disorder. It is preferable to call the developmental disorder *language retardation, developmental language disorder,* or *developmental dysphasia* (Zangwill, 1978). The term *childhood aphasia* should be reserved for those disorders in which children have developed language in a normal fashion but, following brain insult, show a language abnormality. Unfortunately, this reasonable distinction is not universally followed and many developmental language problems are called childhood aphasia.

Some insights into the complexities of developmental language abnormalities have been gained. Discovering and treating congenital deafness are important, and mental deficiency and childhood autism can complicate language development (Rapin and Allen, 1986; Wong and Atwood, 1987; Woods, 1985a). The phenomenology of developmental language disorder has been described and categorized (Allen, Rapin, and Wiznitzer, 1988; Cohen, Volkmar, and Paul, 1986; Rapin and Allen, 1983) and remediation processes have been devised (Cross and Ozanne, 1990). Table 3.3 presents one attempt to differentiate varieties of developmental language disorders.

Children who have begun to develop language may suffer a language disturbance following a cerebral insult that is, at least in overall appearance, analogous to the acquired aphasia of adults (Alajouanine and Lhermitte, 1965; Guttman, 1942; Hécaen, 1976; Ozanne and Murdoch, 1990; Satz and Bullard-Bates, 1981). Several differences characterize the acquired aphasia of childhood, however. First, the degree of hemispheric dominance for language apparently develops with advancing age. The younger the child at the onset of acquired aphasia, the less robust is the hemispheric dominance for language and/or the better the other (nondominant) hemisphere can assume language function. Zangwill (1960) termed this an "equipotentiality" of the two hemispheres for language in the young child. The other hemisphere (usually the right) retains some ability to take over language function through the first 10 or 12 years of life (Lenneberg, 1967) and possibly well beyond (Cummings et al., 1979; Smith, 1966).

Another frequently observed characteristic is that the younger the child at the onset of acquired aphasia, the more rapid and more complete the recovery of language. If the damage involves only one hemisphere, recovery is routinely sufficient for normal language use. Careful testing, however, suggests that language function may never be quite as full in the child who recovers from aphasia secondary to dominant hemisphere damage (Hécean, 1976; Lenneberg, 1967). With increasing age, the time necessary to recover language function increases; a child aged 3 or 4 with an acquired aphasia, although originally mute, may speak within a few weeks or a month, whereas in a child of age 10 or 12 many months may go by before return of significant language function. Obviously, both the rate and

Table 3.3. Developmental Language Disorders

Disorders Affecting Comprehension and Expression

Verbal auditory agnosia (word-deafness)
    Inability to decode language
    Speech onset delayed
    Speech production absent or sparse

Mixed phonological-syntactic deficit
    Comprehension poor
    Speech onset delayed
    Verbal output nonfluent, agrammatic, and poorly articulated

Expressive Disorders

Verbal dyspraxia
    Comprehension good
    Speech onset delayed
    Verbal output nonfluent and poorly articulated

Phonologic programming deficit
    Comprehension good
    Speech onset normal or delayed
    Verbal output fluent but unintelligible

Disorders of Central Processing and Formulation

Semantic-pragmatic deficit
    Comprehension defective
    Echolalia and perseveration common
    Speech onset varies from precocious to delayed
    Verbal output fluent, verbose; syntax and lexicon intact

Lexical-syntactic deficit
    Comprehension poor for complex sentences
    Speech onset usually delayed
    Notable word-finding problems impede sentence formulation
    Verbal output fluent with notable word-finding pauses

Adapted from Allen, Rapin, and Wiznitzer, 1988.

the degree of recovery vary with the severity of cerebral damage and the presence of bilateral damage seriously compromises the recovery. In children the ability of the nondominant hemisphere to assume some or many language functions apparently continues for some time after the onset of aphasia and probably continues well beyond the ages of 5 to 12 years usually suggested in the literature (Krashen, 1973; Lenneberg, 1967). Many young soldiers who become aphasic following brain injury sustained in combat make considerable language recovery; in general, aphasia onset at age 20 to 30 years has a far better prognosis for language recovery than aphasia occurring in the 50- or 60-year-old subject. Before simply accepting advancing age as the key feature, however, attention must be given to the cause of the aphasia (Ozanne and Murdoch, 1990). The most common cause of aphasia in the young is trauma, which in general has a better prognosis for recovery. Vascular and neoplastic problems, which have graver outlooks for language recovery, predominate at later ages. A good general rule is that the younger the age at onset of aphasia, the faster and more complete the improvement, a factor most notable in the young, developing child.

Another significant characteristic of childhood aphasia concerns fluency of verbal output following brain insult. It is widely held that no child with acquired aphasia develops a fluent, paraphasic, jargonistic verbal output; this is not true in the absolute but the vast majority of children with acquired aphasia have a non-fluent verbal output (Lopera, 1992; Satz and Bullard-Bates, 1981). Many are mute initially (a relatively rare event in the adult) and in the early recovery stages of childhood aphasia the verbal output is characteristically slow, sparse, and hypophonic. Nonfluent verbal output characterizes acquired aphasia in childhood regardless of the site of brain insult.

Finally, an additional and exceedingly troublesome problem in the evaluation of acquired aphasia in childhood concerns the stage of language development (Cross and Ozanne, 1990). Both the lexicon and the complexity of available grammatical structure increase with age, a factor of obvious significance when evaluating language loss in the child. Language ability of individual children of any given age varies tremendously based on individual intelligence, language used in the home, language shared with siblings or friends, educational experiences, and individual variations in cerebral development. Chronological age represents only one, often insignificant variable in the language capabilities of a child.

Brain damage sufficient to produce an acquired aphasia not only damages acquired language capabilities but may delay normal language development. Coupled with the age-related individual variability in verbal competency, the additional factors of focal brain injury and subsequently delayed language development produce enormous difficulties for the clinician attempting to correlate the language competency of an aphasic child with normal expectations. The standard procedure is to compare the child's acquired aphasia with normal adult language function, noting all deficits but disregarding those language functions unavailable to or poorly mastered by a child of that age; at best, this represents a crude guess. Demonstrating the amount of language lost by the child and predicting the eventual outcome of an acquired aphasia of childhood is extremely difficult (Cross and Ozanne, 1990).

The pathology underlying childhood language problems deserves separate mention. Language retardation can be the result of a variety of abnormalities. Abnormal language development (developmental dysphasia) and damage early in development when the structural brain changes involve the temporal and/or pari-etal lobes can produce language retardation (and developmental dyslexia) (Gala-burda and Kemper, 1979). Because of the equipotentiality of the hemispheres for language, bilateral cerebral pathology must be conjectured in cases of severe language retardation.

One crucial factor underlying childhood language impairment is that the child cannot learn to use language if language cannot be received or compre-hended. Deafness is an important cause of developmental language disorder (so-called secondary dysphasia). If the deafness is peripheral, corrective measures can be instituted, either a mechanical hearing aid or specific training for language in the deaf. If, however, the deafness is based on a central abnormality, the child will not benefit from sound augmentation and will respond only poorly, if at all, to standard deaf-training techniques. Serious language retardation occurs in the child with central deafness. One of the few carefully studied cases of develop-mental language retardation to come to postmortem showed developmental abnor-mality of the auditory system within the cerebrum producing central deafness and severe language retardation, intractable to available training techniques (Landau, Goldstein, and Kleffner, 1960).

Acquired aphasia of childhood can stem from many different pathological sources, generally analogous to the causes of aphasia in adults (see Chapter 5). The most common etiology of aphasia acquired in childhood is trauma, but other sources such as infection, tumor, or cerebrovascular accident can be seen. Prior to the widespread use of antiobiotics, cerebral abscess in the temporal lobe stem-ming from chronic otitis media was a common cause of childhood aphasia (Smyth, Ozanne, and Woodhouse, 1990). Acquired aphasia is not common in childhood but it does occur; because it occurs within a system that has undergone some degree of language development, some of the characteristics of adult onset aphasia will be found.

The prognosis in cases of developmental language disorder must remain guarded. Effective treatments are limited and potentials for language development are variable. If the child is of reasonable intelligence, advancing age and matura-tion of the nervous system allow many such children to develop compensatory mechanisms to provide some degree of communication. Some techniques for the remediation of inborn language disturbances have been developed and claim some success (Woods, 1985a); the problem remains severe, however, and many chil-dren with language retardation remain permanently disabled.

The prognosis for acquired aphasia of childhood is considerably better. If the child is young and the damage is limited to one hemisphere (e.g., stroke), the undamaged hemisphere may assume dominance for language. Unfortunately, bi-lateral damage (as in, e.g., head trauma, infection, anoxia, metabolic/toxic disor-ders) is common and seriously impairs recovery potential. Prognosis must be guarded in such cases, at least until the clinical course reveals evidence of recovery. Most children who acquire aphasia do regain a useful degree of language function, and many recover a surprising ability to use language competently.

Aphasia in Polyglots

Polyglots, individuals fluent in several languages, present an interesting problem when they become aphasic. Are they equally aphasic in different languages? Which of their several languages will they recover? A tendency for one language to recover better than the others has been recorded with sufficient frequency to warrant opinions and discussion (Albert and Obler, 1978; Paradis, 1977, 1990; Vaid, 1986). Some polyglot aphasics become functional in one language while remaining severely aphasic in their other language(s). Ribot's rule (Ribot, 1883) posited that the language best recovered by the polyglot aphasic would be the mother tongue. Ribot's rule was based on observations that, following brain trauma, information learned early in life is retrieved better than more recently acquired information (similar to retrograde amnesia). Neither the observation nor Ribot's rule is consistently true. A second early postulation concerning the recovery of language by polyglots, often called Pitres's law (Pitres, 1895), states that the language that the patient was consistently using at the onset of the aphasia will be recovered best, even though not the first learned. This rule also fails validation. In fact, both Ribot's rule and Pitres's law are "honored as much by being broken as by being followed" (Hécaen and Albert, 1978).

In discussing the recovery of language function by the polyglot aphasics, Goldstein (1948) emphasized three factors:

1. Some polyglots are truly fluent only in one (usually the mother) tongue, limiting recovery of other previously known languages. Exceptions to this observation are known (Hinshelwood, 1900), but it does apply to many polyglot aphasics.
2. More than one language may recover but the recovery level may be uneven. Goldstein stated that "the patient will try to use the language that appears best for his purposes," possibly to the exclusion of the others. Careful testing of truly polyglot aphasics in their several languages, however, usually reveals that at least some degree of function has been recovered in each (Nilipour and Ashayeri, 1989). In addition, the characteristics of aphasia (e.g., alexia, poor repetition) demonstrated in one language are almost always demonstrable in the other(s).
3. Dialect seriously confuses the picture of recovery by a polyglot aphasic. As a dialect is most often dependent on the motor or phonemic qualities

of verbal output, it may be differentially lost or retained in aphasia, complicating but not truly reflecting, the underlying loss or retention of language.

Goldstein concludes that multiple factors determine the pattern of language recovery of an aphasic polyglot and, in general, recovery will reflect the patient's attempt to achieve the best communication system available.

In an extensive review of the literature on aphasia in bilinguals and polyglots, Paradis (1977) identified six modes of language recovery: (1) *differential:* each language is impaired separately and is recovered at the same or different rate; (2) *parallel:* different languages are similarly impaired and restored at the same rate; (3) *antagonistic:* recovery of one of the languages progresses while the other(s) regress; (4) *successive:* one language does not show any recovery until another has been restored; (5) *selective:* one or more of the languages are not recovered at all; (6) *mixed:* two or more languages are used in some combination. Some of these patterns occur more frequently, apparently influenced by other factors (e.g., the context of the language used, the age at which the language was learned, etc.).

One important factor in determining the first language to be recovered by a polyglot aphasic is the language milieu during recovery. In French Canada, many citizens are bilinguals but in most hospitals only one of the two languages is used; the first language recovered by aphasics in these circumstances is most often the language used by the hospital staff when communicating with the patient (Lambert and Fillenbaum, 1959).

Some observers posit that variations in recovery of separate languages by a polyglot aphasic are based on lesion localization (Bychowski, 1919; Obler and Albert, 1977), a premise emphatically denied by others (Goldstein, 1948; Pitres, 1895). The best examples involve written language, particularly two languages that utilize strikingly different methods of writing (e.g., Indo-European vs. Chinese vs. Arabic) (Obler and Albert, 1977; Sasanuma and Fujimura, 1971; Yamadori, 1975). That lesion localization may be a factor in differential recovery is reasonable but, at most, is only one of multiple factors. Based on present knowledge, the anatomical site of the aphasia-producing lesion does not appear to be the factor of greatest importance in language recovery in polyglot aphasics (Albert and Obler, 1978).

A related but decidedly controversial proposal suggests that brain representation of language may be different in multilinguals. Crossed aphasia in right-handers has been reported to be more frequent in multilinguals (Albert and Obler, 1978; Karanth and Rangamani, 1988), and some authors suggest the possibility that right-hemisphere participation in language is greater in bilingual or multilingual subjects (Gloning and Gloning, 1965/1983). The opposite view, however, has also been proposed (Stark et al., 1977). The idea of greater bilateral hemispheric participation for language in polyglots, although theoretically enticing, has not been conclusively demonstrated (Paradis, 1987; Vaid, 1983).

Zatorre (1989) has argued that little evidence exists to support the idea that the right hemisphere participates in second and subsequent languages in any way significantly different from the first-learned language. Clinical observations tend to support the notion that the left hemisphere controls the first and subsequent languages to the same degree. Experimental evidence is contradictory, confusing, and easily contaminated by methodological problems. Based on extensive study, Paradis (1990) stressed that the clinical evidence indicates that both languages in bilinguals are subserved by the left hemisphere in the same proportion as in monolinguals. Some evidence suggests that interhemispheric organization of the individual languages of polyglots may be different, however (Vaid, 1983).

In summary, aphasia in polyglots offers, in a microcosm, a glimpse of the multiplicity of confusing factors that influence the clinical features of aphasia. No simple or steadfast rule can be set for the recovery of language in a polyglot aphasic.

Aphasia in Illiterates

The study of aphasia in illiterate subjects offers one possible avenue toward discovery of how the acquisition of written language may affect brain organization for language. A number of significant studies have been presented. Critchley (1956) indicated that aphasia was less severe in illiterates and appeared to have a better prognosis than in literate subjects. Cameron, Currier, and Haerer (1971), based on a study of aphasia in individuals of variable reading competency, suggested that language had a more bilateral hemispheric representation in illiterates. In their series, Cameron and colleagues found that reading and writing skill apparently increased the degree of hemispheric asymmetry for language function. Rosselli, Ardila, and Rosas (1990b) found both language and praxis less strongly lateralized in illiterates. Damasio and colleagues (1976), however, were unable to demonstrate that the cerebral organization of language differed in illiterates; they found that regardless of the subject's inability to read and write, severe aphasia occurred following left-hemisphere damage. Two studies of aphasia in illiterates (Lecours et al., 1988; Matute, 1988) focused on whether the acquisition of reading and writing influenced the cerebral organization of language. Their investigations reached similar conclusions: in illiterates, the hemispheric directionality for the representation of language does not differ from literates. Aphasia occurred just as frequently in cases of left-hemisphere damage in illiterates as in literates; however, the aphasia appeared to be less severe in the illiterates, suggesting that a more bilateral representation of language might be present in the brains of illiterates. Thus, although literacy does not change the direction of brain asymmetry for language, it may increase the degree of hemispheric specialization. In the vast majority of humans, language is asymmetrically represented in the brain with the left hemisphere playing the major role. The learning of a new language system (written language) does not change this basic arrangement but may increase (or appear to increase) the degree of asymmetric language representation.

Aphasia in Special Languages

Several special language forms have been presented in the aphasia literature with particular interest given to aphasia for sign language and for Morse code. Deficits in manual communicating systems are known to be associated with left hemisphere damage in deaf subjects (Bellugi, Poizner, and Klima, 1983; Critchley, 1970; Douglass and Richardson, 1959; Sarno, Swisher, and Sarno, 1969) in a manner similar to normal hearing subjects (Mateer et al., 1982). Aphasia for sign language usually indicates left-hemisphere damage, but certain cerebral asymmetries in deaf individuals may be influenced by the use of sign language. Thus, hemispheric asymmetry for processing of different types of information may be observed in deaf subjects who had learned to sign. Those who did not use sign language would not show a cerebral asymmetry. Appropriate cases for study (e.g., acquired aphasia in a congenitally deaf individual) are scarce. The development of hemispheric asymmetry for language in the deaf may be linked to the learning of a language (sign) in a manner analogous to the increased lateralization of language in the literate, but data to support this contention also remains inadequate.

Only two cases of aphasia for Morse code have been reported (Ardila, 1987; Wyler and Ray, 1986). Morse code requires a complex, multiskill ability that includes at least three crucial factors: (1) a linguistic component, (2) a motor component, and (3) an auditory component. The first reported case (Wyler and Ray, 1986) noted that damage in the left temporal lobe produced a deficit in the third component (the ability to detect auditory temporal sequences). The second reported case (Ardila, 1987) was in an individual with a tumor involving the right parietal lobe who showed difficulty with both the linguistic and the motor components (inability to convert language to hand movements and inability to perform skilled manual movements) required for sending Morse code signals. The latter patient was left-handed, a point that further clouds interpretation of hemispheric specialization for Morse code. This question will never be settled, as competency in Morse code has virtually disappeared.

A single-case study of left-hemisphere damage with aphasia in a skilled stenographer reported preserved ability to read and write shorthand despite the subject's alexia and agraphia for normal written language (Landis, Regard, and Serrat, 1980). The possibility that the right hemisphere was dominant for the shorthand written language could be proposed, but not validated, by the findings from this single case.

Summary

In the investigation of language impairment, many factors must be appreciated. Among the more elusive are variations in language function based on degree of hemispheric specialization, age at onset of aphasia, level of literacy, and the language or languages used by the patient before onset of aphasia. Although not explaining (or apparently altering) the characteristic features of an aphasia syndrome, these variations may be significant for the understanding and management of an individual aphasic's problem.

4

Linguistic Analyses of Aphasia

· ·

Aphasia cannot be considered only as a neurological disorder. As a disruption of language, aphasia is also a linguistic disorder. The disruption may be manifested in different aspects of language function—phonological, morphological, syntactic, or semantic—and the aphasia syndromes can be distinguished, at least to some degree, by the linguistic function impaired. Although aphasia rarely involves only a single linguistic component (Blumstein, 1981), the linguistic abnormalities can be related to specific aphasia syndromes. Thus, they need to be analyzed, and this requires familiarity with basic linguistic concepts. Over the years many investigators have developed outlines of the human language system (see Figures 4.1 and 4.2).

Basic Linguistic Concepts

Language function may be viewed as a hierarchy of linguistic units of ascending complexity—features, phonemes, morphemes, and syntagms (Lecours et al., 1983).

A *feature* is an muscular action (or nonaction) of the human buccophonatory apparatus that produces sound. A *phoneme* is the audible production of a group of features capable of conveying meaning, and a *morpheme* is the least combination of phonemes that contains meaning. *Syntagms* are groups of morphemes, appropriately sequenced to provide a unified meaning (Lecours et al., 1983). Figure 4.2 illustrates this linguistic hierarchy as a two-way activity for the encoding and decoding of language material.

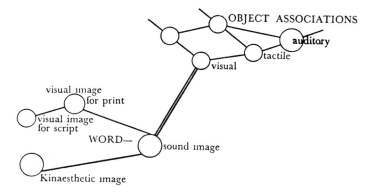

Psychological schema of the word concept.
The word concept appears as a closed complex of images, the object concept as an open one. The word concept is linked to the concept of the object via the sound image only. Among the object associations, the visual ones play a part similar to that played by the sound image among the word associations. The connections of the word sound image with object associations other than the visual are not presented in this schema.

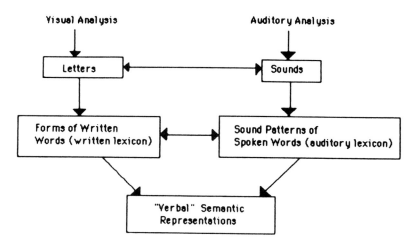

Figure 4.1. Two models to illustrate postulated language processes. The upper scheme is from Freud (1891/1953), the lower scheme from Caplan (1987).

Phonological Analysis

Phonology encompasses both the phonetic and the phonemic systems of the language (Blumstein, 1981). Phonetics pertains to the study of the sound, without reference to meaning or function. Thus, dysarthria (a speech, not a language, disorder) implies a distortion in sound production causing phonetic deviations.

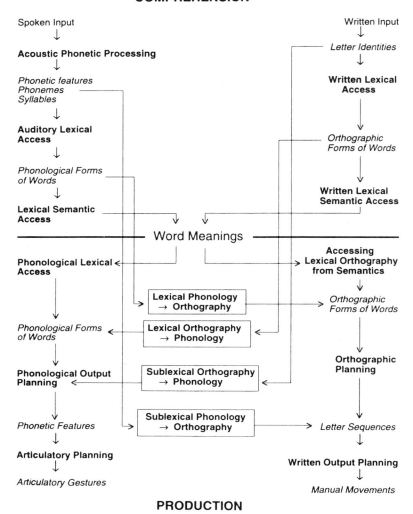

COMPREHENSION

Figure 4.2. Modern attempt to outline all of the potential linguistic actions used to process spoken and written language. (From Caplan, 1993).

Some natural phonetic variations occur during language production, the most important resulting from context. For instance, the /p/ sound is not identical in "pear" (initial position) and "spare" (middle position after /s/); only in the first case is it aspirated. Such variances of the same language sound (phoneme) are considered contextual variations and represent a phonetic, not a phonemic change. Many factors can be responsible for phonetic variations within language sound production and some regional variations deserve mention.

The minimal meaningful unit of sound in language is a *phoneme*. Some phonemes are considered universal (/p/ and /m/ are found in virtually all the known languages of the world) but even these may have different variants in different languages. The number of phonemes in any language is quite limited; English has about thirty-four phonemes and Spanish twenty-three. Some phonemes appear only in a restricted family of languages. The Chinese spoken language has many distinct dialects and the number of different phonemes is high. In fact, although the ideographic characters allow the Chinese written language to be understood by almost all Chinese, many Chinese speakers (even those who are well educated) cannot understand the spoken language of many other Chinese speakers.

Phonemic changes can imply changes in the meaning of two words differing in only a single phoneme and the two are said to represent a minimal pair (e.g., "dear"–"peer"), with the two distinguishing phonemes of the two words (i.e., /d/ and /p/) said to be in opposition because their switch conveys a different meaning (Jakobson and Halle, 1956). Phonemes can be analyzed according to their articulatory or acoustic features. At the level of physical characterization, a feature is an action state of the buccophonatory apparatus resulting from action or nonaction of buccophonatory muscles. In English (as in most Indo-European languages), /p/ and /b/ are different phonemes; in many other languages, however, they are variants of a single phoneme. The /p/ and the /b/ phonemes in the syllable-initial position are distinguished by the articulatory parameter of the voice onset time. They share other features: both are consonants, stops, and bilabial; however, the /p/ is voiceless and the /b/ is voiced; thus, in /b/ the vocal chords vibrate at the release of the stop consonant sound. In Spanish, /r/ and /r/ are two separate phonemes, but English has only one /r/ phoneme; conversely, /b/ and /v/ are two phonemes in English but Spanish has only /b/. According to an International Phonetic Alphabet, phonemic representations are written into virgules (e.g., wall = /wol/), whereas phonetic representation is written in brackets (e.g., wall = [wol]).

Morphological Analysis

Morphology represents the analysis of patterns of word formation (e.g., inflexions, derivations, compositions). It refers to the construction of words in a language. A *morpheme* is the minimal meaningful unit and can be either a word or part of a word. A morpheme can be composed of one phoneme (e.g., the independent article "a") or several phonemes (e.g., the word "cat" has three phonemes: /k/, /a/, and /t/). The *lexicon* is the total stock of morphemes in a language. Usually two different types of morphemes are distinguished: lexical morphemes (or lexemes) and grammatical morphemes. The lexical morpheme refers to the distinguishing root structure of a word. Grammatical morphemes include affixes (bound grammatical morphemes), particles that can be added to a lexical morpheme, and connectors (free grammatical morphemes such as articles, prepositions, etc.). The word "rapid" has a single morpheme (lexical morpheme); the word "rapidly" has two morphemes (one lexical and one grammatical).

Syntactic Analysis

Syntax refers to the rules applied to the construction of phrases and sentences. Words are interconnected in the sentence by means of grammatical connectors. The sequence of words in the sentence (article, noun, adjective, verb, etc.) often carries the specific communication intention (e.g., in "The dog bites the cat" and "The cat bites the dog," the meaning depends solely upon word order). Different languages employ different word orders and vary in how strictly the word order must be followed. English is included among the languages with relatively strict word order (e.g., it is not possible to find acceptable alternative word orders for the sentence "The man walks in the street"). In contrast, Spanish has an extremely flexible word order (e.g., the following word orders are acceptable for the same sentence: "El hombre camina por la calle," "Camina por la calle el hombre," "Por la calle camina el hombre," "Por la calle el hombre camina," "El hombre por la calle camina," "Camina el hombre por la calle"). All of these variations can be found in natural context but the probability differs considerably.

The relationship between two (or more) words in language utterances is a syntagmatic one. "The" is an article, and "House" is a noun, but in the utterance "The house" the two words are in contiguity, holding a syntagmatic relationship. "The house" is a syntagm because both words are interdependent, having a grammatical relationship.

Grammar refers to the rules that govern the structure of language and includes both morphology and syntax. Grammatical errors can be morphological (errors in word formation) or syntactic (errors in phrase structure). Thus, "They goes" is a morphological error; "I look you" is a syntactic error. Both types of errors occur in the agrammatism of aphasia.

Semantic Analysis

Semantics refers to word meanings, and the entire network of meanings of a word represents its semantic field. "Table" has a semantic field that may not include the objects used for seating but "chair" and "table" share a common semantic field in that they are furniture. The characteristics of "table" can vary, however; the word can represent a wooden or metal object that can be large or small, can have one or several legs, etc. The semantic fields of words change during language development and are different among individuals, dependent upon their personal

background. For instance, the word "bear" does not have exactly the same connotations for a child and for a hunter, and "depression" is quite different as used by
a psychiatrist and by an economist. Two separate words with the same meaning
are synonyms; perfect synonymity is virtually nonexistent. The semantic fields of
words differ among languages. The English word "language" does not have the
exact same semantic field as the Spanish word "lenguaje" nor does it cover all
facets implied by the French words "langue" and "langage." In addition, a single
word can have different meanings (homonymy and polysemy); often, one of the
meanings is stronger (or more primary) than the other(s). Most people would first
say that "table" is an article of furniture to put things on, but "table" can also be
used to represent a summary in a technical paper (a homonym).

A hierarchical organization can be outlined for the meanings in words (Buckingham, 1981a; Luria, 1976a,b). "Animal," "bird," and "chicken" exist in a vertical axis: chickens are birds and birds are animals. But "mammals" are also animals and "robins" are also "birds." "Animal" is a superordinate word with regard
to "bird," and "bird" is a superordinate word with regard to "chicken." The opposite of superordinate is hyponym; "birds" and "mammals" are hyponyms of "animal." "Chicken" and "robin" are hyponyms of "bird." "Chicken" and "robin" are
contrast coordinates (Goodglass and Baker, 1976) and comprise a minimal contrastive set (Miller and Johnson-Laird, 1976). Between themselves "chicken" and
"robin" hold a syntagmatic relationship but they can be said to have a paradigmatic relationship with "bird." They are contrastive and, based on a particular situation, "chicken" must be selected in contrast to "robin" (or "parrot," or any other
bird name) as the appropriate word. To select "robin" would represent a paradigmatic error. In some usage, "robin" can be considered a prototypical "bird";
"chicken" is not.

Pragmatics stems from recognition that language has a number of different
uses: to communicate events, to express emotions, to request information, to give
commands, etc. Pragmatics is the study of how language is used in each of the
different contexts.

Prosody (or intonation) is a term used to identify a number of routinely superimposed, suprasegmental aspects that provide additional communication information. Prosody includes stress, pitch, melody, rhythm, the juncture (spacing)
between words, and the intervals and pauses in conversational language, each of
which can convey or emphasize the meaning of a linguistic communication.

Language Deviations in Aphasia

In aphasia any aspect and any level of language can be impaired. Some of the
language deviations are characteristic of particular types of aphasic disorder and

deserve recognition for proper evaluation and management (Ardila and Roselli, 1993b).

Paraphasias

Literal Paraphasias (vs. Phonetic Deviations)

A paraphasia may be an incorrect word or an incorrectly produced word. One type of paraphasia, literal (phonemic) paraphasia, refers to an inappropriate phoneme use. Literal paraphasic errors can be *omissions, additions, displacements,* or *substitutions* of a phoneme. Phonetic-level changes (phonetic deviations) are usually not classed as literal paraphasias because they represent a different level of language disorder, an incompetent realization of the phoneme; the name paraphasia is not applied to errors in phonetic competence which are included with the speech disorders. Phonetic deviations are frequently observed in anterior (motor) aphasia but are not usually present to any significant degree in posterior (sensory) aphasia.

Articulatory Paraphasias

Even when phonemic paraphasias are presumed present in motor aphasic output, they can be the result of phonetic deviations pronounced so that they are wrongly perceived as phonemes by the listener (Buckingham, 1979b, 1989); in this sense they represent phonemic changes for the listener but are phonetic deviations for the speaker (Buckingham and Yule, 1987). A motor articulatory deficit can be misidentified by the listener as a phonemic paraphasia. Luria (1976b) noted that some literal paraphasias in afferent motor aphasia (conduction aphasia) output are perceived as phonemic substitutions but are actually articulatory in origin. Similarly, errors in the selection of the articulatory movements required to produce a phoneme (articuleme) can be misperceived as a deviated phonemic production. Luria suggested that in this situation the patient was not confusing the sounds of the language (phonemic disintegration) but, rather, presenting an apraxic motor misproduction of the articulatory selection.

Verbal Paraphasias

A verbal paraphasia is defined as the erroneous use of a word belonging to an inventory of the language in place of another word that also belongs to one of the language inventories (Lecours et al., 1983). Several different types of verbal paraphasia can be distinguished. First, and least definite, is *formal verbal paraphasia,* a transformation in which the substituting word and the substituted word are similar in form but not meaning (e.g., pear//dare); formal verbal paraphasias may be interpreted as a type of phonemic paraphasia (Lecours et al., 1983).

Morphemic verbal paraphasia refers to the use of an inappropriate word that has been assembled by using morphemes belonging to the language inventory (e.g., "summerly"). The resulting word may be acceptable from the point of view of the language but unacceptable for the context in which it appears. These innovations (creation of a new word by combining existing morphemes in a new way) are particularly observed in Wernicke aphasia (Liederman et al., 1983). When the resulting word is unacceptable from the point of view of the language, the deviations are often called neologisms but are also known as blends, hybrids, and telescopages. Such deviations can be due to: (1) incorrect affixation; (2) simultaneous encoding of two phonologically related lexical items having no semantic similarity; (3) simultaneous encoding of two semantically related words that are not phonologically associated; (4) perseveration or anticipation of part of a word in the sequential string (Buckingham, 1981b).

Semantic verbal paraphasia designates an aphasic transformation in which the desired and the substituted words are close in meaning (e.g., table//chair). Semantic verbal paraphasias that are observed in aphasics can be considered under several different headings: (1) the desired and the substituted words belong to the same semantic field (e.g., lion//tiger); (2) they are antonyms (e.g., big//small); (3) the target word is replaced by a superordinate (e.g., lion//animal). Superordinate substitution is characteristic of much aphasic language output, particularly when there is a word-finding problem. Words with a high level of generality but low content—e.g., thing, stuff, etc.—frequently recur); (4) an environmental proximity between the desired and the substituted words (e.g., cigarette//matches).

Patients may also introduce a word that, in the given context, is neither phonologically nor semantically related to the word that appears to be required (e.g., "It has been colorful to come to the hospital"). This type of deviation has been called an *unrelated verbal paraphasia* (Buckingham, 1979a; Green, 1969).

Syntagmatic Paraphasias

Paraphasias do not necessarily refer only to a single word; substitutions can appear among more complex linguistic units (e.g., the aquarium for the fish//the cage for the lion); the substitution of a meaningful, albeit incorrect, phrase can be called a syntagmatic paraphasia.

Other Linguistic Deviations

Circumlocutions

Substitutions of object description (e.g., snow//soft, white//cold) and instrumental function (e.g., watch//knowing the hour) can be observed in aphasic output. Substitutions of this type, called circumlocutions, occur frequently in posterior (sensory) aphasia.

Anaphors

An anaphor, by definition, is a word that has an antecedent occurring before or after the word to which it refers (Buckingham, 1981a). Aphasics often use anaphors for which a referent is nonexisting (indefinite anaphors). For instance the patient may say "I read it" but the key referent ("book," "letter," or "newspaper") has not been mentioned; "It" is an indefinite anaphor in this situation.

Neologisms

Neologisms have been defined as a phonological form for which it is impossible to recover, with any reasonable degree of certainty, a single item or items in the patient's vocabulary as it presumably existed before the onset of the aphasia (Buckingham and Kertesz, 1976). In other words, it is not possible for the examiner-listener to identify the target word; it is, however, almost always possible to identify its grammatical category based on its inflexion and phrase position. In general, neologisms are combinations of appropriate, reproduceable phonemes that convey no meaning in the speaker's vocabulary. Neologism may, in some cases, be due to a double error: a lexical selection error that, before it reaches phonetic materialization, is distorted phonemically.

Table 4.1 presents a summary of the main language deviations found in aphasia.

Jargon Aphasias

Jargon aphasia (Brown, 1981; Weinstein and Kahn, 1952; Weisenburg and McBride, 1935/1964) is a descriptive term referring to fluent, well-articulated language output that lacks meaning for the listener. The increased bulk of the verbal output and the absence of meaning are based on an overabundance of paraphasias and neologisms. Different types of jargon aphasia can be distinguished: *phonemic jargon, semantic jargon,* and *neologistic jargon* (Kertesz, 1985). All three deviations tend to occur together although one may predominate. Neologistic and semantic jargon are the primary components of a schizophrenic language output that has been termed *word salad,* an apt phrase for the mixture of misused linguistic features produced by the schizophrenic subject. Much more often, however, word salad is based on brain damage (Benson, 1979a).

Agrammatisms

Agrammatism describes a disruption of grammatical structure within language output (Goodglass and Berko, 1960; Kean, 1985; Menn and Obler, 1990; Pick, 1913). Patients with agrammatic aphasia have maximum difficulty in using (and understanding) grammatical morphemes (connectors and affixes) and lesser degrees of difficulty in the use and understanding of lexical morphemes. The disrupted grammatical structure often appears to be telegraphic because of omission

Table 4.1. Language Deviations in Aphasia

Phonetic deviations

Literal (Phonemic) Paraphasias
  Omissions
  Additions
  Displacements
  Substitutions
  Articulatory paraphasias (misperceived as phonemic paraphasias)

Verbal Paraphasias
  Formal verbal paraphasias (phonemic relation)
  Morphemic verbal paraphasias
  Semantic verbal paraphasias (semantic relation)
  Unrelated verbal paraphasias

Syntagmatic Paraphasias

Circumlocutions

Anaphors

Neologisms

Jargon aphasias
  Phonemic jargon
  Semantic jargon
  Neologistic jargon
  Schizophrenic word salad

Agrammatisms

Paragrammatisms

---

of the functional-grammatical markers (e.g., "The big boy went home" becomes "Boy—home"). Although phrase length is significantly decreased, semantic content is maintained; considerable meaning is expressed by the use of a few meaning-rich words. Verbs tend to be incorrectly used and tense, person, and number designations are often omitted (Miceli et al., 1984); nouns are not only the most frequent but the best-preserved language elements in agrammatic output.

Paragrammatisms
Paragrammatism (or dyssyntaxia) is a grammatical deviation characterized by a verbal output that violates the normative rules of morphosyntactic convention (Lecours et al., 1983). Paragrammatism may result from: (1) An overuse of grammatical elements (particularly connectors) associated with a decrease of nouns (lexemes); (2) an erroneous selection of grammatical elements; (3) an absence of defining limits in the sentences, correlated with an excessive verbal output. Pres-

sure to speak (logorrhea), when combined with other features of paragrammatism almost invariably indicates a disorder in the posterior (parietal-temporal) language system.

In acquired reading and writing disorders (alexia, agraphia), deviations similar to those described for oral language can be found. Literal substitutions are called literal paralexias in reading and literal paragraphias in writing. Verbal substitutions become verbal paralexias and verbal paragraphias. The agrammatism and paragrammatism seen in oral production can also be found in writing. Thus, jargon agraphia parallels jargon aphasia.

Linguistic Impairments Characterizing Different Aphasic Syndromes

Separate language features—phonetic, phonemic, morphemic, semantic, syntactic, and pragmatic—can be impaired by brain damage; the different aphasic syndromes tend to have characteristic impairments of selected linguistic features.

In Broca aphasia phonetic deviations are almost invariably observed and may be sufficiently severe that individual phonemes may be difficult to distinguish (the syndrome of phonetic disintegration described by Alajouanine, Ombredane, and Durand in 1939). In addition, the Broca aphasia patient often presents a language disautomatization so that every word is produced individually and with effort. Consonant clusters are reduced and phonological transpositions can be observed (i.e., a previously produced phoneme appears again in an inappropriate position or a phoneme programmed for production later in the verbalization is anticipated). Suprasegmental aspects of language are impaired by the disautomatization, producing a disturbance of prosody with disturbed rhythm, improper inflection, and inappropriate fragmentation of language elements leading to an alteration of melody. This produces the disorder described by Monrad-Krohn (1947) as dysprosody. In some cases, the prosodic disturbance can produce the appearance of a foreign accent (Ardila and Rosselli, 1988b; Monrad-Krohn, 1947).

Phonemic disintegration of language is much more commonly observed in the posterior aphasias (Luria, 1966), producing inappropriate sequences of phonemes and abundant literal paraphasias. In general, patients with Wernicke aphasia show good presentation of inflection and other prosodic qualities. Affixes are often preserved and it is frequently possible for the listener to recognize the target word or at least its linguistic category. Plurals and derivational affixes are maintained, a linguistic competency that is not preserved in Broca aphasia. Agrammatic Broca aphasia patients tend to omit affixes, and when the affixes are used they are often inadequate. In Broca aphasia, sentences are short (often one-word phrases) and there is little or no syntactic structure; words are isolated; there is an absence or striking shortage of grammatical connectors, and word order may be violated. Broca aphasia patients tend to produce grammatical deficits in word composition (morphology) and in sentence structure (syntax).

Difficulty in recognizing the semantic field of a presented word is a particularly characteristic problem for the patient who has one of several types of posterior aphasia, especially anomia (semantic anomia) and the extrasylvian aphasia syndromes (see Chapter 9). Disturbed semantic fields become prominent in classificatory tasks (Ardila, 1983; Gainotti et al., 1986). The patient fails to determine the semantic boundaries of a word and may express surprise that a single word may have a different meaning. Kudo (1987) observed that hierarchical semantical categorization is impaired in all aphasia patients, with subjective category domains more diffuse in aphasics than in normal subjects. Patients with fluent Wernicke aphasia are most affected by disordered semantic fields and often have a profound disintegration of semantic boundaries; the traditional semantic limits of words appear lost to them. The underlying representation of semantic categories is relatively preserved in Broca aphasia, particularly in comparison to the serious disruption seen in fluent aphasias (Grober et al., 1980). Word-finding difficulties and verbal paraphasias, particularly semantic verbal paraphasias, are considerably more abundant in all fluent aphasics.

Patients with left frontal-lobe damage and extrasylvian motor aphasia often have a different problem, a lack of verbal initiative. For these patients, language is not spontaneously available for the communication of external events or internal states, even to express basic biological needs. These subjects appear to suffer an inability to employ the elements of language; the pragmatics of language, the ability to produce narrative discourse, is seriously disturbed and there is a notable hesitancy in the initiation of articulation (Alexander and Benson, 1991; Benson, 1979a).

Table 4.2 presents a summary of the language levels principally impaired in different aphasic syndromes.

The relationships between linguistic impairment and type of aphasia is considerably more complex than suggested by the outline in Table 4.2. Although certain linguistic problems tend to predominate in specific types of aphasia, the relationship is far from specific.

Agrammatism has a strong correlation with Broca aphasia and can usually be distinguished from the paragrammatism found in posterior aphasia. Nonfluent, agrammatic patients show poor comprehension of syntax (Martin, 1987) but this does not mean that syntactic deficits are restricted to anterior, nonfluent aphasics. Auditory syntactic comprehension deficits are found in aphasics with perisylvian area lesions (frontal, parietal, and temporal) and particularly in those cases with

Table 4.2. Level of Language Impaired in Different Aphasic
        Syndromes

LEVEL OF LANGUAGE IMPAIRED	MAIN SYNDROMES IN WHICH IMPAIRMENT APPEARS
Phonetic	Dysarthria
	Broca aphasia
Phonemic	Wernicke aphasia
	Conduction aphasia
Morphemic	Broca aphasia
Syntactic	Broca aphasia
Semantic	Extrasylvian sensory aphasia
	Wernicke aphasia
Pragmatic	Extrasylvian motor aphasia

involvement of Wernicke's area (Naeser et al., 1987). Niemi, Koivuselka-Sallinen, and Laine (1987) found that the paraphasias seen in Wernicke aphasia appear more often in syntactically derived words than in lexically derived words, suggesting that morphosyntactic factors may interfere with word processing in Wernicke aphasia. Patients with Wernicke aphasia present a restricted range of syntactic forms and impairments in their ability to use the syntactic information in a sentence to assign role relations (Martin and Blossom-Stach, 1986) and their ability to combine morphemes is also restricted (Liederman et al., 1983). Luria (1966, 1976a,b) emphasized that in some fluent forms of aphasia, particularly extrasylvian sensory aphasia, the impairment in the ability to comprehend the "communication of relationships" (e.g., "the son's mother"//"the mother's son") will be notable. This disorder could be considered a type of agrammatism but is considerably different from the well-described agrammatism seen in Broca aphasia or the paragrammatism described in Wernicke aphasia (Ardila, Lopez, and Solano, 1989b). Luria points out that difficulty in "communication of relationships" particularly affects grammatical structures that arise late in language acquisition, relationships that represent and demand greater structural complexity (Luria, 1976a).

Language comprehension is restricted or abnormal in some manner in every type of aphasia. Comprehension deficits, however, are qualitatively different among the different aphasia syndromes. Evidence suggests that disorders in comprehension in Broca aphasia happen mainly, if not totally, because the patients do not have complete control of grammatical morphology (Berndt and Caramazza, 1981; Zurif, Caramazza, and Myerson, 1972). In fluent aphasias a number of other factors may lead to language comprehension deficits: phonemic disintegration, disordered semantic fields for words, verbal auditory agnosia, deficiencies in verbal memory, etc. In conduction aphasia language repetition is most impaired and language comprehension is least impaired; patients with conduction aphasia, however, often fail to comprehend long and complex sentences that require active decoding and maintenance of sequential order via internal repetition (Luria, 1966). Patients with extrasylvian motor aphasia (transcortical motor aphasia) may readily understand simple and direct statements but may misinterpret complex, abstract, absurd, or metaphorical statements. Table 4.3 summarizes the primary linguistic deficits characterizing the major aphasia syndromes. Additional descriptions of specific linguistic impairments will be included in the discussions of individual symptom clusters in later chapters.

Cross-linguistic studies may be helpful in clarifying which linguistic disorders are fundamental (i.e., involve all languages) and which depend upon the characteristics of a particular language (Ardila et al., 1989c; Bates et al., 1988). Some aspects of language are universal, so that similar deficits will be readily observed in any aphasic, no matter which language they speak; other aspects appear almost language dependent. Bates, Friederici, and Wulfeck (1987) compared the verbal output of agrammatic aphasic patients who were native speakers of either English, German, or Italian. The array of language deficits was somewhat different across the three languages but some aspects appeared universal. Thus, word order was spared and grammatical morphology was impaired in all three languages. Impairment of grammatical morphology appears to be a funda-

Table 4.3. Main Linguistic Deficits in Aphasia

TYPE OF APHASIA	MAIN LINGUISTIC DEFICITS
Broca aphasia	Agrammatism
Wernicke aphasia	Phonological discrimination deficits; memory deficits for phonological sequence of words
Conduction aphasia	Repetition impairments
Extrasylvian motor aphasia	Pragmatic function of language is altered
Extrasylvian sensory aphasia	Deficits in semantic relationships of words

mental language deficit in agrammatic aphasic patients, regardless of the native language, but the specific details of the breakdown tend to be distinct, dependent on the language of the speaker.

Summary

In summary, general relationships can be established between the type of aphasia and the characteristics of language impairment but these relationships have proved to be complex and multiple. Understanding of language structure is a prerequisite to the linguistic analysis of aphasic language disturbance and represents one key factor for determining clinical distinctions.

5

Brain Damage in Aphasia

· ·

By definition, aphasia is the result of brain damage; therefore, a neuropathology of aphasia exists. Both the type of pathology and the location of the brain lesion are significant to the clinicians caring for an aphasic patient. Techniques that demonstrate lesion type and site are crucial to the neuropathology of aphasia. Several generalizations can be offered (Benson, 1979a):

1. *Aphasia is produced by damage to brain structures.* Neuropathological processes that involve nonbrain portions of the nervous system (e.g., cranial nerves) and secondary neurological dysfunctions such as systemic or psychogenic disorders do not produce aphasic language syndromes. Metabolic and toxic disorders (e.g., hepatic encephalopathy) produce a broad, overall disruption of brain function, not a focal aphasia. Also, because language *loss*, by definition, is a requirement for aphasia, congenital and developmental disorders in which language failed to develop cannot be considered sources of aphasia.

2. *The neuroanatomical location, not the etiology, of the brain damage is the crucial factor in aphasic symptomatology.* Aphasia can follow any type of neuropathology capable of causing structural alterations in the language area of the brain, whether this be in the cortex, the cortical-cortical connections or in certain subcortical regions. It is the neuroanatomical site of damage that determines the individual symptoms or symptom clusters of language impairment.

3. *Consistent aphasia indicates structural pathology involving the language area.*

Aphasia may accompany functional central nervous system (CNS) disorders such as epilepsy, toxic or metabolic confusional states, or migraine aura that are capable of producing focal cortical disorder. In these situations, the aphasia is almost invariably transient and/or overshadowed by other neurologic or behavioral abnormalities.

4. *Identical aphasia syndromes may be produced by different neuropathological states.* The clusters of clinical findings that make up the syndromes of aphasia are not the product of specific types of pathology but rather depend on the portion of the language area involved. Some types of brain pathology, however, more commonly affect certain brain regions and thus the symptom complex of aphasia may provide valuable diagnostic clues for the clinician.

5. *When pathology involves nonlanguage brain areas, aphasic symptomatology will be absent or negligible.* When pathology involves brain regions outside the language area, including most subcortical structures and the entire nondominant hemisphere, language alterations are absent or, if present, minimal and vague.

Despite our stress on anatomical locus in contrast to etiology in the genesis of aphasia, the type of pathology does have significance for the neurologist. The underlying disease process must be recognized and treated along with the language problem; both the type of language therapy offered and the patient's prognosis depend on the basic pathology.

Neuropathological Substrate of Aphasia

A wide variety of disorders that can cause focal damage to appropriate brain areas can produce aphasia. Clinical features (e.g., age of patient, acuteness of onset, type of "neighborhood findings") often provide the clinician with sufficient data

Table 5.1. Five Aphorisms for Brain Damage and Aphasia

---

1. Aphasia is a product of brain damage.

2. It is the neuroanatomical location of brain damage, not the etiology, that determines aphasic symptomatology.

3. When aphasia is prominent, focal structural pathology involving language area structures must be suspected.

4. Different pathological states can produce identical aphasic syndromes.

5. Damage to nonlanguage areas of brain produces little or no aphasic symptomatology.

---

to allow etiologic diagnosis. Variations are considerable, however, and knowledge of disease states beyond mere categorization is often valuable in the understanding and management of aphasia. A number of the more common brain disorders associated with aphasia will be discussed here.

Vascular Disorders

Disorders of cerebral or extracranial blood vessels causing ischemic damage to certain brain areas rank high among the causes of structural alterations to the central nervous system (Romanul, 1970). Vascular disease (stroke), in fact, is the most common cause of aphasia (Tonkonogy, 1986).

Three kinds of cerebrovascular accident (CVA)—thrombosis, embolism, and hemorrhage—are the classic etiologic categories of stroke; although not accurately descriptive of all cerebral vascular conditions that can produce aphasia, the traditional triad will be used in this chapter. Advanced diagnostic techniques have altered the suspected incidence of the three varieties. At one time cerebral hemorrhage was the diagnosis suggested, almost automatically, for most stroke cases. As autopsy studies that include examination of the brain became more common, the favored etiology shifted to thrombosis (Wechsler, 1952). In recent years, concomitant with the increased popularity of great vessel surgery, the diagnosis of embolism has risen to account for as many as one-third of all cerebral ischemic strokes. Currently, brain imaging techniques suggest that the incidence of small vessel lesions deep in the brain, probably occlusive, is much higher than previously suspected.

Whether cerebrovascular pathology produces good case material for the study of aphasia has been debated (Critchley, 1970b; Geschwind, 1965). Many investigators, particularly those who work in neurosurgical centers where trauma and tumor predominate, note that a stroke rarely involves an otherwise normal brain. Widespread vascular insufficiency and/or multiple small infarcts are present in many cases of stroke-induced aphasia (Ring and Waddington, 1968); brain pathology distant from the site of the vascular accident is almost always present. Others dispute this statement, noting that in many carefully studied postmortem cases significant pathology was limited to brain areas served by the involved vessel, producing a sharply focal lesion (Fisher, 1975). There is truth in both statements. Some vascular cases do show multiple areas of ischemic damage, and it becomes difficult to ascribe specific language symptoms to any single lesion locus. Other cases will have a single precisely located lesion so that clinical-anatomical correlation appears firm. Precisely located lesions are of considerable consequence for the student of language; for the clinician, however, the limitation of lesion size is not the major concern. Cerebrovascular disease is common and the underlying etiology of the vascular disorder must be recognized and treated.

Thrombosis

The occlusion of a vessel from a blood clot attached to an overgrown vessel wall was once considered the most common cause of acute cerebrovascular disease (Fisher, 1975), and a stroke was accepted almost automatically as evidence of arteriosclerosis (Weschler, 1952). Classic thrombosis is produced by overgrowth of arteriosclerotic material within the vessel sufficient to occlude the lumen and attract blood materials that clot or produce a subintimal hemorrhage. Although now considered less frequent, thrombosis is still estimated to be the etiology of about two-thirds of all ischemic strokes (Grotta, 1993). Occlusion of a cerebral artery produces immediate cessation of blood flow and subsequent death of brain tissue (ischemic infarction) in the territory supplied by the involved vessel. The resulting neurologic defect (syndrome) reflects the vascular territory involved. Table 5.2 presents the most common aphasic syndromes associated with particular cerebrovascular territories.

Many disease processes other than arteriosclerosis can cause thrombosis. Inflammatory disorders such as giant cell arteritis, syphilitic endarteritis, polyarteritis nodosa, or lupus erythematosus can occlude cerebral vessels. Blood disorders such as polycythemia, leukemia, or sickle cell anemia can produce cell aggregations capable of occluding vessels. Altered cerebral circulation, particularly hypotensive episodes secondary to heart failure, myocardial infarction, cardiac arrhythmia, surgical shock, postural hypotension, dehydration, or even the bradycardia and hypotension of sleep, may allow an already compromised vessel to occlude

Table 5.2. Association between Aphasic Syndromes and Selected Cerebrovascular Territories

CEREBROVASCULAR TERRITORY	APHASIC SYNDROME
Anterior Cerebral Artery Occlusion	Extrasylvian motor aphasia
Posterior Cerebral Artery Occlusion	Occipital alexia
Middle Cerebral Artery Occlusion	
Total	Global aphasia
Orbitofrontal branch	Broca aphasia
Rolandic branch	Broca aphasia, cortical dysarthria
Anterior parietal branch	Conduction aphasia
Posterior parietal branch	Wernicke aphasia, extrasylvian sensory aphasia
Angular branch	Anomia, extrasylvian sensory aphasia
Posterior temporal branch	Wernicke aphasia
Anterior temporal branch	Anomia

fully. Trauma to one of the carotid arteries sufficient to damage the inner lining (intima) can produce subintimal hemorrhage or a tear of the intima that can act as a nidus for cell aggregations; either can lead to occlusion of the involved vessel.

Embolism

Occlusion of a vessel by material floating in the arterial system (embolism) is a frequent cause of stroke. For years most emboli were thought to come from the heart: small bits of mural thrombus dislodged from the cardiac wall during cardiac rhythm changes. With the advent of carotid angiography, it became possible to demonstrate that calcific plaques in the carotid vessels (and other large vessels) were a common source of emboli to the brain. Emboli can form in and migrate from cardiac surgery sites, bacterial endocarditis foci, the vessels of the lungs, or even the great veins by entering arterial circulation after passage through a defect in the heart wall. On rare occasions emboli consisting of fat particles from fractured bones or of tumor-cell aggregates may produce brain infarction. If the involved vessel feeds the language area, embolism can cause aphasia.

Hemorrhage

Bleeding into cerebral tissues is most often associated with hypertension (Hier et al., 1977) but may follow blood extravasation from a ruptured aneurysm, an angioma or an arteriovenous (A-V) malformation. Intracerebral blood collections may also occur in individuals with blood dyscrasia (disease processes producing bleeding tendencies) or arteritis. Anticoagulant therapy is frequently used to manage patients with coronary or cerebrovascular occlusive disease; if not monitored carefully, it can allow bleeding into brain tissue. Intracerebral hemorrhage, based on trauma or tumor (although not vascular disorders by definition) may produce significant cerebral damage. If hemorrhage damages an area of brain that subserves language, an aphasia will result.

Pathophysiology of Vascular Disorders

The degree, site, and type of brain damage produced by cerebral vascular disorders varies considerably. Both thrombosis and embolism occlude vessels and thus produce partial or total ischemia in the tissues receiving vascular supply from the involved vessel; ischemia produces cell death (infarction). Both neurons (gray matter) and myelinated pathways (white matter) can be affected but white matter can withstand ischemia much better than gray matter. Tissue at the center of an infarct tends to be completely destroyed, whereas on the periphery both neurons and white matter pathways may survive. Incomplete ischemia may cause neurons to cease functioning temporarily but not die. Over time, some injured neurons recuperate sufficiently to resume functioning and many white-matter pathways survive to carry impulses again. The tendency for spontaneous recovery so nota-

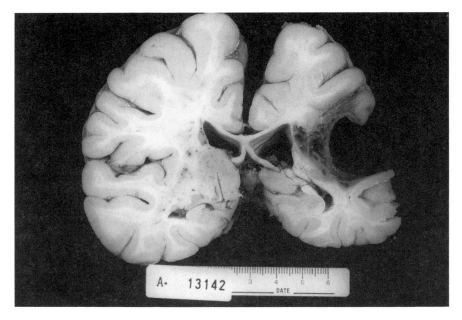

Figure 5.l. Coronal slide of brain showing large post-CVA cavitation in left language area. (Courtesy of H. Vinters, M.D., Division of Neuropathology, UCLA School of Medicine).

ble in aphasia (see Chapter 20) probably stems at least in part from the delayed return to function (measured in weeks) that can follow infarction.

The end result of occlusion based on either thrombosis or embolism is an infarct, a cystic cavity devoid of neurons or white matter and surrounded by a glial scar (see Figure 5.1). In contrast, hemorrhage most often occurs deep in the brain and not only causes local tissue destruction but rapidly forms a mass lesion that compresses surrounding tissues. The mass of extravasated blood may produce sufficient pressure to occlude nearby vessels, adding an ischemic element to the zone of tissue destroyed by the bleed. Initially, intracerebral hemorrhage produces a hematoma, a mass of blood encapsulated by compressed cerebral tissues (see Figure 5.2). The hematoma forms rapidly to produce a maximal disruption of brain function. If the bleeding stops and the patient survives, the mass will shrink, eventually leaving only a cystic cavity with discolored sclerotic walls. Hemorrhage accounts for over one-third of cerebrovascular accidents but only about half of these are intracerebral (Grotta, 1993). Extracerebral (subarachnoid) hemorrhages can also compress language-significant brain areas acutely but are far less likely to produce a permanent aphasia condition.

The clinical picture will vary directly with the vascular territory involved (middle cerebral, anterior cerebral, or posterior cerebral artery) and, to a lesser

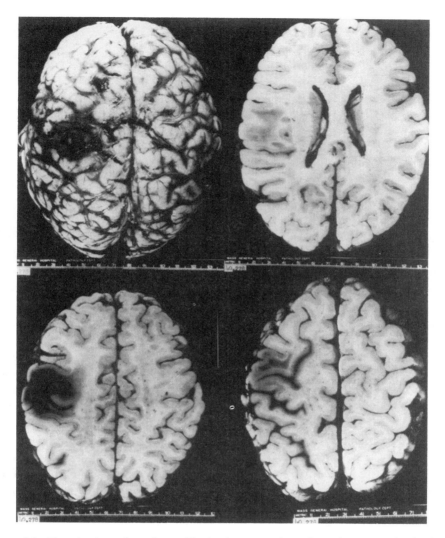

Figure 5.2. Four horizontal sections of brain demonstrating a large hematoma in the language area. (From Levine and Sweet, 1983).

degree, with the type of pathology. The site of an infarct is often located at a distance from the site of vessel occlusion or damage. Emboli tend to affect smaller (often cortical) branches, producing damage near the site of occlusion, whereas thrombi most often involve larger, more centrally located branches and can produce both cortical and subcortical damage at a distance from the site of occlusion. When cerebral infarction involves the border zone territory (see Figure 5.3), ves-

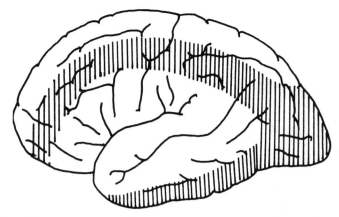

Figure 5.3. Graphic representation of the vascular border zone (vertical hatching) of the left hemisphere. (From Cummings and Benson, 1992).

sel occlusion almost always occurs at a considerable distance, often in the carotid arteries as they course through the neck. In this situation, a compensatory vascular supply, via vessels of the circle of Willis (the arterial ring at the base of the brain), provides supplemental but often insufficient blood flow for the territory fed by the occluded branches (Romanul and Abramowitz, 1961). Although tissues fed by these collateral vessels can survive, those tissues located the farthest out on the vascular tree (the so-called border zone) may become ischemic and infarcted, producing an unusual vascular injury with characteristic language impairments (i.e., extrasylvian aphasia) (see Chapter 9).

The location of pathology—cortical, subcortical, or mixed—reflects the causative vascular pathology and significantly influences any verbal-output disorder produced. Hypertension, hypotension or diabetes more often produce small, deeply situated infarctions (lacunes) and the resulting verbal-output disorder more often features speech disorder (see Chapter 16). Thrombosis involving a major vessel tends to produce a mixed cortical-subcortical infarction whereas emboli, by occluding multiple small terminal branches, may produce either cortical or subcortical damage.

The constituents of the language symptom cluster (the aphasia syndrome) vary, depending on the area of the vascular tree affected, and may provide clues to the type of vascular disease present. The generalizations suggested at the beginning of this chapter (Table 5.1) remain firm. The area of brain that is damaged, not the vessel involved or the specific vascular pathology, determines the aphasic symptomatology. Two patients may have the same pathology at the same location on the same vessel and yet present clinically distinct aphasic symptomatology. The site and the extent of brain infarcted following vascular disease can vary substantially depending on variations in collateral circulation; aphasic symptomatology always reflects the brain area rendered nonfunctional, not the location of vascular occlusion.

Intracerebral hemorrhages most frequently affect one of two distributions. One, usually associated with vascular disease or hypertension, involves subcortical structures such as caudate, putamen, thalamus, internal capsule, or insula. Unique communication impairment syndromes result from the primarily subcortical locus of the hemorrhage (see Chapter 10). The second, hematoma associated with trauma or neoplasm, more often involves more superficial cortical and/or underlying subcortical areas; the resulting aphasia syndromes are quite different, depending on the anatomical locus involved. Identical-appearing hemorrhagic pathlogy that involves different loci will produce different language impairments (Alexander and LoVerme, 1980).

Trauma

Brain injuries during war have produced many cases of aphasia (Conrad, 1954; Kleist, 1934b; Luria, 1947/1970, 1963; Russell and Espir, 1961; Schiller, 1947), as have other types of brain trauma (e.g., motor vehicle accidents, falls). Some authorities think that gunshot wounds cause the most accurately localized brain pathology available for studying aphasia (Conrad, 1954; Critchley, 1970b; Luria, 1947/1970). Others disagree, primarily because the most common types of battle injuries (e.g., from shrapnel, low-velocity missiles, and either open- or closed-head trauma) are almost invariably associated with widespread brain damage. Even high-velocity missile wounds tend to deform numerous intracerebral structures. In most of the head trauma cases evaluated in civilian practice, no break occurs in the dural covering of the brain (closed-head injury); localization in these cases is routinely complicated because multiple, widely spread areas of the brain are involved. The focal neurological signs produced by brain trauma often indicate multiple sites of damage located at a distance from the site of impact (Figure 5.4).

With the many traffic accidents in today's society (at least half of the estimated five hundred thousand cases of traumatic brain injury that occur each year in the United States are due to motor vehicle accidents) and the steadily increasing number of civilian gunshot wound victims, trauma now represents a common cause of aphasia (Levin and Grossman, 1978). Traumatic aphasia is almost routinely complicated by amnesia and often by other neurobehavioral abnormalities (see Chapter 17) that obscure language evaluation. Based on a study of fifty-six closed-head injury cases, Sarno (1980) stated, "The boundaries which usually help identify and classify patients with linguistic deficits after brain damage do not seem to hold to the same degree for the head trauma patients as they do in the stroke population." Although trauma is a common cause of aphasia, the mix-

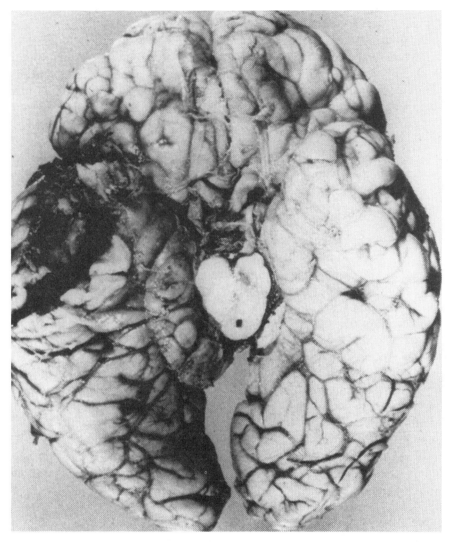

Figure 5.4. Undersurface of fixed brain showing traumatic injury with hemorrhages involving left medial and lateral posterior temporal lobe. (From Adams, Graham, and Gennarelli, 1985).

ture of language impairment with other neurobehavioral disorders often obscures the aphasia symptomatology and frustrates attempts to locate the site of damage related to the aphasia.

In addition to producing direct destruction of cerebral structures, hematomas secondary to brain trauma can complicate the aphasia features. Both extracerebral (subdural or epidural) and intracerebral hematomas can produce acute increases in intracranial pressure. The subsequent symptom pictures tend to be dramatic; although often present, aphasia is overshadowed by other symptoms. On the other hand, aphasia (particularly a mild word-finding disturbance) may be a significant finding in cases of longstanding chronic subdural hematoma. The degree of trauma to the head may be mild (e.g., bumping the head on a cupboard door) and may have been forgotten by the patient, but aphasia may result from the apparently insignificant head injury.

Aphasia is relatively infrequent following closed-head injury (about 2%) (Heilman, Safran and Geschwind, 1971), but is fairly common as a residual of open-head injuries (Conrad, 1954; Luria, 1947/1970; Russell and Espir, 1961; Schiller, 1947). Left hemisphere involvement most often predominates in post-traumatic aphasia, but many cases with the major locus of trauma in the right hemisphere will show language deficits, probably reflecting the widespread nature of the brain injury. In general, the prognosis for recovery from aphasia is better following brain trauma than following stroke, probably due to the younger age of most trauma victims. Persistent posttraumatic language defects are usually coupled with a broad spectrum of other mental impairments.

Neoplasms

Intracranial neoplasms, although not as common as strokes, do produce aphasia (Hécaen and Angelergues, 1964). Those neoplasms that involve brain tissues (e.g., gliomas) tend to infiltrate widely before they cause focal destruction. Early symptomatology in such cases tends to be general (e.g., headache, poor concentration, decreased vigilance) (Hécaen and Ajuriaguerra, 1956). Only late in the course will distinct language disorder be noted (Holmes, 1931; Pool and Correll, 1958).

Intracranial neoplasms may be divided, for discussion purposes, into two major classes—intracerebral and extracerebral. Intracerebral neoplasms include the glioma series (e.g., glioblastoma, astrocytoma, medulloblastoma, oligodendroglioma, ependymoma) and are the most common aphasia-producing tumors (Figure 5.5). In older patients another intracerebral tumor, metastasis from an extracranial cancer, increases in frequency as a cause of aphasia. Intracerebral tumor can cause any type of aphasia (Ausman, French, and Baker, 1981; Luria, Pribram, and Homskaya, 1964) but motor speech disorder is the most common.

Extracerebral brain tumors such as meningiomas usually develop slowly, allowing time for considerable accommodation by the cerebral tissues and causing minimal disruption of function until late in the course. Most of the initial language symptoms produced by intracranial neoplasms are caused by mass effect

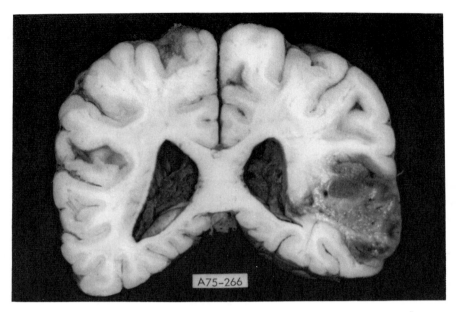

Figure 5.5. Large glioblastoma involving left temporal lobe. (Courtesy of H. Vinters, M.D., Division of Neuropathology, UCLA School of Medicine).

that interferes with blood supply or occludes cerebrospinal fluid circulation. Tumors located outside the brain (extracerebral) include meningioma, craniopharyngioma, pinealoma, acoustic neuroma, neurofibroma, and others. Aphasia is uncommon with extracerebral tumors. When it does occur, distortion or displacement of brain tissues or the compression of a major vessel is most often present (Kertesz, 1985).

The symptoms produced by intracranial neoplasm tend to be vague in the early stages. Only rarely do untreated intracranial neoplasms produce clear examples of the focal aphasic syndromes, but evaluation of the language disorder features of early, untreated intracranial tumors may provide some useful diagnostic information. Thus, a correlation between fluent or nonfluent aphasic output and posterior or anterior locus of tumor has been reported (Rosenfield and Goree, 1975). More often, the language impairment in untreated intracranial tumors remains nonspecific—word-finding problems, slowness in comprehension, and/or hesitancy in verbal output. Untreated tumors may produce language symptoms based on malfunction of brain tissue distant from the site of the tumor. For instance, a tumor located high in the frontal or parietal area can produce downward pressure sufficient to compress temporal-lobe brain tissue against the tentorium (Kernohan and Sayre, 1952). The resulting temporal-lobe herniation can compromise one (or both) posterior cerebral arteries and produce posterior language disorders such as alexia and anomia even though the tumor itself is located at a considerable distance from the brain territory involved.

Aphasic findings have only limited value in the localization of intracranial neoplasm. Neuroimaging studies provide far more accurate localizing data and when clinical examination does reveal language disorder in untreated neoplasms the findings tend to be intermixed with many additional behavioral problems. The common failure to correlate tumor site with traditional sites for language symptomatology has given rise to some of the reports in the aphasia literature refuting the validity of language localization (Critchley, 1970b).

Surgery for cerebral neoplasms, particularly the standard debulking procedure, can provide sharply defined focal language findings. The decompression procedure destroys and removes a pocket of gray and white matter that, although infiltrated or compressed by tumor, had remained functional. The site of the surgical decompression resembles a vascular infarct, in both appearance and disordered function, and may be associated with a precise aphasia syndrome.

Infections

Intracranial infection produces widespread behavioral symptomatology; any language disorder produced by cerebral infection/inflammation will be obscured by many other serious dysfunctions. Currently, the brain infection that most frequently produces aphasia is herpes simplex encephalitis. The initial symptom picture (headache, confusion, fever, and coma) indicates widespread brain abnormality and frequently leads to death; with appropriate diagnosis and treatment, however, many patients with herpes encephalitis now survive. As the stupor clears a severe aphasia is often noted, and anomia may remain as a long-term residual of the brain infection. The language disorder in these patients is almost always obscured, however, by a more generalized pervasive dementia and by a severe inability to learn (amnesia). Although confrontation naming tests will demonstrate the presence of an anomia, the degree of amnesia almost always overshadows the aphasia (Cermak and O'Connor, 1983; Rose and Symonds, 1960) and the word-finding problem tends to recover better than the amnesia. Aphasia is rarely the most disabling symptom and tends to be overlooked. Many other brain infections can produce aphasia (Figure 5.6), almost always accompanied by so many other neurobehavioral problems that aphasia is overshadowed.

One infectious process that can produce a focal aphasia syndrome is intracerebral abscess. In addition to the inflammatory changes that produce systemic malaise and destroy brain tissue, an abscess produces symptoms by direct pressure (mass effect), focal tissue destruction, distortion of the vascular supply and/or obstruction to CSF flow. The acute symptom picture tends to be nonspecific, but following treatment (particularly surgical drainage) a focal aphasia may persist. Before the use of antibiotics was prevalent, temporal-lobe abscess secondary

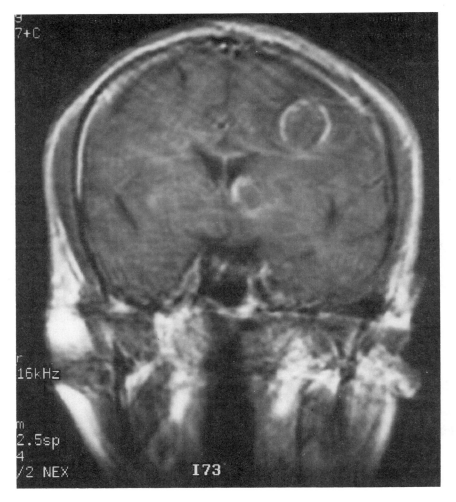

Figure 5.6. CT scan showing a large calcified toxoplasmosis cyst in the left frontal-parietal white matter with a second cyst in the left periventricular area. (Courtesy of B. L. Miller, M.D., Department of Neurology, Harbor-UCLA Medical Center).

to chronic ear infection was a well-known source of aphasia (Lishman, 1987); intracerebral abscess is now rare.

Miscellaneous Causes of Aphasia

Aphasia may occur with many other types of intracerebral pathology but usually only as part of an extensive neurologic and behavioral dysfunction. For instance, *multiple sclerosis* (MS) rarely causes aphasia until late in the course (see Chapter

10) and the language difficulty is most often restricted to a word-finding problem. Most MS subjects who are aphasic also suffer serious amnesia and/or dementia (Achiron et al., 1992). *Huntington's disease* can produce some degree of aphasia but rarely does the language disorder appear significant relative to the other serious neurologic and behavioral problems. In fact, the absence of significant aphasia in the face of severe mental problems represents a significant diagnostic marker of Huntington's disease (McHugh and Folstein, 1975). It was this lack of formal language deficits in disorders such as Huntington's disease, Parkinson's disease, and progressive supranuclear palsy that led to the cortical-subcortical differentiation in dementia categorization (Albert, Feldman, and Willis, 1974; Benson, 1983; Cummings and Benson, 1984; McHugh and Folstein, 1975) (see Chapters 17 and 18).

Aphasia, or at least a relatively focal language impairment, can also result from *epilepsy*. Aphasia may occur with the seizure (ictal) or may appear in the post-ictal recovery period (Ardila and Lopez, 1988; Engel, 1989; Suzuki et al., 1992). Epileptic language disorder is transient, most often lasting only a few minutes, and usually indicates a seizure focus located in the language area of the brain. Aphasia can also occur as a prodrome of migraine headache (Ardila and Sanchez, 1988; Campbell and Caselli, 1991); again, the transient nature of the language impairment is notable.

Aphasia is common in late-life cortical degenerative disorders (e.g., Alzheimer's and Pick's diseases) and may occur in prion disorders such as Jakob-Creutzfeldt disease (Brown et al., 1986; Gorman et al., 1992; Mandell, Alexander, and Carpenter, 1989) or other progressive disorders affecting cortical structures. Chapter 17 discusses some of these problems along with other language alterations associated with aging. Although the degree of language dysfunction in these disorders may be considerable (in advanced stages), there are usually so many other behavioral and neurologic problems present that aphasia represents only a small part of the clinical picture. Considerable investigation of the language symptomatology of degenerative dementia has been carried out in recent years (Balota and Duchek, 1991; Bayles and Kaszniak, 1987; Cummings et al., 1985; Kempler, Curtiss, and Jackson, 1987; Kirshner et al., 1984; Powell et al., 1988; Smith, Chenery, and Murdoch, 1989; Sommers and Pierce, 1990); variations in language disorder have proved valuable as diagnostic aids in dementia (Cummings and Benson, 1986).

One significant variation of degenerative brain disorder is the syndrome called *progressive aphasia* (Mesulam, 1982). Although progressive aphasia is not common, a number of investigators have reported patients with a slowly progressive language impairment but little other evidence suggesting memory, cognitive, or neurobehavioral dysfunction until the terminal stages of the disorder (Kempler et al., 1990; Kirshner et al., 1984; Luzzatti and Poeck, 1991; Mendez and Zander,

1991; Sapin, Anderson, and Pulaski, 1989; Snowden et al., 1992; Wechsler, 1977; Weintraub, Robin, and Mesulam, 1990). Both nonfluent and fluent language disorders have been described in progressive aphasia (Snowden et al., 1992). By most reports, the course of the disorder is slow (measured in years). Appropriate brain imaging studies, particularly PET or SPECT scans, have revealed left hemisphere dysfunction, often relatively focal (Kempler et al., 1990). A few patients with progressive aphasia have come to postmortem and a variety of etiologies have been reported including spongiform degeneration (Kirshner et al., 1987; Shuttleworth, Yates, and Paltan-Ortiz, 1985), Pick's disease (Wechsler et al., 1982), and widespread plaques and tangles (Benson and Zaias, 1991). The variety of neuropathological substrates indicates that progressive aphasia is a syndrome, a cluster of language features that can result from different disease processes (Mesulam, 1987), a premise in agreement with the statements in Table 5.1.

In summary, almost any disorder that affects the language area of the brain can produce language impairment. The type of pathology is not directly consequential to the specific aphasia symptom cluster but does have considerable bearing on the patient's ultimate prognosis. For the clinician the type of pathology is a pertinent factor.

Localization Techniques

Localization of the neuroanatomical site of brain damage in cases of aphasia remains a significant aspect of aphasiology, particularly for the clinician. Over the years many different ways to localize aphasia-producing lesions have been suggested; not all have proved successful. In fact, the localization of aphasia-producing lesions in the living patient was immensely difficult before the recent technical advances in brain imaging. Even with these tools, localization remains less accurate than desirable. Traditionally, aphasia syndromes have been developed by clustering clinical findings and then correlating the resultant syndrome with whatever neuroanatomical information was available. The symptom clusters will be discussed in subsequent chapters. The major techniques currently used to locate the site of brain damage (all successful methods are still used to some degree) will be outlined.

Neuropathology

The postulations of Broca, Wernicke, Bastian, Dejerine, and most other nineteenth-century aphasiologists relied upon direct postmortem anatomical observation of patients who had suffered a demonstrable language impairment. Henschen (1922) abstracted over a thousand cases of aphasia taken from the medical literature with both clinical description of language impairment and anatomical evidence (mostly from postmortem studies) sufficient to allow localization. Many hundreds of additional cases have been published in subsequent years.

Although offering precise anatomical information, autopsy material has a number of drawbacks for aphasia localization. First, and most significant, the patient must have survived the brain insult and recovered to a sufficient degree to allow language evaluation but then must have suffered no additional CNS pathology from the time of the language evaluation until death. Development of a valid, consistent aphasic syndrome requires a significant period for stabilization of brain function; weeks or even months may pass before the aphasia features are solidified sufficiently for precise interpretation. Many subjects disappear from follow-up or suffer additional cerebral pathology that obscures neuroanatomical correlation. Many cases in the literature, particularly those reported in the nineteenth century, died before developing a well-delineated clinical picture. Therefore, interpretations of brain-language correlations based on these subjects tended to be misleading.

Despite obvious problems, necropsy material remains important for localization in cases of aphasia. Postmortem study provides, at least potentially, a far more exact anatomical localization than any other currently available technique and many investigators still consider autopsy material to be the gold standard for aphasia localization.

Neurosurgery

Surgical excision of intracranial (particularly intracerebral) pathology can produce aphasia. The anatomical area involved is recorded as accurately as possible in the surgical notes so that any residual aphasia may be studied long after the surgery is performed and any resulting language syndrome has stabilized. Important studies of aphasia have utilized neurosurgical material (Hécaen and Angelergues, 1964) and postoperative neurosurgical cases remain good sources of anatomical correlation material.

A different neurosurgical approach to the study of language function was initiated by Penfield (Penfield and Roberts, 1959) and has been carried forward by Ojemann (Ojemann, 1983; Ojemann and Ward, 1971). In these studies, dealing primarily with epileptic subjects and with the patient awake during the intracranial surgical procedure, various brain areas were stimulated; if the area studied included a portion of the language area, significant alterations in language function could be elicited. Focal stimulation studies of cerebral cortex (and related subcortical structures) in these investigations and the subsequent surgery (Figure 5.7) have yielded important observations of language function.

Surgical correlation studies of brain-language functions also have significant

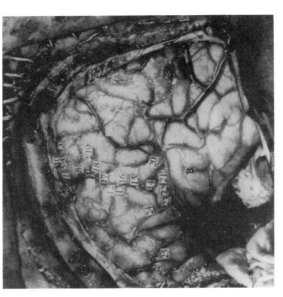

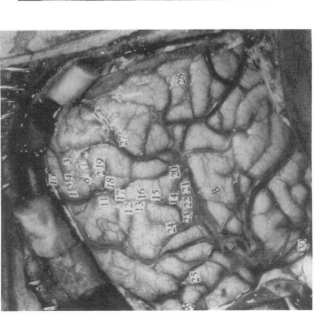

Figure 5.7. Before (*left*) and after (*right*) photographs of a left-temporal-lobe resection performed for seizure control. (From Penfield and Roberts, 1959).

drawbacks. Anatomical landmarks may be difficult to identify, and distortion of structures in the surgical field by edema, bleeding, contusion, or mass pressure hampers exact localization. Variations in the gyral pattern among individuals add to the difficulty of precise localization. Finally, only the surface of the cortex can be visualized; limited information is available concerning the extent and effect of subcortical pathology or of infiltration beyond the surgical area. Even direct brain stimulation studies of the type performed by Penfield, Ojemann, and others that monitor effect on the awake subject are open to question. First, a strong, non-physiological stimulation is needed to produce a response; second, almost all stimulation studies are performed on individuals with abnormal neural circuitry based on chronic epilepsy. Disturbances of language function demonstrated under these circumstances may not be reliable indicators of normal language processing.

Posttrauma Skull Defects

In the past, many influential studies correlated language impairment with damage to brain structures caused by trauma by using the site of damage to the skull as the indicator of underlying brain damage. Marie and Foix (1917), Luria (1947/1970), Schiller (1947), Conrad (1954), and Russell and Espir (1961) correlated aphasic symptoms or syndromes with the site of skull damage. The procedure is appealingly direct. Following recovery from the head injury, the language impairment features can be evaluated and these data correlated with the location of skull damage as demonstrated by direct palpation and/or simple skull X ray.

Many problems hinder the use of the skull defect site to locate aphasia-producing pathology. The skull defect may be far removed from the area of injured brain. In particular, low-velocity missiles and shrapnel bits tend to be deflected in a nonlinear path within the skull. Studies attempting to trace the intracranial path of a missile from the site of entrance to the site of exit have reported remarkable variations (Levin, Benton, and Grossman, 1982; Russell, 1947). The amount of injured brain cannot be determined from external observation. In fact, the degree of skull damage has little correspondence and may even have an inverse relationship to the amount of damage to the brain itself (Levin et al., 1982).

Despite significant problems, most studies of aphasia resulting from penetrating skull injuries do demonstrate symptom cluster localizations consistent with traditional aphasia studies (Luria, 1947/1970; Marie and Foix, 1917; Russell and Espir, 1961; Schiller, 1947). Even Conrad (1954), who interpreted his findings in cases of brain trauma as solid proof of a single language function (Gestalt) and used his data to argue against the earlier localization studies, demonstrated clear differences in language symptomatology dependent on the anterior or posterior location of left-sided skull defects.

Neurologic Examination

Many aspects of the neurologic examination demonstrate "neighborhood signs" which are often invaluable for localizing the site of brain pathology. Unfortunately, neurologic examinations are often performed poorly and/or reported inadequately. A good examination, including a complete neurobehavioral evaluation, is a complex, time-consuming task; most physicians are neither trained to perform nor able to invest the time needed to carry out such an exam. In addition, clinical-anatomical correlations of many higher brain functions (e.g., visual imagery, unilateral attention, praxis, frontal control mechanisms) remain even more primitive than corresponding aphasia-anatomical correlations (Farah, 1990; Heilman, Valenstein, and Watson, 1985a,b,c; Stuss and Benson, 1986; Mesulam, 1990). Basic neurologic findings (e.g., hemiparesis, sensory loss, visual-field defect), although relatively nonspecific, do provide valuable localizing information.

Visual Sensory Examination

A visual-field defect represents damage along a well-localized neural system. A full hemianoptic-field defect suggests involvement of the geniculo-calcarine pathway deep in the parietal or occipital lobe. A defect involving the superior quadrant of vision indicates posterior temporal lobe pathology (involving Meyer's loop of the geniculo-calcarine tract), whereas an inferior quadrantant field defect most often indicates damage to pathways deep in the parietal lobe (Kelly, 1985). Many neurobehavioral studies have used unilateral visual attention disorders to aid localization of the causative lesion (Bisiach and Luzzatti, 1978; De Renzi, 1985; Mesulam, 1985). When language functions are disturbed (particularly reading and naming), impaired information from visual-field examination often proves pertinent. Many investigators have produced elegant studies of visual transmission and visual processing, both normal and pathological, and have correlated their findings with lesion localization studies (Damasio and Damasio, 1989; Damasio, Damasio, and Van Hoesen, 1982; Farah, 1990; Grüsser and Landis, 1991).

Motor Examination

Paralysis can provide important localizing information. A spastic paralysis that involves the entire side of the body (hemiplegia), suggests a deep lesion involving the internal capsule or the motor pathways rostral or caudal to this landmark. When weakness is limited to a single limb, either cortical pathology or a small discrete subcortical white-matter lesion is probable (Adams and Victor, 1989). Crural paralysis, weakness that involves the leg and shoulder but not the arm or face, characterizes midline frontal pathology, usually based on involvement of the anterior cerebral artery. Weakness greater in the proximal (shoulder, hip) than distal musculature suggests infarction of the border zone between the middle cerebral artery and the anterior and/or the posterior cerebral artery territories (Bogousslavsky and Regli, 1986). Infarction in the territory of the middle cerebral artery tends to produce a "predilection" weakness that involves antigravity muscles (flexors of the upper extremity, extensors of the lower extremities) (Adams and Victor, 1985; Brust, 1985) more than other musculature.

Sensory Examination

Unilateral loss of pain and/or temperature sensation suggests pathology at the level of the thalamus or even deeper. When pain sensibility is near normal but other (cortical) sensory examinations such as position sense, double simultaneous stimulation, two-point discrimination, graphesthesia, and stereognosis are abnormal, pathology involving either the parietal cortex or pathways connecting the parietal lobe with the thalamus can be suspected. Aphasia plus a "deep" sensory loss (hemianalgesia) suggests a large wedge-shaped lesion, usually an occlusion of the middle cerebral artery near its origin from the internal carotid artery. Cortical sensory loss plus aphasia suggests occlusion of one or more distal branches of the middle cerebral artery. Both aphasia rehabilitation strategies and prognosis differ based on the level of brain involvement indicated by the sensory testing.

A relatively rare but striking sensory disturbance called the "pseudothalamic" pain syndrome provides some localization information (Benson, 1979a). Patients with this disorder suffer unilateral impaired cortical sensory functions and eventually (usually several months post-CVA) complain of discomfort and paresthesias in the affected limbs. Deep pain sensation is basically intact but finer sensory discrimination such as position sense and localization are disordered. The pain, although aggravating, is not the severe torture that characterizes the thalamic pain syndrome (Botez, 1985; Dejerine and Roussy, 1906; Mauguiere and Desmedt, 1988); for instance, the degree of discomfort in the pseudothalamic syndrome is not increased by manipulation or palpation of the involved limb. The discomfort is, however, consistent and disturbing. When the pseudothalamic pain syndrome is associated with aphasia, pathology in the white matter just below the parietal operculum can be suspected; conduction aphasia is the most common language impairment associated with pseudothalamic pain.

Motor Praxis

The demonstration of ideomotor apraxia in an aphasic subject may provide localizing information (Geschwind, 1965; Heilman, 1993). Liepmann (1900, 1905) described several varieties of ideomotor apraxia and postulated anatomical-clinical correlations that have been confirmed. Liepmann's anatomical correlations are presented in Chapter 17.

Many additional findings from a full neurobehavioral evaluation have localizing value. Such diverse entities as acalculia (Grafman, 1988; Grafman et al., 1982;

Spiers, 1987), constructional disturbance (Benton, 1967; Gainotti, 1985; Luria, 1964; Warrington, 1969), dressing disturbance (Botez, 1985; Brain, 1941), visual agnosia (Farah, 1990; Grüsser and Landis, 1991), prosopagnosia (Damasio, 1985; Meadows, 1974), verbal learning disorder (Rausch, 1985), the Gerstmann syndrome (Gerstmann, 1931; Benton, 1961, 1991) and many others co-occur with aphasia and help define and localize an aphasic syndrome. Pertinent neurobehavioral problems commonly demonstrated in aphasics will be presented in Chapter 17.

Brain-Imaging Studies

Although the neurologic exam, basic background information (such as the occurrence of stroke or tumor), and, of course, the ultimate localization from postmortem evaluation remain significant, most brain localization information is now obtained from brain imaging. The advent of modern brain-imaging techniques has greatly enhanced the ability to localize aphasia-producing lesions in the living subject (Damasio and Damasio, 1989). Data from these brain imaging studies have, almost without exception, firmly supported the established syndrome localization.

Isotope Brain Scan
The first noninvasive localization technique used for aphasia study was the isotope brain scan. Following injection of an isotope, counts of radioactivity were made over brain areas (primarily lateral). In selected pathologies and with appropriate timing, focally increased radioactivity indicated the location of the pathology (Figure 5.8). Howes and Boller (1978) utilized postmortem material to demonstrate that the isotope brain scan provided reasonably accurate lesion localization information. Early studies of aphasic subjects, utilizing isotope brain scan studies (Benson and Patten, 1967; Kertesz, Lesk, and McCabe, 1977), demonstrated the location of lesions in living individuals with aphasia and, in general, provided support for the traditional anatomical-behavioral correlations (Karis and Horenstein, 1976).

Cerebral Blood Flow and Metabolism Studies
Considerably improved isotope techniques have been developed and most have proved useful in aphasia research. Cerebral blood flow studies (Knopman et al., 1982, 1984; Soh et al., 1978; Warach et al., 1992) have evolved as better radiopharmaceuticals and better scanning methods became available. The most widely used of these techniques, single-photon emission-computed tomography (SPECT), uses relatively stable isotope products to demonstrate cerebral blood flow and, to a lesser degree, perfusion of metabolites (Holman and Hill, 1987).

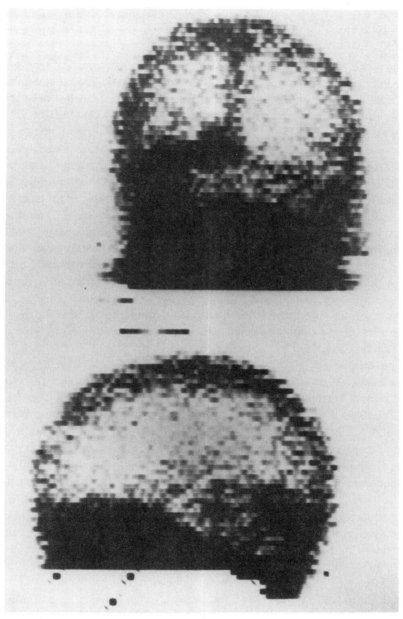

Figure 5.8. Isotope brain scan illustrating left-posterior-cerebral-artery-territory damage in a patient with occipital alexia. (From Benson and Tomlinson, 1971).

Resolution with SPECT techniques, however, is relatively poor (considerably less exact than the original isotope brain scans) and few pertinent aphasia localization studies have been performed with SPECT scans.

Far more exciting has been the use of positron isotopes. Positron emission tomography (PET) (Phelps et al., 1979) provides relatively precise neuroanatomical delineation based on variations in glucose metabolism and has been used extensively in the study of aphasia (Metter et al., 1981, 1984, 1988). Unfortunately, static isotope studies (those demonstrating lesion location) often failed to support the classical anatomical-behavioral correlations. The extent of the lesion (area of hypometabolism) demonstrated by PET scan tends to encompass large areas of cortex (Figure 5.9). In the largest and best-studied series, Metter and colleagues (1990) correlated (F18)-fluorodeoxyglucose scans (PET scans) with data from the Western Aphasia Battery (Kertesz, 1982) and the Porch Index of Communicative Ability (Porch, 1967) in forty-four aphasic subjects. No significant correlation could be made between the aphasia syndrome diagnosed (Broca, conduction, etc.) and the region of hypometabolism. At most, the PET demonstrated a difference between fluent aphasia (temporoparietal hypometabolism) and nonfluent aphasia (frontoparietal hypometabolism). Based on PET correlations, Metter and co-workers suggested that dominant hemisphere temporoparietal hypometabolism was responsible for the language deficit, a turn toward the holistic view of language function proposed by Marie and his followers.

Dynamic isotope studies have been designed to reveal brain areas with increased blow flow or alterations of metabolic rate when the subject performs certain activities (Larsen, Skinhøj, and Endo, 1977; Larsen, Skinhøj, and Lassen, 1978; Peterson et al., 1988). With improved scanning instruments, better isotopes, and statistical monitoring techniques, rapid alterations of brain activity can be demonstrated (Mazziotta et al., 1983). Thus, the brain areas activated in reading (Ingvar and Schwartz, 1974), tonal recognition (Mazziotta, et al., 1982), automatic data recital (Larsen, Skinhøj, and Endo, 1977), and other language-associated activities have been studied. Complex techniques utilizing both multiple and single subjects, multiple repetitions of a single action, subtraction of non-stimulation from stimulation scans, and an array of statistical maneuvers have been devised and have provided additional correlation data (Cohen and Book-heimer, 1994; Howard et al., 1992; Woods, Mazziotta, and Cherry, 1994). To date, the dynamic isotope studies remain somewhat artificial laboratory exercises. Although the results suggest that information of potential significance concerning the neuroanatomical basis of selected language functions might be demonstrated, the techniques have yet to provide useful data for aphasia research.

Computed Tomography

The most revolutionary advance in brain imaging was the introduction of computed tomography (CT) in 1972 (Oldendorf, 1980). The technique developed rap-

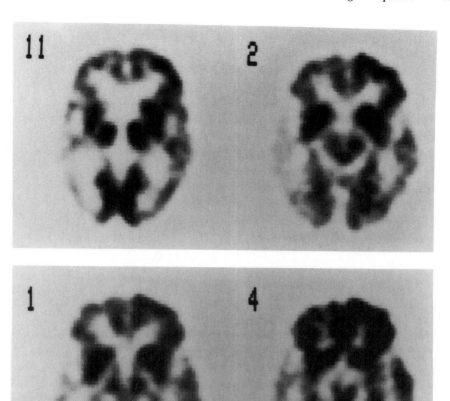

Figure 5.9. FDG positron emission-computed tomographic scans illustrating left temporal hypometabolism in a patient with Wernicke aphasia.

idly to become the standard technique for the demonstration of brain abnormality. Based on data from differential penetration of X-ray beams processed through complex computerized mathematics, a tomographic image of the brain can be produced. CT scanning provides noninvasive and relatively accurate localization technique for some types of aphasia-producing lesions.

The CT scan is particularly valuable for demonstrating the location of structural damage produced by stroke and, to lesser degrees, for localization of trauma or tumor. In the mature cerebrovascular case (at least six weeks post-CVA; CT scans performed earlier may appear normal, as in Figure 5.10), the lesion may be

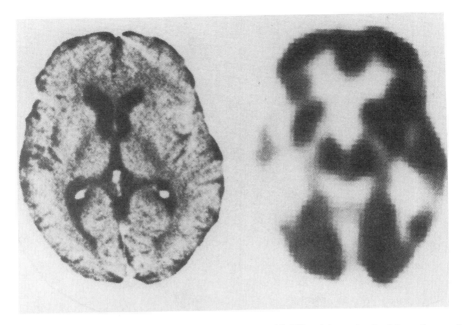

Figure 5.10. Composite views of brain of a patient with Wernicke aphasia. Note that early post-onset CT scan *(left)* does not show the lesion which is clearly demonstrated on the PET scan *(right)*.

accurately plotted and can provide useful anatomical information for correlation with the symptom picture. CT demonstration of aphasia-producing lesions has been extensively studied (Alexander and Benson, 1991; Alexander, Naeser, and Palumbo, 1987; Damasio and Damasio, 1989; Kertesz, Harlock, and Coates, 1979; Naeser and Hayward, 1978).

The CT scan has several drawbacks. In many instances, the lesion is not clearly demarcated and the scan can provide, at best, only an indefinite approximation. Even when the scan shows a sharply outlined lesion, the angulation of the tomographic image can produce localization distortion. Considerable variation in the relationship of neuroanatomical structures can be produced by slight differences in head position in the scanning apparatus. Angulation must be carefully monitored to provide anatomical accuracy (Damasio and Damasio, 1989); correction factor schemes are available (Damasio and Damasio, 1989; Naeser, 1983). When used in a research setting, the CT scan provides excellent information for localization purposes. In the hands of most radiologists and clinicians, however, localization is no more than approximate. If one keeps these limitations in mind, the CT offers valuable aphasia localization information with no risk to the patient.

Magnetic Resonance Imaging

A more recent addition to the armamentarium of brain imaging is the magnetic resonance image (MRI). This tool was introduced in the early 1980s and its use has spread rapidly, almost to the level of essential adjunct to the neurological evaluation. MRI remains an expensive technique, however, and does not enjoy the almost universal availability of the CT scan. Operating on an entirely different physical principle that uses an extremely powerful magnetic field to alter electrical fields in the brain which can then be monitored electronically, the MRI also produces computerized images (slices) of brain tissues. Not only can images be obtained in horizontal patterns (as in the CT) but, through electronic reconstruction, various other anatomical sections (coronal, sagittal, horizontal, specially angled) can also be generated. The MRI can reveal small intracerebral lesions, not only of vascular (Kertesz et al., 1987) but also of demyelinating or posttraumatic etiology. Because of this greater sensitivity, the MRI is of value for many aspects of clinical-pathological investigation (Kertesz et al., 1988) though it has not yet produced significant information for the localization of aphasia that was not previously available from CT scan studies (Damasio and Damasio, 1989).

Computer techniques now permit the combination (coregistration) of data from MRI and isotope scans (PET and SPECT) to generate a three-dimensional view of aphasia-producing lesions (Mazziotta et al., 1990; Watson et al., 1993). Whether the technique of coregistration can yield additional data of consequence for delineating the neuroanatomical basis of language is yet to be determined.

Summary

The localization of aphasia-producing lesions has advanced tremendously in the past several decades, particularly with the advent of noninvasive techniques that can produce accurate anatomical localizations (Mazziotta, 1994). With one exception, all imaging techniques have demonstrated anatomical localizations for the varieties of aphasia that are similar to the findings of the nineteenth-century clinical-pathological correlation studies. The exception has been the clear demonstration of subcortical aphasia (see Chapter 10), an entity that was unknown, or only vaguely suspected, before the advent of CT scanning.

6

Assessment of Aphasia

· ·

Although the delineation of language competency demands a repeatable means to characterize and gauge the dysfunction, formal aphasia assessment techniques were late in development. All early reports of aphasia merely describe the communication disturbance (Benton and Joynt, 1960). The first attempts to measure language competency were made by individual clinicians (almost always physicians) who reported techniques used to test and/or treat a single individual. A number of pertinent techniques were described (e.g., the Three-Paper Test of Marie), some of which remain in use. Purely clinical evaluations of aphasia became increasingly sophisticated and have remained a major assessment technique.

The first widely disseminated report of a standardized procedure for testing aphasia appears in the volume *Aphasia and Kindred Disorders* (Head, 1926). Head presented detailed descriptions of his language evaluations, including a number of novel tests. Following this work, Weisenburg and McBride (1935/1964) developed a relatively comprehensive battery of tests for aphasic language evaluation. Their group of tests represents the first attempt at a psychometric aphasia battery as they were the first to use completely standardized procedures and to compare the subject's test results with those of normal subjects. After World War II several new aphasia batteries were introduced (Eisenson, 1954; Schuell, 1955, 1957; Sklar, 1966; Wepman, 1961), which varied in comprehensiveness but were reasonably similar in approach. Both aphasia investigators and language therapists continue to use selected items from several of these tests to assess their patients. New test items and test batteries are still being introduced but most language therapists prefer to use selected test items from several batteries.

Three different strategies for aphasia evaluation will be presented here. The first will outline a clinical approach for assessing aphasia that is flexible, practical, and informative. Second, a number of tests to assess specific functions of language (the psychometric approach) will be described. Finally, a brief overview of some of the more widely used batteries for aphasia assessment will be presented. The clinical and psychometric approaches should not be considered contradictory; they are complementary in practice. The simple bedside examination is most useful for a quick diagnostic impression or for serial clinical aphasia assessments. For planning a rehabilitation program or for conducting language research, a quantitative, standardized, and more detailed appraisal of aphasia is needed.

Clinical Testing for Aphasia

Bedside testing for aphasia is the method most widely used by physicians. This informal appraisal of language probes several specific aspects: (1) Expressive language; (2) Repetition of spoken language; (3) Comprehension of spoken language; (4) Naming; (5) Reading; (6) Writing.

Expressive Language

The evaluation of aphasia traditionally begins by monitoring the spontaneous or conversational verbalizations made by the patient. Although many clinicians merely describe pertinent features of aphasic output, others suggest subdividing the output, most often into fluent or nonfluent types. This dichotomy was clearly described in 1864 by Hughlings Jackson (1932) who divided his aphasic patients into two groups—those who couldn't speak, and those who produced lots of words but made mistakes. The terms *fluent* and *nonfluent* were coined by Wernicke (1874) and have been used by many investigators for over a century. Unfortunately, these terms are not fully accurate descriptions and tend to mislead inexperienced examiners. Formal studies have probed the validity of this dichotomy by outlining specific verbal output criteria, noting frequency of combinations of various output features and correlating these clusters with the neuroanatomical locus of pathology. In general, the clinical observations that correlate nonfluent output with anterior lesions and fluent output with posterior lesions have been supported (Benson, 1967; Poeck, Kerschensteiner, and Hartje, 1972; Wagenaar, Snow, and Prins, 1975).

Nonfluent aphasic output has several striking characteristics that make it relatively easy to define. The key feature is *decreased output,* often fewer than 10 words per minute. Any output of less than 50 words per minute appears abnormally sparse and provides an easily noted abnormality. A second feature is *in-*

creased effort; when attempting to produce a word, the nonfluent aphasic patient struggles, often visibly, utilizing facial grimaces, body posturing, deep breathing, hand gestures, and so forth in attempts to aid or augment output. A third common characteristic is *dysarthria;* when verbal sounds are finally produced, they are often poorly articulated and difficult to understand. A quick test to determine if a sound represents an aphasic dysarthria is to attempt to imitate the sound produced by the patient. It is extremely difficult for the normal speech apparatus to imitate the nonfluent dysarthric output of an injured vocal apparatus (Alajouanine, 1956). A fourth noteworthy characteristic of nonfluent aphasic output is *decreased phrase length* (Goodglass, Quadfasel, and Timberlake, 1964); most responses by nonfluent aphasics are limited to a single word and even with clinical improvement, phrase length tends to remain short. The combination of features just described leads to an unmelodic, dysrhythmic, incompetently inflected verbal output called *dysprosody* (Monrad-Krohn, 1947) that represents a fifth distinctive characteristic. The major features defining prosody include melody, inflection, rhythm, and timbre of the verbal output. Goodglass and colleagues (1964) found abnormal speech prosody to be the single most distinctive feature for differentiation of nonfluent (anterior) from fluent (posterior) aphasia. All five of these characteristics need not be present for an aphasia to be considered nonfluent, but some degree of sparse output, short phrase length, and dysprosodic speech are present in almost every nonfluent aphasic patient.

One additional, often diagnostic, feature of nonfluent aphasic speech is noteworthy. Even though few words are produced, the output often conveys considerable information. Most words produced are nouns, action verbs, or descriptive adjectives—semantically rich words that convey a great deal of information. In contrast, there is a notable decrease (even absence) of syntactical (grammatical, functor, filler) words; exceptions are syntactical words included in short stereotyped phrases uttered as a single unit (e.g., "come in"). Nonfluent aphasic patients often communicate considerable information despite severely limited verbal production. The one-word sentence or "telegram-style" speech that omits all grammatical structures, a feature called *agrammatism,* is a striking characteristic of nonfluent aphasia. In addition to omitting syntactically specific language structures (prepositions, articles, adverbs, and even many adjectives and verbs), the agrammatic aphasic patient will have difficulty handling relational words (e.g., big/small, nearer/farther), plurals, pronouns, possessives and verb tense (Goodglass and Berko, 1960).

When most profound, nonfluent aphasic output may be limited to reiteration of a single word or syllable (e.g., a constant repetition of "good-bye," "Jesus Christ," "zu-zu," "ba-ba," or others), a condition termed *verbal stereotypy* (Alajouanine, 1956). Over time, patients with this limitation may develop control of the melody and inflection of the phrase and thus communicate well beyond the lan guage content of the stereotypy. Variations in nonfluent aphasic output are vast, ranging from an isolated utterance to a subtle decrease in syntactical competence, but the major features are clearly distinguishable from those of fluent aphasia (see Table 6.1).

Fluent aphasia has verbal output features that are almost directly opposite those of nonfluent aphasia. The quantity of verbal output ranges from low-normal to supernormal levels. Some fluent aphasic patients have been shown to have an output of over 200 words per minute and most fall within the normal range of 100–150 words per minute (Howes and Geschwind, 1964). Speech production in fluent aphasia demands little or no effort and articulation is normal. Phrases are of normal length (5 to 8 words) and a normal or at least acceptable prosodic quality is noted.

The most striking characteristic of fluent aphasic output concerns lexical content. Frequent *pauses* occur in the output of most fluent aphasics but are qualitatively distinct from the pauses that occur between each utterance in the nonfluent aphasic patient. The patient with fluent aphasia easily articulates a series of words but tends to pause when a semantically meaningful word is needed. If the word is not readily retrievable, the patient may attempt to substitute a descriptive phrase. The description may depend upon another unavailable specific word, necessitating yet another descriptive phrase. This "circling around" produces a wordy but meaning-poor output called *circumlocution*. Frequently the patient will substitute a generalization ("it," "thing," "them," etc.) for an unavailable word but often the output is continued with the key word omitted.

Fluent aphasic patients can produce long sentences containing so few substantive words that almost no information is conveyed, an output called *"empty speech,"* a significant identifying characteristic of fluent aphasia. Most pauses in

Table 6.1. Fluency in Aphasia

CHARACTERISTIC OF OUTPUT	NONFLUENT APHASIA	FLUENT APHASIA
Quantity	Sparse (less than 50 wpm)	Normal (100 to 200 wpm)
Effort	Increased effort	Normal ease of production
Articulation	Dysarthric	Normal
Phrase length	Short (1 to 2 words/phrase)	Normal (5 to 8 words/phrase)
Prosody	Dysprosodic	Normal
Content	Excess of substantive words	Lacks substantive words
Occurrence of paraphasia	Rare	Common

Adapted from Benson, 1967.

fluent aphasia output reflect the deficiency of meaningful, substantive words (the words that dominate nonfluent output). Errors in use of grammatical structures may be noted; fluent aphasics may produce incorrect verb tenses, use inappropriate conditional clauses or prepositional phrases, produce disturbed word order or misuse prefixes, suffixes, and inflections. This output characteristic has been termed *paragrammatism* (Lecours et al., 1983; Pick, 1913).

One additional feature of fluent aphasic output deserves emphasis, the occurrence of *paraphasia* (Goodglass, 1993; Ryalls, Valdois, and Lecours, 1988). (See Chapter 4 for discussion of linguistic qualities of paraphasia). For clinical purposes, paraphasia may be defined simply as a substitution within language. Paraphasias are common in aphasia and can help differentiate fluent from nonfluent output. Although phonemic substitutions do occur in nonfluent aphasia (Blumstein, 1973), they appear in a substrate of poorly articulated output and often represent dysarthric misproduction. The poorly articulated substitutions of nonfluent aphasia contrast with the substitutions of well-produced but incorrect language components of fluent aphasia. Although some fluent aphasics may be aware of some of their paraphasias, most remain unaware of most of their substitutions. When an aphasic patient produces a rapid verbal output, liberally laced with paraphasic substitutions and deficient in meaningful words, the output becomes incomprehensible and has been termed *jargon aphasia* (Alajouanine, 1956; Brown, 1981; Lecours and Lhermitte, 1969).

Both formal and informal studies demonstrate that the verbalizations of most aphasics fall into one of the two subtypes—fluent or nonfluent. The anterior/posterior neuroanatomical distinction for the locus of the lesion in the two varieties of aphasic output has been described for over a century and fully confirmed by numerous clinical investigations (see Chapter 14).

Repetition of Spoken Language

The ability of an aphasic patient to repeat words presented by the examiner represents a significant but often overlooked language function. Repetition is relatively easy to test at the bedside and can usually be judged on a simple pass/fail basis. Starting with simple tasks such as repetition of digits (e.g., one, twenty-six, three-seventy-four, and so on) and commonly used words (e.g., "house," "automobile"), the complexity of the repetition tasks can be increased to the level of complex sentences (e.g., "When the tired businessman returned home he found the house filled with his son's friends"), multisyllabic words (e.g., "constitution," "congressional investigating committee"), and phrases featuring multiple relationships and/or complex syntactic structures (e.g., "When he gets here we can ask him if he was really there," or "No ifs, ands, or buts").

Many aphasic patients have difficulty repeating exactly what the examiner has said, even at an elementary level. Although the difficulty in repetition often reflects, rather accurately, problems of verbal output or language comprehension, for some aphasics repetition is considerably more difficult than their other language problems (Berndt, 1988b). In contrast, some aphasics are unexpectedly good at repetition despite obvious problems in spontaneous output, language comprehension, or both.

A strong, almost mandatory, tendency to repeat spontaneously what has been said by the examiner is called *echolalia* and, when present, is of diagnostic significance. When fully developed, echolalia can encompass long phrases and entire sentences; the echoed phrase may be the only output the patient can offer and may be followed by a string of unrelated words (jargon), with the patient apparently unaware of what is being produced. Most patients with echolalia show the completion phenomenon (Stengel, 1947); thus, if cued with a recognizable phrase that is incomplete (e.g., red, white and _____; grass is _____), the echolalic patient will automatically supply the correct word. Even more dramatic is the ability of some echolalic patients to continue and even complete poems or nursery rhymes initiated by the examiner. A related problem, *echoing*, may be difficult to distinguish and is sometimes considered interchangeable; close observation, however, makes it is clear that echoing represents a totally different disturbance. In the echoing phenomenon, the patient will repeat a single word or short phrase just uttered by the examiner, almost always inflected as a question, and almost invariably indicating a need to reinforce a poorly understood bit of language. Echoing is a classic characteristic of the deaf and, when present in aphasia, echoing indicates the patient's insecurity with language comprehension (i.e., a request for confirmation).

Comprehension of Spoken Language

The ability to comprehend conversational language is difficult to assess. Both bedside clinical evaluations and formal, standardized tests of language comprehension may prove inadequate for such assessment (Goodglass, 1993); both may produce misleading results. The traditional clinical method for probing comprehension competency is to monitor the patient's response to verbally presented commands. The aphasic patient's ability to carry out complex commands, particularly several unrelated motor actions performed in sequence, indicates a considerable degree of intact comprehension, but even correct response to verbal commands is open to misinterpretation; the examiner's nonverbal language (e.g., gesture, voice inflection) may provide sufficient information for the aphasic patient to respond correctly. Although some aphasic patients may carry out selected verbal commands while failing to comprehend any other spoken or written language, their failure to carry out commands does not necessarily indicate an inabil-

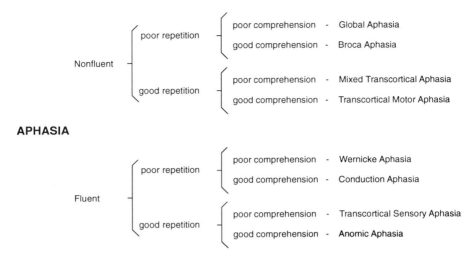

Figure 6.1. Algorithm for demonstration of aphasia syndromes based on observations of fluency, repetition, and comprehension.

ity to decipher language stimuli (Bachman and Albert, 1988); both apraxia (disturbance of the ability to carry out motor activities on verbal command—see Chapter 16) and sequencing disturbance (an inability to maintain the steps of a serially ordered, multistep command) can seriously interfere with motor performance tasks.

To obviate problems in motor response, comprehension tests that require minimal motor movement can be presented. Yes/no questions are one example. Some aphasic patients, however, cannot consistently handle the simple motor movements for yes or no responses, thereby producing undecipherable, perseverative, or mixed responses; the examiner cannot automatically accept their response failure as a failure of language comprehension. A second approach to comprehension testing that demands only limited motor activity requests the patient to point to objects about the room, or in an array, when the examiner says the name of the object. If the patient successfully accomplishes pointing to single named objects, the test can be made increasingly complex by offering vague functional descriptions of the object or demanding that the patient point to a series of objects in the sequence recited by the examiner. Some aphasic patients, despite understanding the words, fail even the elementary motor task of pointing, a failure that inaccurately exaggerates the patient's language-processing problems.

Comprehension of spoken language is rarely an all-or-none (pass/fail) phenomenon. Some aphasics comprehend commonly used words but fail to understand low-frequency words. Others comprehend concrete, meaningful, real-world names but fail to understand relational or syntactical structures such as prepositions, possessives, verb tenses, etc. Some aphasics can comprehend an individual word but fail to understand the same word when it is part of a sequence; thus, they may correctly point to the door, the window, and the floor when the names are presented individually but fail when asked to point to the same three in sequence (Albert, 1972; Luria, 1966). A patient's ability to comprehend fluctuates; an initial comprehension failure often improves if the same general topic is maintained but then decreases when the topic is changed. Comprehension also depends on familiarity of context; for example, after demonstrating poor comprehension during formal testing, an aphasic patient may demonstrate considerable appreciation of conversational material with the spouse. Conversely, some aphasics will obey a command (e.g., "Point to your nose") but fail similar requests after two or three commands are presented in sequence and then fail the original request. Their limited comprehension ability appears to have fatigued.

Most aphasics do understand some spoken language; conversely, almost all have at least some problem with comprehension. It is almost never correct to state that comprehension is "absent" or "normal" in aphasia. Abnormalities of language comprehension should be described as accurately as possible in both quantitative and qualitative terms. It should be remembered that *most aphasics comprehend better than test results indicate.*

Naming

Almost without exception, aphasic patients will have some difficulty in naming, word-finding (Goodglass and Geschwind, 1976—see Chapter 14). Aphasic word-finding problems have been given many different names; the most commonly used term is *anomia.*

Testing for anomia is comparatively easy. Objects can be shown and the patient asked to give their name; failure to name the object indicates a word-finding problem. Given this failure at word finding, many examiners follow by offering, verbally, a multiple-choice list of names including the correct one; this is *not* a test of naming but, rather, represents a test of the patient's auditory comprehension (the name is presented by the examiner). It is the patient's failure to produce the name on confrontation that demonstrates a naming disorder. It is better that the examiner follow by offering a prompt, or cue. The initial phoneme of the object's name may be presented (phonemic prompting) (e.g., a whispered /p/ when a pen is shown) or an open-ended sentence in which the missing word would be appropriate (contextual prompting) (e.g., "You write with a _____").

Testing of word-finding ability is important in aphasia evaluation, and word-finding tests should be included in all aphasia examinations. Eight informally presented tests of naming capability can offer a wealth of useful diagnostic information:

1. Auditing the patient's conversational speech for word-finding problems (e.g., empty speech) and noting whether the defect stems from word production problems (e.g., faulty articulation, paraphasia) or an inability to retrieve the correct word
2. Testing the ability to name items on visual confrontation from the following categories: objects, body parts, colors, geometric shapes, numerals, letters and actions
3. Testing the ability to name items presented tactilely
4. Testing the ability to name from auditory stimulation (e.g., jangling keys)
5. Testing the ability to name illness-related items (e.g., thermometer, bedpan)
6. Testing the ability to name objects from a verbal description of their function
7. Monitoring the ability to benefit from cues (prompting) when naming is failed
8. Testing the ability to produce lists of names in a specified category (e.g., animals, articles of furniture) or words beginning with a specified letter of the alphabet.

By utilizing results from these tests, plus neighborhood neurologic and aphasic signs, the examiner can demonstrate varieties of anomia and suggest neuroanatomical correlations (see Chapter 14).

When analyzing word-finding disturbances it must be remembered that the nonfocal cerebral abnormalities that produce dementia and confusional states can also produce word-finding problems. Although almost invariably present in aphasia, anomia is not an absolute indication of a focal brain disorder.

Reading

Alexia, the loss of the ability to read (comprehend written language) following brain damage, either with or without disorder of spoken language, is relatively easy to evaluate, at least in a crude manner; if quantified results are required, however, standardized test material is necessary. Simply presenting the written name of a body part or a room object for the patient to identify can be performed easily at bedside. If the patient is successful at this level, the examiner can then present more-difficult written material, including phrases or sentences dependent on low-frequency or relational (syntactic) words. A more challenging bedside test of reading ability probes the patient's comprehension of printed paragraph-length material from a newspaper or magazine. The patient's recognition of words spelled aloud by the examiner is another way to assess reading ability (Geschwind, 1962; Howes, 1964). Most patients with a parietal-temporal alexia will fail to recognize words spelled aloud, whereas those with occipital alexia will comprehend relatively well (see Chapter 11).

The most common misconception in the testing of reading ability is to equate the ability to read out loud with the ability to comprehend written material. Thus, most aphasics with nonfluent verbal output disturbances fail when asked to read aloud, but some of them may comprehend written language adequately. The opposite can also occur—some aphasic patients can read aloud flawlessly but comprehend little or nothing of what they have read. The ability to read aloud and the ability to comprehend written language should be tested separately; only loss of the ability to comprehend written language is called alexia.

Writing

Virtually every aphasic has some difficulty in writing (agraphia). A good initial test of writing ability is to request that the patient write his own name; many aphasics succeed. The ability to sign one's name is probably the most overlearned writing skill and many aphasic patients with severe agraphia can produce their own signature readily but fail at writing any other words. Assessment of writing ability must not stop at the level of signature production. Testing of the patient's ability to write words and sentences to dictation and the ability to produce written sentences on command (e.g., "Describe your job") should follow. In nonhemiplegic patients, writing can be tested in each hand, comparing the ability to copy written words with the ability to produce similar words to dictation (Bogen, 1969). Five aspects of writing ability deserve specific attention: (1) mechanics, (2) syntax, (3) semantic content, (4) spatial distribution, (5) ability to spell. Multiple variations of acquired writing disorder combined with extensive variations in a patient's premorbid writing competency makes any consistent demonstration of exact clinical-anatomical correlations for agraphia quite difficult. Some clinicians suggest that tests of writing ability can act as accurate screening devices for language disturbance, but many studies (Benson and Cummings, 1985; Leischner, 1969; Roeltgen, 1985) have shown that variations in acquired writing disorder can represent basic motor control defects as well.

In summary, the clinical testing of aphasia is a flexible, nonstandardized operation that constantly undergoes reorientation. Therein lies both the weakness and the strength of the process. An experienced examiner can perform a clinical evaluation on the aphasic patient's language in only a few minutes and, by focusing on the primary problem, obtain an in-depth view of the language impairment that is often more accurate and more exact than that which is obtained through formal aphasia batteries or research techniques. However, even in the best hands, the results of clinical testing are subject to inconsistent interpretations based on theoretical bias or narrow approach. When performed by inexperienced examiners the clinical evaluation can be misleading. The need for rigid, standardized testing techniques is obvious. Nonetheless, most techniques utilized in formal aphasia batteries and even those designed for performing research in language dysfunction had their origins in clinical (bedside) testing.

Tests of Specific Language Functions

A great diversity of test procedures is available to assess selected language functions (e.g., language comprehension, language production, naming); many have been put into rigid and accurately reproducible formats. These tests are not designed to provide total coverage of aphasic phenomena but they do furnish indepth, often replicable determinations of a particular aspect of disordered language. They provide a valuable adjunct to clinical language evaluation. A few of these tests will be described below.

Language Comprehension Tests

The Token Test (De Renzi and Vignolo, 1962) has become one of the most extensively used tests of language comprehension. The test consists of twenty tokens in two shapes (circles and squares), two sizes (large and small) and five colors (red, green, yellow, blue, and white) which are arranged in front of the patient. Sixty-two commands are given in five levels of increasing difficulty. Initial commands include two semantic categories (e.g., "Touch the red circle"); second-level commands demand understanding of three semantic categories (e.g., "Touch the large white square"); the third and fourth levels present sequences of two (e.g., "Touch the blue square and the white circle") and three (e.g., "Touch the small white square and the large red square") semantic categories. Spatial relationships are tested in the final level (e.g., "Put the blue circle under the white square").

The Token Test has been widely used in the assessment of aphasic comprehension (Boller and Vignolo, 1966; Lezak, 1995) and many modifications have been introduced (Benton and Hamsher, 1976, 1978; Boller and Vignolo, 1966; Spellacy and Spreen, 1969; Spreen and Benton, 1969, 1977). De Renzi and Faglioni (1978) developed a short version (thirty-six items) and studied the effects of age and education on Token Test scores. They recommended adjustment of scores for education (3–6 years of education earn one point, 10–12 years subtract one point, 13–16 years subtract two points, more than 17 years subtract three points) and proposed a 29–point cutoff score. The shortened version of the Token Test is presented in Table 6.2.

Table 6.2. Token Test—Shortened Version

Part 1. All twenty tokens
  1. Touch a circle
  2. Touch a square
  3. Touch a yellow token
  4. Touch a red one
  5. Touch a black one
  6. Touch a green one
  7. Touch a white one

Part 2. The small tokens are removed:
  8. Touch the yellow square
  9. Touch the black circle
10. Touch the green circle
11. Touch the white square

Part 3. The small tokens are replaced:
12. Touch the small white circle
13. Touch the large yellow square
14. Touch the large green square
15. Touch the small black circle

Part 4. The small tokens are removed:
16. Touch the red circle and the green square
17. Touch the yellow square and the black square
18. Touch the white square and the green circle
19. Touch the white circle and the red circle

Part 5. The small tokens are replaced:
20. Touch the large white circle and the small green square
21. Touch the small black circle and the large yellow square
22. Touch the large green square and the large red square
23. Touch the large white square and the small green circle

(continued)

Table 6.2. Token Test—Shortened Version (*Continued*)

Part 6. The small tokens are removed:

24. Put the red circle on the red square

25. Touch the black circle with the red square

26. Touch the black circle and the red square

27. Touch the black circle or the red square

28. Put the green square away from the yellow square

29. If there is a blue circle, touch the red square

30. Put the green square next to the red circle

31. Touch the square slowly and the circles quickly

32. Put the red circle between the yellow square and the green square

33. Touch all the circles, except the green one

34. Touch the red circle—no—the white square

35. Instead of the white square, touch the yellow circle

36. In addition to touching the yellow circle, touch the black circle

From De Renzi and Faglioni, 1978.

Picture Vocabulary Tests

Although word-finding problems usually affect all categories of words, there are some instances in which aphasic patients have selective difficulty producing names in one or more categories (Kremin, 1988). Thus, their ability to name nouns is usually more severely impaired than their ability to name letters and numbers (Goodglass et al., 1966); in some cases naming in specific categories (e.g., colors, body parts) may be failed while other categories are handled successfully.

Naming ability is the language function most sensitive to the effects of aging (Bayles and Kaszniak, 1987) and is invariably seen in patients with dementia of the Alzheimer type (Bayles, 1982; Cummings and Benson, 1983, 1992). Some investigators suggest that naming disorder is the single language disorder best correlated with the severity of dementia (Skelton and Jones, 1984).

A number of formal tests of naming ability have been developed. Kaplan, Goodglass, and Weintraub (1978) devised the Boston Naming Test (BNT), which consists of sixty line drawings ranging in difficulty from easy, high-frequency items to difficult, rarely used words. The items are relatively unambiguous in that the items have no commonly used alternative names. If the subject fails to name on visual confrontation, the examiner can present a description of the item (contextual cue), and if the subject still fails, a phonological cue can be presented. The maximum score is 60.

Norms for the BNT have been established for children, normal adults, elderly, and aphasics (Borod, Goodglass, and Kaplan, 1980; Goodglass and Kaplan, 1983; LaBarge, Edwards, and Knesevich, 1986; Van-Gorp et al., 1986). High test-retest reliability was reported by Huff et al. (1986). Two normative studies using the BNT in elderly subjects (LaBarge, Edwards, and Knesevich, 1986; Van Gorp et al., 1986) agreed that naming ability remains fairly stable until individuals are in their seventies, after which a variable but significant decline occurs.

Another frequently used test of naming ability, the Peabody Picture Vocabulary Test (PPVT) (Dunn, 1965b), has been standardized for children (ages $2\frac{1}{2}$ to 18) and is particularly useful for measuring developmental or acquired aphasia. The test consists of 150 picture plates that have four line drawings of objects. The subject is asked to identify (by pointing to) the item when the name is given by the examiner. When this test procedure is reversed (name the item pointed to), the test can be used to quantify naming ability. The level of difficulty in the PPVT ranges from elementary to challenging. The ease of subject response makes the PPVT particularly valuable for testing severely brain-damaged subjects.

Verbal Fluency Tests

Fluency was the term originally suggested for a measure of the number of words a subject can produce within a particular category in a limited span of time (usually one minute) (Milner, 1964). Two categories are routinely sampled: semantic (words belonging to a particular semantic group such as animals or fruits), and phonological (words beginning with a particular letter of the alphabet). Factors such as age, sex, and level of education are known to influence performance on category naming (Ardila and Rosselli, 1988b; Benton and Hamsher, 1976; Rosselli et al., 1990; Wertz, 1979).

For normal subjects, the number of different words beginning with a particular letter that can be produced in one minute is twelve or more. Accommodation must be made for age, educational level and gender. Category naming is found to be abnormal in patients with left frontal-lobe damage (Benton, 1968) and cortical dementia (Benson, 1979c); in addition, almost all aphasics have difficulty producing names in a selected category.

The *FAS*, a verbal fluency test requesting production of three word lists based on the initial letters *F*, *A*, and *S*, was developed for the Multilingual Aphasia Examination (Benton and Hamsher, 1978—see aphasia test batteries below); extensive normative values were obtained. Frequency ranges were subsequently established for several languages (English, French, German, and Spanish).

One subtest of the Stanford-Binet Intelligence Battery (Terman and Merrill, 1973) requests the subject to name as many animals as possible in a specified time. This test was included as part of the Boston Diagnostic Aphasia Examina-

Table 6.3. Verbal Fluency: Animal Names Produced in One Minute

SCHOOLING	AGE				
	56–60	*61–65*	*66–70*	*71–75*	*>75*
0–5 years	12.82	12.21	11.21	11.28	9.45
6–12 years	16.00	15.93	13.39	12.70	10.95
>12 years	16.10	16.15	15.81	13.77	11.72

From Ardila, Rosselli, and Puente, 1994.

tion (Goodglass and Kaplan, 1972, 1983—see aphasia test batteries below). Normative data indicate that 10-year-old subjects produce an average of twelve different animal names in one minute and adults average about sixteen. The score can be affected by age, educational level, and gender. Table 6.3 presents some normative data for verbal fluency tests.

Many additional specialized tests probe various aspects of language processing; most have been devised to scrutinize an individual language function. This has been particularly true in model-based linguistic research in which tests are designed to prove or disprove a theoretical construct. Most such investigations are inadequately validated and many prove difficult to administer and/or interpret in clinical settings. Some of these tests, however, probe sensitive areas and can be included in either clinical or formal aphasia assessment batteries. Many additional tests of individual language functions will probably be developed in the future.

Aphasia Test Batteries

Following the initial report of Head (1926), Weisenburg and McBride (1935/1964) produced a battery of tests specifically designed to define the language qualities of aphasic patients. Although never widely used, the Weisenburg and McBride approach, a consistent battery of language tests, was the harbinger of a new era in aphasia assessment. Over the next fifty years a number of batteries were devised to assess aphasia; some have been standardized to a greater or lesser degree; some have been widely utilized. Although overall similarity is obvious, significant differences exist. No single test vehicle or battery of tests has proved best; all or parts of each assessment battery reported here have been favored and used in contemporary practice. Almost every aphasic patient entering a formal aphasia therapy program will have part or all of one or more batteries administered and the results will help shape the patient's therapy program. Some currently popular test batteries will be mentioned and their more distinctive characteristics described but none will be outlined in detail.

Early Aphasia Batteries

One of the earliest widely used battery of tests for assessing language impairment was Examining for Aphasia (Eisenson, 1954), a medium-length test in two divisions—expressive and receptive. Eisenson's battery was widely used and many of the techniques initiated in this battery were enlarged, modified or otherwise altered by other investigators for use in subsequent batteries. Two long, rationally formulated aphasia batteries were devised in the 1950s. The Language Modalities Test for Aphasia (LMTA) (Wepman, published in 1961) and the Minnesota Test for the Differential Diagnosis of Aphasia (MTDDA) (Schuell, 1955, 1957, 1965) were developed at about the same time but had significant differences in composition. The MTDDA was specifically designed to classify aphasic patients into one of five categories indicating prognosis for language recovery, and it offers an extensive evaluation of five language disorders: (1) auditory disturbances, (2) visual language (reading) disturbances, (3) speech and oral language disturbances, (4) visual motor (writing) disturbances, (5) disturbances in numerical relations and arithmetical processing. The MTDDA is long and difficult to administer but provides extensive data for characterizing aphasia. Both the LMTA and the MTDDA have subtests of considerable value for evaluating aphasia. Many aphasia therapists utilize subtests from one or both batteries, either in isolation or in combination with other test material. Although the MTDDA was devised by an aphasia therapist to guide therapists in planning treatment, and the LMTA was devised by a psychologist and emphasizes psychological characteristics, subtests of the LMTA have proved helpful to aphasia therapists and the MTDDA has been used extensively in psychological research programs. The LMTA, slightly modified, is included as the language test in the popular Halstead-Reitan Neuropsychological Battery (Reitan and Wolfson, 1985).

Later Aphasia Batteries

Spreen and Benton published the Neurosensory Center Comprehensive Examination for Aphasia (NCCEA) (1969, 1977), an extensive, carefully validated battery consisting of twenty language subtests plus four visual and tactile subtests. The language subtests evaluate comprehension, production, reading, and writing skills, including word fluency, digit repetition, visual object naming, description of object use, tactile object naming, sentence repetition, sentence construction, object identification, oral reading of names and sentences, reading of names and sentences for meaning, object name writing, writing to dictation, copying sentences, and articulation. The scores indicate response correctness, are corrected for the subject's age and educational level, and then are converted into percentile scores to indicate relative performance level. The NCCEA is a powerful tool for differentiating aphasics from nonaphasics and, through multiple discriminant analyses, provides correct classification in over three-fourths of cases (Spreen and Risser, 1981).

Benton and Hamsher developed the Multilingual Aphasia Examination (1976, 1978), an aphasia battery modeled on the NCCEA, that is equivalent in different languages (English, French, German, Italian, Spanish). The battery assessed eight areas: visual naming, sentence repetition, digit repetition, word fluency, spelling, oral spelling to dictation, writing to dictation, and block-letter spelling. A speech rating scale and a version of the Token Test probing auditory and reading comprehension of words, phrases, and sentences is included. Some of the subtests have alternate versions for retesting.

Batteries that measure the subject's ability to communicate in general rather than assess ability in a specific language subfunction have been devised. The prototype, a still widely used battery, is the Functional Communication Profile (FCP) (Sarno, 1969). This battery relies on observations by an evaluator; there is relatively little attempt to quantify. The observations are readily classified, however, even by untrained personnel, and formal studies utilizing this battery demonstrate good interobserver reliability. Although not a standardized vehicle, the FCP has proved useful for qualitative judgments, particularly in measuring rapid changes in the subject's communication. The FCP probes five categories: Movement, Speaking, Understanding, Reading, and Other. Scoring is on a nine-point scale, based on the examiner's estimation of the patient's current ability in relation to premorbid ability in a particular area. Histograms are constructed to illustrate the patient's communication profile. Pragmatically, the FCP is of value for assessing functional communication capability and can be used to chart evolution of a patient's language competency.

The Assessment of Communicative Activities Relevant to Daily Living battery devised by Holland (1980) is a more complete probe of both verbal and nonverbal communication. Results from this battery provide considerable information concerning the pragmatic aspects of communication and the battery has proved useful in rehabilitation planning.

The Porch Index of Communicative Ability (PICA) (Porch, 1967), a comparatively simple and eminently quantifiable test of language disability, has attained a significant status among current aphasia testing techniques. The PICA includes eighteen 10-item subtests: four verbal, eight gestural, and six graphic. The PICA takes less time to administer (approximately one hour) than any of the comprehensive aphasia batteries and can be repeated with excellent test-retest reliability.

Although the PICA is easy to administer, the scoring system is intricate and demands that the examiner have formal training in its administration and scoring. The PICA offers excellent quantitative data concerning selected language functions but comparatively little qualitative information. For instance, there is little evaluation of the subject's spontaneous or conversational speech, limited testing of praxis, and limited recognition of complicating neurologic or behavioral factors. The value of the PICA lies in the ability to provide serial measurements of a patient's language recovery. Proponents claim that the eventual prognosis of a case of aphasia can be predicted by using the subject's initial PICA score and noting recovery curves recorded on repeated administrations. Unfortunately, if therapy is directed toward the tasks included in the test, PICA scores can be improved considerably, even if there has not been any real improvement in the patient's functional competency. This trap can be easily avoided, however.

The Boston Diagnostic Aphasia Examination (BDAE) (Goodglass and Kaplan, 1972, 1983), a widely used battery for the diagnosis of aphasia, is an extensive, in-depth assessment. The battery has been translated into several languages. Borod, Goodglass, and Kaplan (1980) obtained normative data for the battery test for an English-speaking population; a second English edition has been published which includes some minor procedural changes, a revised scoring system, Z-scores changed to percentiles, and norms for neurologically normal adults (Goodglass and Kaplan, 1983).

The BDAE has ten sections (plus an optional "spatial and computational" section), as listed in Table 6.4. Each section is tested and scored separately. A five-point Severity Rating Scale can be established and the results presented in two profiles: (1) summary profile (raw scores and two percentiles for each section and subtest); (2) rating-scale profile based on the eight most informative areas (melodic line, phrase length, articulatory agility, grammatical form, paraphasia in running speech, repetition, word finding, and auditory comprehension). Typical profiles for the different aphasia syndromes have been demonstrated and diagnostic algorithms suggested (see Figure 6.1). The spatial and computational section of the BDAE includes drawing to command, stick memory, building with three-dimensional blocks, finger gnosis, right/left discrimination, map orientation, arithmetic, and clock setting subtests, and it provides general information on related neurobehavioral disorders.

The Western Aphasia Battery (WAB) (Kertesz and Poole, 1974; Kertesz, 1979, 1982), a shorter language test, originally modeled on the BDAE, classifies language disorders into classical aphasia syndromes (Broca's, Wernicke's, etc.) and ranks the severity of the subject's language impairment with four language and five performance subtests. The four language subtests (spontaneous language, comprehension, repetition, and naming) are used to classify the aphasic syndrome. The subject's overall performance in these four subtests yields an Aphasia

Quotient (AQ). The supplementary performance subtests include reading and writing, praxis, calculation, and construction (e.g., drawing, Ravens Progressive Matrices). The subject's performance on the combined language and performance subtests provides a Cortical Quotient (CQ). Spontaneous language is evaluated both by the subject's responses to questions (e.g., "How are you today?") and by the subject's ability to describe items. Two ten-point rating scales are used: (1) information content; (2) fluency (which includes grammatical competence and occurrence of paraphasias). Comprehension is assessed with yes/no questions, word recognition tests, and sequential commands. Testing of repetition includes fifteen items that are scored as Correct, Phonemic Error, or Semantic Error. Tests of naming include object naming (without tactile or phonemic cues), word fluency, sentence completion, and responsive speech. Standardization of the WAB, based on the results from a large sample of aphasic patients, has been provided (Kertesz, 1979, 1982).

The Aachen Aphasia Test (AAT), originally developed in Germany (Willmes et al., 1980), includes a detailed evaluation of spontaneous language and multimodal input-output assessment. The AAT has had considerable acceptance in the German-speaking world and has been used in a number of research studies (Huber, Poeck, and Willmes, 1984); currently the AAT is being adapted for other languages.

Paradis (1987) published the most comprehensive and detailed of current test batteries, the Bilingual Aphasia Test (BAT). Parallel forms exist for more than forty languages. The BAT is designed to determine whether a subject's performance in one language is better than in another, to what extent, and in what language skill and/or level of linguistic structure. Although not constructed to discriminate between types of aphasia, it has been used as a screening instrument and typical profiles for different aphasia types have been proposed. The BAT explores different levels of language (phonemic, phonological, morphological, syntactic, lexical, semantic) and language use (comprehension, repetition, judgment, propositionizing, reading, writing) in four modalities (auditory, visual, oral, and digitomanual).

The BAT consists of three parts: Part A is a detailed history of the subject's bilingualism; Part B, administered in the patient's primary language, analyzes the competency of language use; Part C tests pairs of languages spoken by the subject by exploring his ability to translate from one language to the other.

Although only a few research results have been reported (Paradis, 1993), the BAT appears to be the most comprehensive language assessment vehicle currently available for aphasia evaluation. Its long length limits clinical use, however, and almost all research performed with the BAT remains in the area of bilingualism. The BAT is a potentially powerful instrument for research purposes and may come into more general clinical use.

Table 6.4. Separate Scored Sections of the Boston Diagnostic Aphasia Examination

Fluency	Paraphasia
Articulatory rating	Neologistic
Phrase length	Literal
Verbal agility	Verbal
Auditory Comprehension	Extended
Word discrimination	Automatic speech
Body part identification	Automatized sentences
Commands	Reciting
Complex ideational material	Reading comprehension
Naming	Symbol discrimination
Responsive naming	Word recognition
Confrontation naming	Comprehension of oral spelling
Animal naming	Word-picture matching
Body part naming	Reading of sentences and paragraphs
Oral reading	Writing
Word reading	Mechanics
Oral sentence	Serial writing
Repetition	Primer level dictation
Words	Written confrontation naming
High-probability sentences	Spelling to dictation
Low-probability sentences	Sentences to dictation
	Narrative writing
	Music
	Singing
	Rhythm

From Goodglass and Kaplan, 1972, 1983.

Summary

Many different instruments for the formal testing of aphasia are currently available. Each test or battery has proved useful for some phase of the aphasia evaluation; no single one has been accepted as clearly superior to all others. Depending on the use of the results, (clinical assessment, research, rehabilitation), certain tests or collections of tests will be of most value. Most aphasia batteries are administered by language therapists, many of whom are familiar with different batteries and often select subtests from several to assess the clinical situation. Although most of the batteries are standardized, their use in current clinical practice is not.

II

SYNDROMOLOGY

7

Classifications of Aphasia

· ·

At least since the time of Wernicke's original publication, clinicians have indulged in the intellectual exercise of separating varieties of aphasia on the basis of their observations of clusters of language symptoms. The lists of different aphasic syndromes devised since Wernicke's time represent one of the more confusing aspects of the investigation of language impairment. Much of the confusion stems from the use of different terms to represent a single cluster, terms that reflect the linguistic qualities under evaluation or the investigator's academic bias or literary creativity. Although each term adds to the confusion, the most pernicious of all the misunderstandings stem from misuse of the term *syndrome*.

To the clinically naive, an aphasic syndrome may appear to be a fixed group of language findings invariably present when the syndrome is diagnosed. In practice, however, two individual aphasics almost never show identical or even closely similar aphasia symptoms. The variability in symptom pictures has been interpreted negatively by some investigators who think that the syndromes of aphasia lack validity. Despite this recurring element of doubt (Caplan, 1987; Caramazza, 1984; Schwartz, 1984), descriptions of language disorders clustered as syndromes have remained relatively stable since the days of Wernicke and Lichtheim (Benson, 1988b). Numerous alternative classification schemes—with different psychological, linguistic and/or philosophic bases as well as severity ranking systems and speech/language therapy needs—have been proposed (see Lecours, Tainturier, and Boeglin, 1988, for a detailed review of alternative classifications of aphasia). Most of these schemes are valid but all have their own limitations. Although also limited and imperfect, the syndrome classification originally developed by the nineteenth-century continental investigators remains basically accurate, replicable, and clinically useful. Jackson (1868/1915) correctly observed that the neurologic and behavioral characteristics of a brain-damaged patient represent function of the undamaged parts of the brain. It is the patient's residual capabilities, compensating for those functions impaired by brain damage, that produce the phenomenologic picture. It is the resulting cluster of features that clinicians recognize and that—when the symptoms relate to language—has led to the traditional classifications of the aphasia syndromes.

Background

The variety of syndromes presented in the literature has made aphasia one of the most overclassified disorders in neurology. This variety of classifications and terminology has proved to be confusing. A single term may represent strikingly different clinical syndromes in two equally serious approaches. The "chaos" decried by Head (1926) was a direct reference to the many classifications devised in the first fifty years of aphasia investigation. Following Marie (1906a,b,c), many aphasiologists accepted that there was only a single cortical function that they called language (Head, 1926; Goldstein, 1948; Marie and Foix, 1917; Schuell, Jenkins, and Jimenez-Pabon, 1964) but found that they needed some explanation for the distinct symptom clusters of aphasia. Some plan for differentiating and classifying variations in the symptom complexes of aphasia appeared mandatory.

A popular and invitingly simple method of classifying the aphasias is in terms of dichotomies. One dichotomy, still widely used, is the original sensory/motor division made by Wernicke. Most sensory activities (including auditory reception) are carried out in posterior cortical areas whereas most motor activities (including motor speech) emanate from anterior cortex; sensory/motor language problems are thus linked to a basic neuroanatomical localization scheme that holds true for other brain activities. Although it can claim utility, the sensory/motor division is unsatisfactory in that it fails to depict many features that obviously distinguish variations of aphasia.

Probably the most widely used dichotomy for classifying aphasia is the expressive/receptive division that highlights the two most obvious clinical disorders. This division was originally made by Weisenburg and McBride (1935) and, although basically correct, it is also inexact. Very few aphasic patients are completely free of receptive difficulties and virtually no aphasic is entirely without expressive problems. To acknowledge the common mixture of clinical findings, a third, mixed category—expressive-receptive aphasia—was added by Weisenburg and McBride. Unless carefully (and somewhat artificially) used, however, this category can describe almost all types of aphasia.

Several other dichotomies proposed in recent decades—fluent/nonfluent (Benson, 1967), coding/decoding (Jakobson, 1956), and anterior/posterior (Goodglass and Kaplan, 1972)—also fail to match the many language variations that characterize aphasia symptomatology. In a purely linguistic approach, Jakobson (1964) separated paradigmatic and syntagmatic language disorders, and a similar division was suggested by Luria (1976a,b), but like all other dichotomies it fails to reflect much of the richness of aphasia symptomatology.

By contrast, Marie (1906a,b,c) argued that there was only one type of aphasia, the "sensory" aphasia described by Wernicke. He asserted that all language defect syndromes consisted of "aphasia" (an inability to decode and formulate language) and that the other observed differences (e.g., motor speech disorder, alexia) were based on neighborhood motor or sensory dysfunctions. The combination of focal neurologic dysfunction with the basic "aphasia" was thus considered the source of the clinically varied symptomatology noted in actual practice (Schuell, Jenkins and Jiminez-Pabon, 1964). In Marie's non-classification scheme, expressive disorders were attributed to motor speech problems (anarthria) or some other primary motor disability. Only the presence of word-finding defect or comprehension disorder indicated a disorder of the language function.

Jakobson (1964) strongly contested Marie's holistic view of aphasia, and most contemporary aphasiologists now use multifactorial organizational systems of variable complexity to categorize language and its disorders. Despite the continuing confusion over classification and terminology, Howes (1964) observed that the discussion of aphasia types among experienced investigators reveals considerable agreement on most salient points. As Lecours, Tainturier, and Boeglin (1988) noted, "anyone with experience in clinical aphasiology will acknowledge . . . that certain symptom complexes seem to be shared by subgroups of patients."

Table 7.1 lists a number of the most common classifications found in the aphasia literature. Some have played influential roles in clinical practice and related language research. But the possibilities for confusion can be easily appreciated from the variety of labels for the same syndromes. Most aphasiologists would agree that the language disorder characterized by a nonfluent, agrammatic, dysprosodic verbal output represents a single symptom complex regardless of whether it is called Broca aphasia, efferent motor aphasia, agrammatic aphasia, or something else.

A number of the classifications in Table 7.1 are widely accepted in different parts of the world. Luria's classification predominates in Russia and Eastern European countries, whereas variations of the Wernicke-Lichtheim scheme prevail in the English-speaking world and in Western Europe (Benson and Geschwind, 1971; Kertesz, 1979). Luria's system is based on language features that are impaired, whereas the Wernicke-Lichtheim system tends to emphasize neuroanatomical distinctions (e.g., anterior/posterior, cortical/transcortical/subcortical).

Table 7.1. Classifications of Aphasic Syndromes

BROCA 1861	WERNICKE 1881, LICHTHEIM 1885	PICK 1913	HEAD 1926	WEISENBURG & MCBRIDE 1935	KLEIST 1934	GOLDSTEIN 1948	BRAIN 1961
Aphemia	Cortical motor	Expressive	Verbal	Expressive	Word-muteness	Central motor	Broca
Verbal amnesia	Cortical sensory	Impressive	Syntactic	Receptive	Word-deafness	Sensory	Pure word-deafness
—	Conduction	—	—	—	Repetition	Central	Central
—	Transcortical motor	—	—	—	—	Transcortical motor	—
—	Transcortical sensory	—	Nominal	—	—	Transcortical sensory	—
—	—	—	—	—	—	Mixed echolalia	—
—	—	Amnesic	Semantic	Amnesic	Amnesic	Amnesic	Nominal
—	Total	Total	—	Expressive receptive	—	—	Total
—	Subcortical motor	—	—	—	Anarthric	—	—

BAY 1964	WEPMAN 1964	LURIA 1966	BENSON & GESCHWIND 1971	HÉCAEN & ALBERT 1978	KERTESZ 1979	BENSON 1979
Cortical dysarthria	Syntactic	Efferent motor	Broca	Agrammatic	Broca	Broca
Sensory	Jargon, pragmatic	Sensory	Wernicke	Sensory	Wernicke	Wernicke
—	—	Afferent motor	Conduction	Conduction	Conduction	Conduction
Echolalia	—	Dynamic	Transcortical motor	Transcortical motor	Transcortical motor	Transcortical motor
—	—	—	Transcortical sensory	Transcortical sensory	Transcortical sensory	Transcortical sensory
—	—	—	Isolation speech area	—	Isolation	Mixed transcortical
Amnesia	Semantic	Semantic amnesic	Anomic	Amnesic	Anomic	Anomic
—	—	—	Global	—	Global	Global
—	—	—	Aphemia	Pure motor	—	Aphemia

Adapted from Benson, 1979a.

Luria's classification is also widely used in Latin America (Ardila, 1981, 1984a; Azcoaga, 1984; Cairo-Valcarcel, 1985), but both the Luria and the Wernicke-Lichtheim systems are used in the Far East (Gao and Benson, 1990; Sasanuma et al., 1971).

The syndromes that identify motor (Broca) and sensory (Wernicke) aphasia carry the names of the investigators credited with the initial descriptions; these terms are almost universally recognized. Conduction aphasia was proposed as a potential syndrome by Wernicke (1874), and a relevant clinical-pathological correlation for the disorder was presented by Lichtheim (1885). Transcortical aphasia was identified as a separate type of disorder on the basis of a theory of mental function (Lichtheim, 1885; Wernicke, 1881); the term is now used to denote preserved ability to repeat in an otherwise aphasic patient. All of these terms stem from the work of European investigators in the late nineteenth century.

Luria (1966, 1973) took a different approach. He originally listed six different types of aphasia (efferent or kinetic motor, afferent or kinesthetic motor, acoustic-agnosic, acoustic-amnestic, semantic, and dynamic), but in later writings (1976a,b) he added a seventh (amnesic aphasia). Originally, he had been uncertain whether amnesic aphasia represented an independent syndrome or should be subcategorized with acoustic-amnestic or semantic aphasia, but eventually he came to see amnesic aphasia as a distinct clinical disorder. Luria's classification and the names he proposed were based on the level of language disrupted: phonemic discrimination (acoustic-agnosic), lexical memory (acoustic-amnestic), lexical selection (amnesic), understanding the relationships among words (semantic), kinesthetic activity (afferent motor), performance of skilled movements required for production and sequencing of speech elements (efferent motor) and verbal initiative (dynamic).

Although Luria classified aphasia types by linguistic features, he identified consistent clinical-anatomical correlations and was one of the originators of the lesion superimposition method to chart the brain areas that are critical for particular clusters of language disorder (Luria, 1947/1970). The superimposition technique has been widely adopted for clinical-anatomical correlations (Benson and Patten, 1967; Conrad, 1954; Kertesz, 1979, 1983; Kertesz, Lesk, and McCabe, 1977; Metter et al., 1981) and is now used in CT and MRI scan investigations (Kertesz, Harlock, and Coates, 1979; Naeser, 1983; Damasio and Damasio, 1989). Although based on different approaches, the two categorization schemes (anatomical and linguistic) are fundamentally the same.

The newer, more sophisticated imaging technology that is now available and the equally radical advances in language analysis continue to provide finer distinctions in both aphasic syndromology and anatomical localization, but no new classifications of aphasia based on locus of brain damage or novel symptom clusters have appeared. Different subtypes have been distinguished, however, for virtually all aphasic syndromes. This is true for conduction aphasia (Benson et al., 1973; Caplan, Vanier, and Baker, 1986; Caramazza, Basili, and Koller, 1981; Feinberg, Gonzalez-Rothi, and Heilman, 1986; Kertesz, 1979, 1985; Shallice and Warrington, 1977), transcortical sensory aphasia (Alexander, Hiltbrunner, and Fischer, 1989; Coslett et al., 1987; Kertesz, 1982, 1983), transcortical motor aphasia (Ardila and Lopez, 1984; Freedman, Alexander, and Naeser, 1984; Rubens and Kertesz, 1983), Wernicke aphasia (Brown, 1981; Huber et al., 1975; Kertesz, 1983, 1985; Lecours and Rouillon, 1976) and Broca aphasia (Alexander, Benson, and Stuss, 1989; Levine and Sweet, 1983). Thus, ongoing investigations make it increasingly clear that the traditional aphasia syndromes do not represent rigid, invariable symptom clusters; variations in symptoms are so plentiful as to be the rule.

To add to the confusion, a single type of aphasia may have distinctly different loci of pathology. Both conduction aphasia and transcortical motor aphasia are examples of this inconsistency.

Two different neuroanatomical sites of pathology underlying the symptom cluster called conduction aphasia have long been recognized; one is suprasylvian (parietal) and the other subsylvian (temporal) (Benson et al., 1973; Damasio and Damasio, 1980; Kleist, 1934a; Lichtheim, 1885). On clinical grounds Luria (1966, 1970) suggested that the classic conduction aphasia syndrome actually represented two different language defects. His "afferent motor aphasia" resembled the parietal type of conduction aphasia in which altered structure of word sounds in the articulatory unit (articuleme) was a prominent feature. He included the temporal type of conduction aphasia within his category of acoustic-amnestic aphasia and considered it a consequence of verbal memory defect. Kertesz (1979, 1985) also defined two types of conduction aphasia: (1) efferent, featuring greater expressive difficulties and suggesting an anterior lesion; (2) afferent, with fewer phonemic alterations but more comprehension problems and a more posterior location of pathology. Similar distinctions have been made by Shallice and Warrington (1977), Caramazza, Basili, and Koller (1981), and Caplan, Vanier, and Baker (1986). Most of these investigators considered the efferent variation to result from disorganization of phonemic content during the repetition of words, and a parietal and/or insula site has been proposed (Damasio and Damasio, 1982, 1989). The efferent variation has been considered a disorder of verbal memory, particularly the problem noted in the repetition of long sequences; a temporal lobe origin was postulated. Based on study of three cases with atypical anatomical sites, however, Mendez and Benson (1985) offered a disconnection explanation of conduction aphasia. This diversity of opinion indicates that conduction aphasia represents a cluster of symptoms (a syndrome), not a specific language dysfunction with a focal neuroanatomical correlation.

Goldstein (1948) noted that transcortical motor aphasia (TCMA) could have

two different clinical presentations; in one, the ability to repeat was better preserved than the ability to speak spontaneously, whereas in the other the greatest
difficulty was in initiating articulation. Both disturbances produced the same clinical picture. The TCMA cluster of language findings has been noted following
damage to either the left supplementary motor area (Alexander and Schmitt,
1980; Kertesz, 1979; Rubens, 1975, 1976) or the dorsal lateral prefrontal cortex
anterior to Broca's area (Hécaen and Albert, 1978; Walsh, 1978). On the basis of
language findings alone, the two varieties of TCMA can be considered similar,
one produced by damage to tissues anterior to or superior to Broca's area and the
other following damage to the left supplementary motor area. Associated behavioral disorders, not language disability, distinguish the two varieties. In the Luria
scheme (1966, 1976a,b), the term *dynamic aphasia* was introduced to represent a
syndrome of verbal processing disorders (apathy, lack of initiative, poor programming, inability to create a scheme of verbal expression) that resemble transcortical
motor aphasia.

A somewhat similar division into two varieties has been suggested for Wernicke aphasia (Hier and Mohr, 1977; Kertesz, 1983, 1985). Since the time of
Lichtheim (1885) it has been recognized that Wernicke aphasia is not a single,
cohesive aphasic syndrome (Alajouanine, 1956; Hécaen and Albert, 1978;
Henschen, 1922; Huber et al., 1975; Lecours et al., 1988; Luria, 1966, 1976b).
Several subtypes of sensory or Wernicke-type aphasia have been described; these
have been called word-deafness, phonological jargon or semantic jargon, based on
differences in the language impairment. One of the terms, semantic jargon, is
sometimes categorized as a form of amnesic or anomic aphasia (Luria, 1966; Hécaen and Albert, 1978; Brown, 1972) or a variation of transcortical sensory aphasia
(Benson, 1979a; Kertesz, 1983). In this book only two types of Wernicke aphasia
will be distinguished, and the semantic jargon variety will be included with the
extrasylvian aphasias. In this scheme, the major distinction in Wernicke aphasia
centers on the prominence of either word-deafness or word-blindness. Obviously,
mixtures predominate.

Somewhat similar, symptom-based subdivisions have been proposed for
Broca aphasia (Alexander, Benson, and Stuss, 1989; Mohr, 1973) and subcortical
aphasia (Alexander and Benson, 1991; Damasio et al., 1982; Naeser et al., 1982;
Wallesch, 1985).

Proposed Classification of Aphasia

Although many clinical variations of the aphasia syndromes have been described
in recent years, most can still be contained within the original classification
schemes, representing subdivisions rather than new aphasia syndromes. Some of

the traditional names for the aphasia syndromes are frankly inappropriate, however, as they are based on either anatomical or theoretical constructs that are no longer acceptable. This is particularly true of transcortical aphasia in which the language disorder is not "transcortical" but rather is the result of extrasylvian (beyond the perisylvian central language area) damage/dysfunction, a localization that has been repeatedly confirmed (see Chapter 9). Would it not be more appropriate to rename this aphasic subgroup *extrasylvian aphasia,* a term stressing the distinction between perisylvian and extrasylvian aphasic syndromes?

Table 7.2 presents the classification of aphasic syndromes based on cortical involvement that will be followed in this volume. Two primary anatomical divisions are proposed: (1) pre-Rolandic or post-Rolandic language area; (2) perisylvian or extrasylvian language area. Chapters 8 and 9 will present the basic clinical-anatomical and linguistic features that characterize these divisions. Whenever possible, terminology from the Luria functional linguistic scheme or the more recent neurolinguistic and psycholinguistic approaches will be introduced. Chapter 10 will discuss the influences of subcortical damage on language, including the so-called subcortical aphasias.

Table 7.2. Proposed Classification of the Aphasias

PRE-ROLANDIC LANGUAGE AREA	POST-ROLANDIC LANGUAGE AREA
Perisylvian	
Broca aphasia-type I (triangular syndrome)	Conduction aphasia (parietal-insular syndrome)
Broca aphasia-Type II (triangular-opercular-insular syndrome)	Wernicke aphasia-Type I (posterior insular-temporal isthmus syndrome)
	Wernicke aphasia-Type II (superior and middle temporal gyri syndrome)
Extrasylvian	
Extrasylvian motor aphasia-Type I (left dorsolateral prefrontal syndrome)	Extrasylvian sensory aphasia-Type I (temporo-occipital syndrome)
Extrasylvian motor aphasia-Type II (supplementary motor area syndrome)	Extrasylvian sensory aphasia-Type II (parieto-occipital and angular syndrome)

Finally, we acknowledge that a different approach—a linguistic classification with anatomic correlation—would be reasonable. Such schemes are available (Caplan, 1987; Margolin, 1991) but the linguistic approach has proved difficult to use because of the ongoing generation of both new terminology and new schemes to model linguistic activity. The anatomical structures used to anchor the clinical descriptions in this book have proved relatively stable for over a century and entail less terminological confusion.

Summary

Through all the cacophony of aphasia classification and its terminology, one basic fact remains—the number of distinguishable aphasia syndromes is limited and has not changed. Many different terms are applied to the same symptom clusters (see Table 7.1) but correlations of the salient clinical features and the underlying neuroanatomical defects have remained stable. The ongoing cacophony is based on the wide variations in terminology that have been proposed.

8

Perisylvian Aphasic Syndromes

· ·

The first three aphasic syndromes presented in Table 7.2—Broca aphasia, Wernicke aphasia, and conduction aphasia—have two notable similarities in common. First, the sites of brain pathology consistently described are located in the vicinity of the sylvian fissure of the dominant hemisphere; second, one clinical finding, difficulty in the repetition of spoken language, is prominent in each syndrome. The three perisylvian language impairment syndromes constitute the earliest-described and the best-recognized types of aphasia. In this chapter, the basic clinical findings for each syndrome will be outlined, variations within the typical symptom cluster will be discussed, and the neuroanatomical site most commonly involved will be described.

Broca Aphasia

A frontal language disorder was originally postulated by Gall and was the first focal language impairment to be firmly established. Initially termed *aphemia* by Broca (1861a,b), the term *aphasia* was used by Trousseau (1864) to define the language defect described by Broca. *Aphasia* was eventually accepted, but only after considerable controversy (Henderson, 1990). After Wernicke's (1874) demonstration of a language deficit that was clinically different from the one originally described by Broca, aphasia became the common name for all acquired language disorders, prefaced by a term such as Broca or Wernicke to distinguish the clinical syndromes. Broca aphasia (modern terminology tends to omit the possessive mark) is also known as efferent or kinetic motor aphasia (Luria, 1966, 1970), expressive aphasia (Hécaen and Albert, 1978; Pick, 1913; Weisenburg and McBride, 1935/1964), verbal aphasia (Head, 1926), or syntactic aphasia (Wepman and Jones, 1964). *Broca aphasia* remains the most widely accepted term for the syndrome (Benson and Geschwind, 1971; Brain, 1961; Nielsen, 1936), but the term is often used to refer to any basically nonfluent aphasia. Many of the variations among nonfluent language disorders seem to represent important linguistic and anatomic distinctions; in fact, some investigators question whether Broca aphasia actually exists as a specific disorder (Alexander, Benson, and Stuss, 1989). Nonetheless, the term, and the overall symptom cluster, are so well-known (see Table 8.1) that *Broca aphasia* will be used in this chapter to signify one of the basic symptom complexes of aphasia.

Broca aphasia is characterized by a nonfluent verbal output (see Chapter 6) that is sparse, poorly articulated, consists of short phrases (usually limited to one or two words), and is produced with effort. The output contains an excess of semantically significant words with a concomitant deficiency or even absence of syntactical structures and affixes (agrammatism). The product is a telegraphic-style verbal output. Nouns are best preserved, followed by adjectives and verbs;

Table 8.1. Characteristics of Broca Aphasia

Basic Language Characteristics	
Conversational language	Nonfluent
Comprehension of spoken language	Relatively normal
Repetition of spoken language	Abnormal
Pointing to named objects	Relatively normal
Naming	Abnormal
Reading	
Aloud	Abnormal
Comprehension	Often abnormal
Writing	Abnormal
Associated Neurological Signs	
Motor system	Often hemiparetic
Articulation	Abnormal
Cortical sensory function	Normal or abnormal
Praxis	Apraxia of left limbs
Visual fields	Normal
Visual gnosis	Normal

grammatical connectors are most impaired. The verbal output may be limited to a single, often reiterated word or expression (verbal stereotypie [Alajouanine, 1956]). In most cases, however, the comparatively rich substantive output enables the patient with Broca aphasia to communicate some ideas. While a common finding, agrammatism may not be notable in an individual case of Broca aphasia. In addition, alterations of rhythm, inflection, melody, and pitch tend to distort the output, a defect called dysprosody (Monrad-Krohn, 1947). Occasionally, the findings of nonfluency may be mild, with the only notable problem being an alteration of prosodic quality that produces an unnatural sounding output that is easily misperceived as a foreign accent. The combination of linguistic defect and articulation disorder has given rise to many descriptive terms (phonemic disintegration, cortical dysarthria, verbal apraxia, etc.). Any single or even several of these descriptive features may be missing in individuals who will still be considered to have Broca aphasia. Although the fully developed syndrome of Broca aphasia includes the verbal output features noted above, variations which omit one or several output features are so common as to be the rule rather than the exception.

Over the past two decades one feature of nonfluent aphasia output, agrammatism, has received considerable emphasis. The establishment of syntax as a major element in the study of language (Chomsky, 1957; Jakobson, 1956) and in language disorders (Goodglass, 1993; Goodglass and Berko, 1960; Goodglass et al., 1972) led to new theories of language disruption and new techniques for observation. Agrammatism is characterized by an overabundance of content words (nouns and verbs) and a relative decrease in functor words and grammatical word endings. The result is a sparse but information-rich "telegraphic" verbal output. A central disruption of the syntactic parsing component of the language system, a disorder of the neural parsing mechanism, came to represent the key feature of Broca aphasia (Berndt and Caramazza, 1980; Schwartz, Linebarger, and Saffran, 1985). The theory of a central syntactic mechanism has not been fully accepted (Kolk, Van Grunsven, and Keyser, 1985) but the intense investigation of agrammatism has contributed to understanding of the unique language features that characterize Broca aphasia.

A widely used construct to explain the abnormal verbal output of Broca aphasia has been termed "apraxia of speech" (Rosenbek, Kent, and LaPointe, 1989). Defined as a neurogenic phonologic disorder impairing the selection, programming, and execution of normally sequenced volitional speech sounds (Wertz, LaPointe, and Rosenbek, 1984), apraxia of speech is distinguished from dysarthria by the absence of motor speech organ paralysis and is viewed as a motor selection disorder distinct from the language impairment (aphasia). The defining characteristic of apraxia of speech is the relatively normal pronunciation of serial (automatic) speech contrasted to the dysprosodic, poorly articulated nature of volitional speech (Kearns, 1990). Even staunch advocates of the concept acknowledge, however, that almost all subjects showing apraxia of speech will also be aphasic (at least some degree of agrammatism and anomia) and/or dysarthric (Darley, 1968; Wertz, LaPointe, and Rosenbek, 1984). Cases of pure apraxia of speech are rarely encountered in the clinic and the concept remains popular only among a group of language therapists (Canter, Troost, and Burns, 1985; Darley, 1968; Martin, 1974; Wertz, LaPointe, and Rosenbek, 1984). Nonetheless, the basic findings of apraxia of speech (effortful, groping articulatory movements, dysprosody, articulatory inconsistency and difficulty in initiating articulation) depict the major problems in verbal output that characterize Broca aphasia.

In the patient with Broca aphasia, comprehension of spoken language is better than verbal output, but it is rarely normal, particularly with regard to comprehension of grammatically significant structures. Some degree of comprehension defect is almost invariably demonstrable and several characteristics of the comprehension problems can be useful for diagnosis. Although most patients with Broca aphasia can readily point to individual items or body parts named by the examiner, when asked to point to these same items in a specific sequence they often fail at the level of only two or three items. Whether this represents a disturbed ability to manage a sequence or a defect in auditory span is argued (Albert, 1972; Fuster, 1989; Warrington and Shallice, 1969). Whatever the underlying explanation, inability to point to named objects sequentially is a common, in fact almost constant, comprehension defect in Broca aphasia. In addition, many patients with Broca aphasia have difficulty understanding relational words (e.g., bigger/smaller, up/down, within/without) and often have problems comprehending grammatical (syntactical) language structures (Schwartz, Saffran, and Marin, 1980). The same words that Broca aphasia patients tend to omit from their verbal expression prove difficult for them to understand (Caplan and Hildebrandt, 1988; Zurif, Caramazza, and Myerson, 1972). In addition, many patients with Broca aphasia have a problem extracting the meaning provided by word order in a sentence (e.g., the difference between "mother's brother" and "brother's mother"). They understand individual words but fail to realize the temporal constraints of language processing. To the examiner the defects in grammatical output appear more severe than the problems of grammatical comprehension; this apparent difference may merely reflect the relative infrequency of sentences in which the meaning is conveyed by grammatical structures rather than substantive words. The patient with Broca aphasia does comprehend much of what is said, particularly when the information is presented in a relatively grammar-free context. Although the ability to comprehend is abnormal, it is considerably more intact than the ability to express.

Repetition of spoken language is always abnormal in Broca aphasia. Phonetic and phonemic distortions, omissions, iterations, and simplifications of syllabic clusters occur regularly. Despite obvious output abnormalities, repetition is usually superior to spontaneous verbal output and at times repetition can be considered close to normal. Careful evaluation usually shows typical defects. One dramatic difficulty, present in many Broca aphasia subjects, is a selective impairment in the repetition of syntactic grammatical and linguistic structures, the same words that these subjects omit from their spontaneous verbal output. Thus, when a patient with Broca aphasia is asked to say "the young school boy" he may produce only "boy"; with considerable coaxing "young boy" or possibly "school boy" will be presented; "the" will be consistently omitted, even if strongly and repeatedly cued. The problem becomes even more pronounced when the patient is requested to repeat sentences with substantive words plus modifiers (e.g., "the boy took his dog for a walk in the park"); characteristically, Broca aphasia patients merely repeat the substantive words ("boy-dog-park").

The patient with Broca aphasia usually produces considerably better verbal output when asked to present overlearned serial speech such as counting, reciting the alphabet, or naming the days of the week or the months. Articulation is often dramatically improved during these semiautomatic verbal tasks. Although patients with Broca aphasia articulate well when reciting an overlearned series, they may often fail pronunciation of the same words in a repetition task. When singing familiar melodies, the Broca aphasia patient's verbal output may be greatly improved but there is little or no carryover of this improved pronunciation into their spontaneous verbal output.

Naming is always poor in Broca aphasia. The patient is much better at pointing to a named object than at presenting the name of the object following visual presentation. However, confrontation naming in these patients is often better than expected given the extreme paucity of substantive words (names) that are presented in their conversational speech. Problems in articulation (phonetic deviations) occurring during tests of naming may resemble phonemic paraphasias (Buckingham, 1989) but the resulting output is often sufficiently close to the target word to be accepted as correct. Most Broca aphasia patients accept cues (prompting) during tests of naming, appearing to use the cues to overcome problems in initiation of articulation or in pronunciation. The Broca aphasia patient who fails to name an object on presentation may name it readily when the initial syllable is pronounced (or whispered) or even when the lip movements necessary for the initial syllable are demonstrated by the examiner. An open-ended sentence in which the target name is the final word (e.g., "you pound a nail with a _____") often aids the Broca aphasia patient in name production. For some patients the ability to benefit from cues is so marked that it is obvious that the entire naming problem represents word production disturbance, not loss of knowledge of the names. More often, however, their success with prompting is only partial, suggesting that Broca aphasia can produce a combination of articulatory and lexical impairments.

Most patients with Broca aphasia have great difficulty (often total failure) reading aloud. Most also have difficulty comprehending written material (Benson, 1977). Reading comprehension is considerably better than reading aloud but most patients with Broca aphasia find reading difficult and avoid it (see Chapter 11 for additional description of the reading problems of Broca aphasia).

Writing (with either hand) is impaired in Broca aphasia patients. Their written words are made up of oversized, poorly formed letters and contain multiple misspellings and letter omissions. Grammatical function words are routinely omitted or misspelled. In these patients, although the nondominant (usually left) hand often performs better than the paralyzed (dominant) hand, their writing with the nondominant hand is inferior to that produced by nonaphasic individuals writing with their nondominant hand. The deficit is noted in writing to dictation, in attempts to write spontaneously and even in the patient's ability to copy written material. Spontaneous writing (e.g., description of the weather or their job) is virtually impossible (see Chapter 12 for additional discussion of aphasic agraphia). Many Broca aphasia patients can produce more written language with their hemiparetic dominant hand than with the nonparetic, nondominant hand if a device to hold the pen allowing the patient to write with the right wrist is introduced (Brown, Leader, and Blum, 1983; Leischner, 1983). This observation suggests that the poor writing performed by the nondominant hand reflects not only the patient's aphasic agraphia but that some degree of disconnection (ideomotor apraxia) adds to the aphasic disorder.

The neurologic examination almost invariably provides diagnostically useful findings in cases of Broca aphasia; however, considerable variation in the degree and type of disability is found. Most frequently (in over 80% of Broca aphasia patients), the patient will show some degree of right-sided motor weakness, often a full right hemiplegia or significant hemiparesis. If the defect is incomplete, the paresis is usually maximal in the upper extremity with lesser involvement in the lower extremity. Hyperactive reflexes and abnormal pathological reflexes (e.g., Babinski sign) are frequently present on the involved side. Ideomotor apraxia (an inability to carry out, on command, a task that can be performed spontaneously—see Chapter 16) frequently involves the "nonpathological" left limbs (sympathetic apraxia). Sensory abnormality is not consistently found but occurs with fair frequency. When found, the sensory loss may be severe, including loss of both pain and cortical sensory functions, suggesting deep extension of damage. If a severe hemisensory defect is present at the onset of aphasia but clears within days or a week, a unilateral inattention syndrome (neglect) rather than a true sensory loss may be suspected (Heilman, 1979). Visual sensory findings vary tremendously in Broca aphasia. A conjugate deviation of the eyes to the left or a significant degree of right-gaze paresis may be demonstrated at the onset but this usually disappears within a few days or a week. Conjugate deviation of the eyes appears to be associated with unilateral inattention that involves all three major sensory systems (vision, hearing, feeling), a hemisensory state. A lesser degree of right gaze paresis can often be demonstrated for several months following the initial insult, and lesser degrees of hemisensory dysfunction (e.g., poor performance on double simultaneous stimulation tests) can also persist.

Based on initial language and neurological findings and the subsequent recovery course, two variations of the Broca aphasia syndrome have been suggested. For simplicity, the two syndromes will be described simply as Broca aphasia-Type I and Broca aphasia-Type II.

Broca Aphasia-Type I

When damage is limited to the cortex and immediate subcortical structures (Figure 8.1b), only mild defects of articulatory agility and prosody plus reduced word-finding ability are observed. Hemiparesis is minimal and nondominant limb apraxia may be absent or limited. This restricted form will be referred to as Broca aphasia-Type I; this disorder has also been called aphemia, little Broca aphasia, or Broca's area aphasia (Alexander, Benson, and Stuss, 1989; Bastian, 1887; Mohr, 1973). Initially the patient with Broca aphasia-Type I tends to be mute and shows hemiparesis; the paresis (except for the lower face) rapidly clears and speech returns progressively but will be effortful and slow with abnormal articulation and prosody. Some patients with Broca aphasia-Type I show a rapid improvement in articulation and prosody, rapid normalization of repetition and rapid disappearance of phonemic paraphasias (Alexander, Naeser and Palumbo, 1990; Mori, Yamadori, and Furumoto, 1989; Tonkonogy and Goodglass, 1981). Although these patients can produce an occasional long phrase, phrase length is usually shortened; syntax is restricted (simplified) and occasionally incorrect; a full picture of agrammatism, however, is not observed. Language comprehension is good except for complex, syntax-dependent material. Written language defects parallel those of spoken language. In the later stages, individuals with this problem are often said to be "recovered" Broca aphasics.

Broca Aphasia-Type II

Broca aphasia that persists is usually based on more extensive lesions with damage that extends to include the opercula, the precentral gyrus, the anterior insula, the periventricular white matter, and/or the white matter deep to the dominant posterior inferior cortex (Figure 8.1a) (Alexander and Benson, 1991; Damasio, 1981; Kertesz, 1985; Mazzochi and Vignolo, 1979; Mohr et al., 1978). Figure 8.1 illustrates variations in the degree of pathology that produces the two versions of Broca aphasia. Persistent Broca aphasia will be referred to here as Broca aphasia-

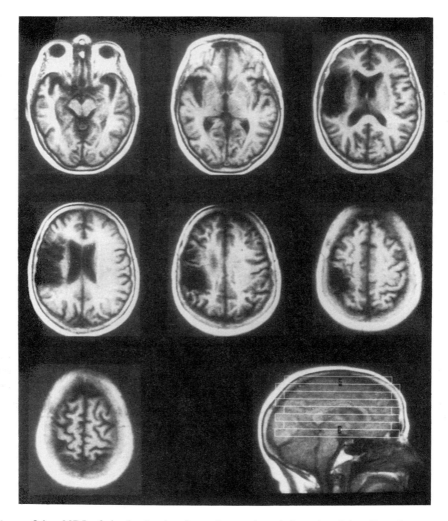

Figure 8.1a. MRI of the brain showing a large, deep infarct involving Broca's area, the internal capsule, and the basal ganglia (causing big Broca aphasia). (From Damasio and Damasio, 1989).

Type II. In this disorder, extension into the deep white matter causes damage to many pathways connecting the anterior regions of the lateral frontal cortex to nearby or distant areas. Four complicating impairments can be distinguished (Alexander, Benson, and Stuss, 1989): (1) impairment in motor system outflow, manifested as dysarthria; (2) deficit in the motor activating system, manifested by initial muteness and subsequent slowness and hesitancy in verbal output; (3) restricted grammatical ability; (4) lexical deficits. Naeser and colleagues (1989)

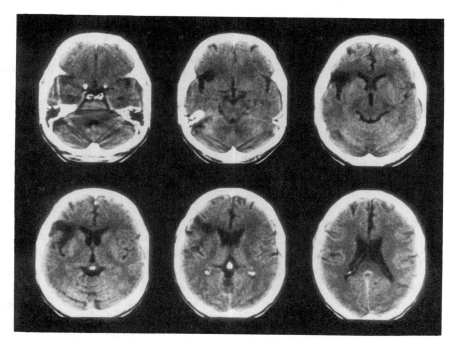

Figure 8.1b. CT brain scan of patient with a small lesion involving Broca's area (causing little Broca aphasia). (From Damasio and Damasio, 1989).

maintain that the degree of extension into the deep white matter governs the capacity for recovery of spoken language.

In summary, Broca aphasia is widely recognized as a cluster of deficits involving language and basic neurologic functions that occurs following damage to the anterior (frontal) elements of the dominant-hemisphere language system. Considerable variation in symptoms and degree of impairment exists and appears directly linked to both the specific locus and the extent of brain damage. Traditionally, the term *Broca aphasia* has been used to designate any anterior aphasia. Detailed evaluation of language defects and other related disorders, however, provides information that allows separation of distinct subtypes that reflect the site of brain damage and extent of language impairment and provide data leading to proper treatment and prognosis.

Conduction Aphasia

Conduction aphasia has also been called *Leitungsaphasie* (Wernicke, 1874), afferent or kinesthetic motor aphasia (Luria, 1966, 1947/1970), central aphasia (Goldstein, 1948), efferent conduction aphasia (Kertesz, 1985), repetition aphasia

(Kleist, 1934b), repetition conduction aphasia (Warrington and Shallice, 1969), or conduction aphasia (Benson and Geschwind, 1971, 1985; Hécaen and Albert, 1978; Hécaen, Dell, and Roger, 1955; Kohn, 1992).

Originally postulated as a distinguishable language disorder by Wernicke (1874), conduction aphasia remains one of the more controversial of the aphasic syndromes. It is traditionally characterized as an aphasia with relatively fluent spontaneous verbal output, good comprehension, and poor repetition with literal paraphasias contaminating both spontaneous verbal output and repetitions of spoken language (Benson, 1979a; Kertesz, 1979, 1985). Benson and colleagues (1973) suggested three basic and five secondary characteristics for conduction aphasia. The three basic characteristics were (1) fluent, paraphasic (usually literal) conversational speech; (2) near normal comprehension; (3) significant disturbances of repetition. The five secondary characteristics, not seen in all cases, were (1) naming disturbances (ranging from literal paraphasic contamination to total inability to produce the appropriate word); (2) disturbed reading with graphic comprehension considerably better than the ability to read aloud; (3) disturbed writing varying from mild spelling difficulties to profound agraphia; (4) ideomotor apraxia (buccofacial and limb); (5) elementary neurological abnormality (cortical sensory loss and some dominant-side hemiparesis). Although any or all of the five secondary findings may be absent, when the three basic characteristics are present a diagnosis of conduction aphasia is warranted.

The most distinctive feature of the conduction aphasia syndrome is the repetition abnormality, the mechanics of which defect have been explained in several ways. The oldest and most robust explanation has been couched in terms of a disconnection of language comprehension (sensory) from language production (motor) (Damasio and Damasio, 1983; Geschwind, 1965; Kleist, 1934a; Mendez and Benson, 1985; Wernicke, 1874). Some investigators prefer to interpret conduction aphasia as an apraxic defect (Ardila et al., 1990; Brown, 1972, 1975; Luria, 1966, 1976a; Vinarskaya, 1971). Given the latter interpretation, conduction aphasia could be interpreted as a verbal apraxia, an ideomotor apraxia of speech (Brown, 1975a), or as a kinesthetic apraxia of speech (Luria, 1976a). Katz and Goodglass (1990), in an extensive review of a unique case of conduction aphasia, demonstrated that their subject had serious problems in the repetition of semantically important words; they suggested calling the disorder deep dysphasia and theorized that a major disturbance in semantic processing was an important feature. They suggested that most patients with conduction aphasia have primary disturbance in phonemic memory processing; in contrast, their subject was relatively competent in phonemic memory processing but showed a major deficit in semantic memory processing. Whether the latter disorder is universally present in conduction aphasia but hidden by the phonemic processing disorder remains unknown.

That several mechanisms might be capable of producing deficient repetition suggests that different types of conduction aphasia could be proposed; an efferent/ afferent distinction (Kertesz, 1979, 1985) and a repetition/ reproduction distinction (Caplan, Vanier, and Baker, 1986; Warrington and Shallice, 1969) have been suggested. The efferent or repetition disorder suggests involvement of phonemic organization and representation of words and is correlated with parietal and insular damage. The afferent or reproduction type implies involvement of auditory-verbal short-term memory, a disruption of the repetition of long sequences of verbal material; an association with temporal lobe damage has been proposed for this latter type (Caramazza et al., 1981). Luria (1976a) found that the language disorder referred to as conduction aphasia covered two distinct linguistic defects. He proposed the term *afferent motor aphasia* to represent the efferent or repetition parietal type mentioned above, and he considered the major problem to be the patient's inability to analyze, manipulate, or otherwise control the composition of movements required to produce language sounds (articulemes), a kinesthetic apraxia of speech. The afferent or reproduction type of conduction aphasia is usually associated with short-term verbal memory deficits, a problem included in Luria's description of acoustic-amnestic aphasia.

Compared to patients with other aphasia syndromes, patients with conduction aphasia produce a particularly high number of literal paraphasias, a disruption that is highlighted in language repetition tasks. Their spontaneous output is variable; in some patients, language output is fluent with normal phrase length and effortless production; in others, conversational speech shows nonfluent, broken, effortful, paraphasia-laden output and frequent word-finding pauses. The conduction aphasia patient may produce one or several sentences easily, then arrive at a point where a particular (usually semantically significant) word is needed and be unable to continue. Superficially speaking, this output may appear nonfluent, but when all output characteristics are considered, more of the characteristics of fluent than of nonfluent aphasia are noted (see Table 6.1). Table 8.2 summarizes the principal language characteristics of conduction aphasia.

Although conduction aphasia patients produce some phonetic deviations and some verbal paraphasias, most switches in oral language correspond to the proposed definition of literal paraphasia (Kohn and Goodglass, 1985). Literal paraphasias are best observed during repetition and can be brought out most strongly by nonword (logotome) repetition (Benson et al., 1973). Other important verbal output problems deserve emphasis. Conduction aphasia patients will often present multiple approximations of the target word that improve with repeated self-corrections *("conduit d'approche")*, demonstrating a preserved acoustic image of the word. Furthermore, the patient, when listening to the examiner, easily distinguishes correctly pronounced from incorrectly pronounced words. Although the conduction aphasia patient may be unable to repeat a word when spoken by

Table 8.2. Characteristics of Conduction Aphasia

Basic Language Characteristics	
Conversational language	Fluent, paraphasic
Repetition of spoken language	Abnormal
Comprehension of spoken language	Good to normal
Pointing to named objects	Good to normal
Naming	Abnormal
Reading	
Aloud	Abnormal
Comprehension	Good to normal
Writing	Abnormal
Associated Neurological Signs	
Motor system	Mild, often transient hemiparesis
Articulation	Normal
Cortical sensory function	Often normal
Praxis	Buccofacial and bilateral limb apraxia
Visual fields	Normal
Visual gnosis	Normal

the examiner, a moment later the patient may produce the same word without effort during spontaneous conversation.

Although the conversational output in conduction aphasia is most accurately described as fluent (Simmons, 1990), the quantity of words produced is notably less than the output in Wernicke aphasia. The patient with conduction aphasia not only produces fewer words but has more and longer pauses. Most frequent are hesitations for word-finding or for the repeated attempts to produce a word because of excessive literal paraphasias. The output often has a broken, dysprosodic quality that can be easily misinterpreted as expressive aphasia. As already noted, a number of features differentiate the output of conduction aphasia from that of Broca aphasia. First, some full, grammatically complex phrases are easily and correctly produced by patients with conduction aphasia. Although many such phrases are clichés (e.g., "I don't know if I can," "What did you say?"), they are far too variable to be classed as stereotypies. In addition, the phonetic deviations that characterize Broca aphasia are distinguishable from those of conduction aphasia. In Broca aphasia most phonetic deviations occur in the context of severe dysarthria, whereas in conduction aphasia phoneme production is good, most often providing accurate pronunciation of an incorrect phoneme. Literal paraphasia is far more characteristic of conduction aphasia than of Broca aphasia.

Several general rules covering the phonological switches (alterations) of conduction aphasia have been proposed by Ardila and colleagues (Ardila et al., 1989b; Ardila and Rosselli, 1990b): (1) *simplification:* phonemes tend to be replaced by more primary, easily produced language sounds. Jakobson and Halle (1956) noted that phonemes acquired earlier in life (and simpler to articulate) tend to replace later acquired phonemes (e.g., /r/, /l/); (2) *switches in the manner and point of articulation* represent about 90% of the paraphasias of conduction aphasia; (3) *consonant changes* are maximal (almost 95% of the total number) whereas vowel switches are minimal. In contrast, vowel changes are considerably more frequent in the paraphasic substitutions (up to six times) in other fluent aphasics (Wernicke and extrasylvian) and are even twice as frequent in Broca aphasia; (4) *articulatory simplification:* phoneme substitutions represent about 70% of literal paraphasic errors, phoneme deletions about 25%. Phoneme additions are uncommon and phoneme exchanges are virtually nonexistent. The types of switches and the responsible mechanisms are the same in spontaneous verbal output and in repetition; in repetition, however, particularly of logotomes, the frequency is higher. The patient with conduction aphasia often performs automatic speech exercises (e.g., counting) adequately if given a start. Similarly, words are often produced better in singing than in conversational output.

Comprehension of spoken language is unexpectedly good in conduction aphasia. In many patients comprehension appears virtually normal and in the others the difficulty is most often limited to the understanding of complex grammatical structures or statements that contain multiple key words or phrases (Heilman and Scholes, 1978). In general, the patient's comprehension of spoken language is fully adequate for normal conversation, better even than most Broca aphasia patients. A significant degree of comprehension disturbance makes the diagnosis of conduction aphasia questionable.

In contrast to their normal comprehension, patients with conduction aphasia have notable difficulty repeating spoken language. The dramatic difference between comprehension and repetition represents the most dramatic feature of the conduction aphasia syndrome and is often considered the key finding (Kleist, 1934b; Simmons, 1990). The repetition is characterized by approximations contaminated by literal paraphasias, but if asked to repeat numbers or color names, conduction aphasia patients may produce verbal paraphasic substitutions. Their repetition is often poorer than their ability to produce the same words in conversational speech. When unable to correctly repeat a word or phrase the patient with conduction aphasia may produce an excellent paraphrase (e.g., when asked to say the word "rifle" an aphasic soldier said, "Riffe . . . riddil . . . oh hell, I mean gun"). Similarly, after totally failing to repeat a word or phrase, the patient may easily produce the same word or phrase in conversation.

Conduction aphasia patients present a distinctive dissociation between pointing and naming. Pointing tasks (e.g., "Show me the _____") are easy for them. Naming tasks, in contrast, tend to produce abundant literal paraphasias, as much or even more than during repetition. In some of these patients, word-finding defect (anomia) appears to be entirely based upon paraphasic substitutions; true inability to find a word does occur in conduction aphasia, however.

Testing of reading ability in conduction aphasia patients often demonstrates a striking dichotomy. Characteristically, these patients have a serious problem reading out loud, rapidly breaking down to a severely paraphasic output. In contrast, these same individuals can comprehend most material read silently. Many patients with conduction aphasia fail when asked to read aloud a three- or four-word sentence, but they can easily read (silently) an entire newspaper, a novel, or even a scientific textbook with good comprehension. Some conduction aphasia patients, however, do show reading impairment (Green and Howes, 1977); extension of the aphasia-producing lesion into the parietal lobe (angular gyrus) has been suggested to explain these instances (Simmons, 1990).

Writing is invariably disturbed to some degree in conduction aphasia, often to a significant degree. Most of these patients can write some words and produce well-formed letters but spelling tends to be poor because of omissions, reversals, and substitutions of letters. Words in a sentence may be misplaced or omitted. Luria (1966) called this afferent motor agraphia, noting a parallel between the errors in oral and written language, and postulated a common underlying mechanism. In addition, some of the graphic errors of conduction aphasia may represent an apraxic agraphia (Ardila and Rosselli, 1990b).

The neurological examination in conduction aphasia patients varies considerably. In some, virtually no neurologic abnormality can be demonstrated. In other cases, however, elementary neurologic abnormality is clearly present. Unilateral paresis may be totally absent, mildly present, or be significant. Weakness characteristically involves the face and arm to a greater degree than the leg. Sensory findings also vary but at least some sensory loss is present in most cases. The impairment tends to involve cortical sensory functions (e.g., position sense, stereognosis, two-point discrimination, etc.), but pain appreciation is often fully normal (Benson, 1979a). Late in recovery from conduction aphasia, however, some patients may develop a unique pain syndrome. Called "pseudothalamic pain syndrome" (Benson, 1979a), the disorder suggests a resemblance to the classic thalamic pain syndrome described by Dejerine and Roussy (1906). Pseudothalamic pain is a constant but much less intense pain than that characterizing the Dejerine-Roussy syndrome and is not exacerbated by external stimuli. Patients with pseudothalamic pain syndrome show cortical sensory loss and may have mildly decreased pain realization, paresthesias, and/or mild hyperalgesia (Benson, 1979a). In contrast, some individuals with conduction aphasia show pain asymbolia (Geschwind, 1965), a situation in which the patient shows much less response to pain stimuli than would be anticipated. The decreased realization of pain is bilateral even though the known neuropathology is limited to the left hemisphere.

Variations may also be found in the visual system of patients with conduction aphasia. Most often there is no involvement of the extraocular movements and the visual fields are full, but some conduction aphasia patients do show a quadrantanopia or even a hemianopic visual-field defect. The variable visual-field loss probably reflects involvement of sites neighboring the locus of the pathology that underlies conduction aphasia.

Ideomotor apraxia is usually present in conduction aphasia patients (Goodglass and Kaplan, 1983). When asked to perform buccofacial or limb movements the patient may fail, even while insisting that they know the requested movements. The patient may make an inappropriate movement that nevertheless demonstrates comprehension of the command. Incorrect, extraneous movements on command (parapraxia) appear to parallel the paraphasias that contaminate their repetition of spoken language. The common association of literal paraphasia with buccofacial apraxia in conduction aphasia suggests that conduction aphasia may be considered a verbal apraxia, an inability to perform the movements required for speaking despite normal oral musculature (Ardila and Rosselli, 1990b; Luria, 1976a). Thus, errors of verbal output in conduction aphasia would correspond to apraxic-type errors in commanded movements. In such an interpretation, conduction aphasia represents a "segmentary ideomotor apraxia" or "ideomotor apraxia of speech" (Brown, 1975a), or a "kinesthetic apraxia of speech" (Luria, 1976a). A number of investigators have emphasized the association between buccofacial apraxia and conduction aphasia (Benson et al., 1973; De Renzi, Pieczuro, and Vignolo, 1966; Geschwind, 1965) and the co-occurrence of literal paraphasia and buccofacial apraxia (Poeck and Kerschensteiner, 1975; Tognola and Vignolo, 1980). Common underlying mechanisms can be surmised.

Brain damage in cases of conduction aphasia most often involves the left parietal lobe (lower postcentral and supramarginal gyri) and the insula (see Figure 8.2) (Ardila, Rosselli, and Pinzon, 1989; Benson et al., 1973; Damasio and Damasio, 1980, 1983; Green and Howes, 1977; Kertesz, 1979, 1985), but there is disagreement regarding the exact location. One traditional explanation (Damasio and Damasio, 1980; Geschwind, 1965) suggests involvement of the dominant-hemisphere arcuate fasciculus, a band of white matter originating in the posterior temporal lobe and coursing forward via the superior longitudinal fasciculus to the motor association cortex of the frontal lobe. Involvement of the arcuate fasciculus (most often deep in the supramarginal gyrus) could thereby produce separation of the sensory and motor language areas (as originally suggested by Wernicke in 1874) (see Figure 8.2). In this postulate, conduction aphasia represents a disconnection of an intact verbal auditory sensory area from an intact motor speech area (Geschwind, 1965; Lichtheim, 1885). Some investigators, however, suggest that involvement of the supramarginal gyrus, the lower part of the central gyrus, and/or the insula, not the underlying white-matter defect, is the essential finding in conduction aphasia (Dubois et al., 1973). In this view, it is damage to the cortex (neuronal area), not the white-matter connection, that is pertinent. A number of aphasiologists (Canter, Troost, and Burns, 1985; Kempler et al., 1988; Kertesz, Lesk, and McCabe, 1977; Levine and Calvanio, 1982) propose a middle-ground explanation based on a language continuum from Wernicke's area to Broca's area and postulate that conduction aphasia occurs with damage to the center of this continuum. Mendez and Benson (1985) presented three cases with the clinical characteristics of conduction aphasia but with lesions distant from the language-dominant hemisphere parietal-insular area; they postulated that disconnection of an intact right-hemisphere temporal-lobe language comprehension area from an intact left-hemisphere motor language area could produce the syndrome of conduction aphasia. Kleist (1934b) and others (Benson et al., 1973) had reported similar cases. The explanation of the language disorder in conduction aphasia remains controversial; it appears possible that more than one explanation exists to explain the variety of symptoms that can accompany the syndrome.

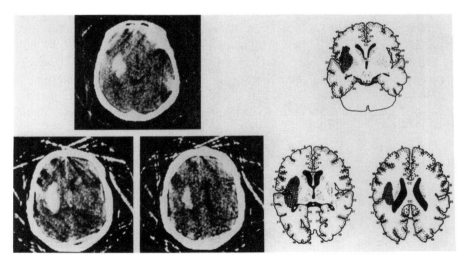

Figure 8.2. CT scan demonstrating hemorrhage in the deep white-matter tissues that connect Wernicke's area with Broca's area—the site of the arcuate fasciculus—producing conduction aphasia. (From Damasio and Damasio, 1980).

Although the theoretical interpretations remain debatable (Goodglass, 1993; Strub and Gardner, 1974) and the site of pathology for conduction aphasia is variable, the syndrome is fully recognizable, occurs rather commonly (between 5 and 10% of cases examined at the Boston VA Aphasia Research Center—Benson, 1979a) and offers important information for clinicians and linguists.

Wernicke Aphasia

Wernicke aphasia is the second most widely recognized of all aphasia syndromes, but variability in the symptom cluster has led to a variety of other names, including sensory aphasia (Wernicke, 1874), receptive aphasia (Weisenburg and McBride, 1935/1964), central aphasia (Brain, 1961), acoustic-amnestic aphasia (Luria, 1966), verbal agnosia (Nielsen, 1936), and others. Although the syndrome is widely accepted and at one time was considered the only true aphasia, it is easily overlooked, even by competent clinicians. When mild or incomplete, the disorder can go unrecognized, glossed over or misinterpreted as a psychological problem. Table 8.3 lists the major language findings that identify Wernicke aphasia.

Table 8.3. Characteristics of Wernicke Aphasia

Basic Language Characteristics	
Conversational language	Fluent, paraphasic
Comprehension of spoken language	Abnormal
Repetition of spoken language	Abnormal
Pointing to named objects	Abnormal
Naming	Abnormal
Reading	
Aloud	Abnormal
Comprehension	Abnormal
Writing	Abnormal
Associated Neurological Signs	
Motor system	Normal
Articulation	Normal
Cortical sensory function	Normal
Praxis	Normal
Visual fields	Normal or superior quadrantopia
Visual gnosis	Normal

The verbal output in Wernicke aphasia is fluent with a normal, or even an excessive, number of words produced per minute. In fact, the most prolific output of words produced in any of the aphasia syndromes occurs in Wernicke aphasia. Patients with Wernicke aphasia often augment their verbal output, adding additional syllables to the ends of words or additional words or phrases at the ends of sentences. The output can become so excessive that the patient speaks nonstop unless forcefully halted by the examiner. The phenomenon of excessive output is called logorrhea or "press of speech" and is almost diagnostic of Wernicke aphasia. Jakobson (1964) interpreted the excessive output of Wernicke aphasia to represent a loss of the boundaries of sentences; the sentences become endless. Wernicke aphasia patients need little effort to produce their verbal output, the length of uttered phrases is normal (five to eight words), they have no problems with either articulation or prosody and most of their utterances have an acceptable grammatical structure. Excessive use of grammatical words, a phenomenon called "paragrammatism" (Lecours and Rouillon, 1976), may be noted. The content of the verbal output, however, is almost invariably deficient in meaningful words; despite the plethora of words produced by the Wernicke aphasia patient, ideation is not effectively conveyed, a phenomenon appropriately termed "empty speech."

Another phenomenon almost invariably present in the verbal output of Wernicke aphasia patients is paraphasia. The language substitutions may be literal or verbal, and even neologisms (made up of multiple superimposed phonemic substitutions) can be seen. When the patient produces an excessive number of words interlocked with multiple paraphasic substitutions, the output becomes incomprehensible, a gibberish termed "jargon aphasia" (Brown, 1981; Lecours and Rouillon, 1976). Jargon aphasia output usually contains all three types of paraphasic deviations in variable quantities. Although this type of output is characteristically present in early Wernicke aphasia, it tends to decrease or disappear so that not all Wernicke aphasics produce jargon. *Jargon aphasia* should be used only as a descriptive term, not as a distinct language syndrome.

Despite the dramatic features of the fluent output, the verbal output abnormalities are not the most definitive characteristics of Wernicke aphasia. Rather, Wernicke aphasia is best characterized as a disturbance of the comprehension of spoken language. When the comprehension disorder is severe, the patient understands absolutely no spoken language; more often it is partial, with the patient retaining some ability to understand single words, phrases, and even sentences. Many patients with Wernicke aphasia have a problem discriminating phonemes (phonemic perception) (Luria, 1966). In particular, the ability to discriminate phonemes that vary only by one feature (e.g., /b/ and /p/) may be deficient (e.g., "pah" and "bah" cannot be distinguished).

Patients with Wernicke aphasia often understand several words when first tested, then fail to comprehend additional words. Even the words initially understood will not be comprehended if they are immediately retested. This striking phenomenon, rapid "fatigue" of the ability to understand, parallels the comprehension problems noted in an individual attempting to understand a second, poorly mastered language. Although the Wernicke aphasia patient often appears to be following a particular language topic, if the topic is changed his understanding ceases; it takes time to establish the new topic. As a rule, understanding can be maintained only for short intervals and requires apparent effort by the patient. Interference such as extraneous noises, movements, or background conversation seriously hampers understanding.

Lesser (1978) postulated four varieties of comprehension impairment: (1) impaired reception of speech sounds, (2) disturbance of central linguistic knowledge, (3) inability to appreciate concepts, a disorder in the mental manipulation of language, (4) disconnection of some process between the ear (primary reception) and the appropriate response mechanism. To a greater or lesser degree, all four varieties occur in Wernicke aphasia but may vary considerably in degree, leading some investigators to propose subdivisions of Wernicke aphasia.

Patients with Wernicke aphasia, while failing some comprehension tasks, do better in others. There is considerable variability between patients on what task is performed successfully or failed. Most patients with Wernicke aphasia fail to carry out a verbally commanded limb or buccofacial activity although they can readily imitate the activity. In contrast, many Wernicke aphasia patients who fail to comprehend conversation or to follow any other command successfully perform requested actions involving the entire body, such as standing, bowing, swinging a baseball bat, posing like a boxer, or doing a waltz step. Retention of the ability to comprehend whole-body commands, although not universal, is sufficiently common in Wernicke aphasia to warrant attention. The phenomenon is probably best explained as nondominant-hemisphere language comprehension.

Repetition of spoken language is invariably abnormal in Wernicke aphasia, usually in a degree corresponding to the comprehension disturbance. Thus, a patient who understands little or nothing will repeat little or nothing; if an occasional word or phrase is understood, repetition will be successful at about the same degree.

When asked to name objects, body parts, etc. on visual confrontation, patients with Wernicke aphasia often fail completely or produce grossly paraphasic responses. These patients may perform better at pointing to objects named by the examiner than at confrontation naming, particularly if a limited number of objects are placed in front of the patient in an array. Even when the patient can successfully point to objects in an array when the name is presented, they often fail if given only a description of the object or its function (e.g., "an instrument denoting the passage of time") or if several object names are presented serially. Some patients who produce copious verbal output, liberally laced with paraphasias, will produce a neologistic or paraphasic facsimile of the target name. Semantic substitutions in naming tasks in Wernicke aphasia patients are common, as are circumlocutions (attempts to describe rather than name the object).

Reading is usually disturbed in Wernicke aphasia patients and the degree of the disturbance may parallel their problem in spoken-language comprehension. Many examiners, however, have noted variations in the comprehension defect in Wernicke aphasia, dependent on whether language is presented to them orally or in written form (Hécaen, 1969 ; Hier and Mohr, 1977). Some patients show the greatest disturbance in the comprehension of spoken language (word-deafness) whereas others have more difficulty comprehending written language (word-blindness), a bipolar tendency which can be used to categorize subtypes of Wernicke aphasia. When auditory comprehension and repetition are relatively superior, the aphasia-producing lesion tends to be more posteriorly placed, evidently sparing some auditory cortex and pathways; when reading comprehension is better than auditory comprehension, lesions tend to be more anteriorly placed in the posterior temporal lobe (classical Wernicke's area), apparently sparing some essential visual-language pathways (Alexander and Benson, 1991; Hier and Mohr, 1977).

Writing is always abnormal in Wernicke aphasia but the writing output is strikingly different from the agraphia of Broca aphasia. The Wernicke aphasia patient uses the dominant hand, and the output consists of properly formed, legible letters combined to appear like real words; the letter combinations, however, are often meaningless (jargon agraphia). Some correctly produced words may appear amid the unintelligible combinations. In some instances the patient's written output may resemble his paraphasic spoken output. If the patient can be encouraged to sound out his words as he writes them, the similarity may be notable.

Most patients with Wernicke aphasia show no deficits on routine neurologic examination. A transient paresis may last a few days at the onset of the disorder, and some degree of persistent cortical sensory disturbance may be present. Both conditions indicate extension of the basic pathologic lesion of Wernicke aphasia. Careful testing may demonstrate a superior quadrantanopia, indicating involvement of Meyer's loop, the portion of the geniculo-calcarine fibers that fan out through the posterior-superior temporal lobe. The superior quadrantanopia may be the only basic neurologic deficit notable. A complete absence of conspicuous neurologic disorder is common and can lead to diagnostic misinterpretation. For instance, the presence of a nonsense language output without evident focal neurologic deficit suggests delirium, psychosis, or dementia. Many patients in the acute stages of Wernicke aphasia have been given a diagnosis of and received treatment for schizophrenia or other acute psychotic disorder, primarily based on their poor social (language) contact and the absence of elementary neurological findings.

Behavioral impairments are common, often dramatically so, in patients with Wernicke aphasia. These patients tend to be unaware of their own deficit and register a pathological unconcern. This blasé attitude can produce additional, serious problems. Wernicke aphasia patients often misinterpret their own problems and suspect that family members, friends, doctors, nursing staff , and others are the real cause of their comprehension difficulty. They accuse others of not listening carefully or of speaking in a code; this can lead to a suspicious, paranoid attitude producing an agitated, even dangerous behavior. In some patients the paranoid behavior is severe, but lesser degrees based on unawareness and unconcern are far more common. The unconcerned behavior is meaningful for diagnosis and often proves disastrous for attempts at aphasia rehabilitation (see Chapter 19 for additional comments).

Many pathological entities can produce Wernicke aphasia. Cerebrovascular accidents (either embolic or thrombotic) or intracerebral hemorrhage that involves the posterior temporal lobe are most common. Trauma or tumor in the temporal lobe can produce a Wernicke aphasia. Before antibiotics were available to treat otic infections, many cases of Wernicke aphasia were produced by abscess in the left temporal lobe.

The location of brain pathology leading to Wernicke aphasia has been demonstrated frequently. Wernicke's original localization, based on autopsy findings (1874), has been reconfirmed by many case studies with the site of brain damage demonstrated by autopsy, surgical intervention, CT scan, MRI, or isotope brain imaging (see Figure 8.3) (Damasio and Damasio, 1989; Kertesz, 1979, 1983, 1985). The full syndrome of Wernicke aphasia indicates damage to the posterior-superior temporal regions of the dominant hemisphere (the superior and middle temporal gyri), with extension into the supramarginal/angular gyrus region and/or the lateral-temporal-occipital junction area commonly present (Damasio, 1981; Kertesz, 1983). Subcortical lesions that interrupt the afferent connections to the temporal cortex (temporal-isthmus damage) are also known to produce the Wernicke aphasia symptom complex (Alexander, Naeser, and Palumbo, 1987).

Although the syndrome of Wernicke aphasia almost invariably indicates dominant-hemisphere posterior-superior temporal-lobe damage, the opposite is not true. As noted in the discussion of conduction aphasia, a patient's entire temporal-lobe auditory processing area may be destroyed without serious impairment of language comprehension. Bihemispheric auditory-verbal competency must be accepted as an explanation in such cases; the nondamaged right-hemisphere auditory processing area is evidently capable of language interpretation in these patients. Non-right-handedness is often present in these cases but some otherwise apparently right-handed (left-dominant) individuals can comprehend language with the right temporal region.

Wernicke's area, the brain region involved in Wernicke aphasia (see Figures

5.9 and 5.10), lies adjacent to the primary auditory cortex (Heschl's gyrus); the primary auditory cortex may or may not be involved in Wernicke aphasia. The variations in the symptom pictures of Wernicke aphasia are based, to a considerable extent, on the location and extent of the pathology in the temporal lobe. Posterior extension probably produces symptoms associated with extrasylvian (transcortical) sensory aphasia, anomia, and probably some degree of visual agnosia. Most aphasics with the clinical findings of Wernicke aphasia are found to have structural damage that involves a considerably larger territory than the dominant-hemisphere auditory association cortex. Broad discrepancies in the boundaries of Wernicke's area have been reported in the literature (Bogen and Bogen, 1976).

Based on the anatomical and clinical variability attributed to Wernicke aphasia, two distinct types will be distinguished in this volume. For convenience, they will be referred to simply as Wernicke aphasia-Type I and Wernicke aphasia-Type II.

Wernicke Aphasia-Type I

The distinguishing characteristic of Wernicke aphasia-Type I is the presence of greater difficulty understanding spoken language than written language. This language syndrome results from damage to the posterior insula–temporal isthmus region and is also known as acoustic-agnosic aphasia (Luria, 1966, 1947/1970, 1976a), word-deafness (Gazzaniga et al., 1973; Kleist, 1934a), verbal auditory agnosia (Vignolo, 1969), a subtype of Wernicke aphasia as proposed by Kertesz (1983, 1985), and a subtype of sensory aphasia as defined by Hécaen and Albert (1978). In Wernicke aphasia-Type I, word-deafness is of a greater degree than word-blindness.

Word-deafness refers to an inability to identify the sounds of language despite intact hearing and preserved ability to identify meaningful nonverbal sounds (Hécaen and Albert, 1978); failure to discriminate the meaningful components of spoken language is the key language feature. In "pure" cases of word-deafness, both reading aloud and reading comprehension are preserved and written communication is both easier and more accurate than oral communication. The patient's language interpretation is not disrupted (as demonstrated by intact written language competency), but damage to the auditory sensory channel makes reception and, therefore, comprehension of spoken language almost impossible. Spontaneous writing is normal but writing to dictation is impossible because of the patient's inability to discriminate the dictated words and repetition of spoken language is severely impaired for the same reason. As the patient is unable to discriminate the verbal sounds of language (phonemes), pure word-deafness can be correctly classed as an auditory verbal agnosia (Schnider et al., 1994; Vignolo, 1969).

Since the first documented demonstration of word-deafness (Liepmann and Storch, 1902), the disorder has traditionally been associated with a lesion deep in the left temporal lobe, often including the posterior insula and/or the temporal isthmus. This topographic description has been generally accepted (Benson, 1979a; Kertesz, 1985) and published cases (Kertesz, 1983) corroborate the presence of deep temporal involvement that includes the posterior insula and adjacent temporal isthmus. A number of reported cases of pure word-deafness, however, have a distinctly different site of pathology. Hécaen and Albert (1978) related word-deafness to subcortical lesions, and an extensive literature (Auerbach et al., 1982; Barrett, 1910; Bonvicini, 1929; Henschen, 1925) correlates word-deafness with bilateral pathology involving the midportions of the temporal lobes. Auerbach and colleagues (1982) postulate that this area in the temporal lobes is necessary for the maintenance of the serial order of language components, an auditory span function. Damage in this area obviates recognition of all but the most elementary auditory language.

Alexander and Benson (1991) distinguish three types of word-deafness: In the first type, the patient's verbal output is fluent, may be grammatically correct or show paragrammatism, and tends to be mildly paraphasic and empty. Reading comprehension is normal or near normal but the written output may be abnormal and resembles the patient's speech. Damage involves the left superior temporal gyrus, including the left primary auditory cortex, with at least partial damage to connections to the posterior-superior temporal gyrus, presumably disrupting auditory processing and leading to paraphasia and mild anomia. Their second type is similar to the first but shows greater disturbance of auditory perception. In this condition the patient fails to recognize any sounds (e.g., musical instruments, natural noises, etc.), suffering a full auditory agnosia (Motomura, Yamadori, and Mitani, 1986; Spreen, Benton, and Fincham, 1965). If bilateral posterior temporal damage is present (Coslett, Brashear, and Heilman, 1984) and if the lesions are sufficiently extensive, the patient will suffer a full cortical deafness. The third suggested type of word-deafness also features bilateral pathology, but the dominant hemisphere lesion is restricted to auditory cortex or auditory pathways without involvement of the posterior-superior temporal gyrus (Auerbach et al., 1984; Metz-Lutz and Dahl, 1984). In this disorder, the patient will show an impairment in temporal (time-dependent) competency, an inability to recognize sequential sounds presented rapidly by the examiner.

Wernicke Aphasia-Type II

The second widely accepted subtype of Wernicke aphasia features a greater degree of word-blindness than word-deafness. If alexia is severe but comprehension of spoken language is relatively well preserved and repetition near normal, the disorder is better classed as a posterior extrasylvian disorder (see Chapter 9). In many instances, however, patients with Wernicke aphasia-Type II suffer distinct problems in auditory comprehension and repetition of spoken language, even though these are not as intense as the patient's difficulty comprehending written language. Wernicke aphasia-Type II can be considered a word-blind version of Wernicke aphasia (Hécaen and Albert, 1978; Hier and Mohr, 1977). The site of the aphasia-producing pathology in Wernicke aphasia-Type II tends to be more posterior, primarily affecting angular gyrus but with encroachment on the posterior temporal (Wernicke's area) cortex and/or the pertinent cortical-cortical pathways of the posterior temporal region.

A combination of the variations of Wernicke aphasia is recognized as a separate entity by many investigators and has been called impressive aphasia (Pick, 1931), receptive aphasia (Weisenburg and McBride, 1935/1964), sensory aphasia (Goldstein, 1948; Hécaen and Albert, 1978), acoustic-amnestic aphasia (Luria, 1966, 1947/1970), and phonemic jargon (Kertesz, 1985) but is most often referred to as Wernicke aphasia (Benson, 1979a; Benson and Geschwind, 1971, 1985; Graham, 1990; Kertesz, 1985). The verbal output is fluent with a normal or excessive number of words (logorrhea) produced with normal articulation and prosody. The grammatical structure of the verbal output is adequate but it can contain an excess of grammatical morphemes (paragrammatism). The verbal output shows a decreased number of meaningful, substantive words (empty speech) and an excessive number of paraphasias (usually semantic, but neologisms are not uncommon). The patient's comprehension of spoken language is always defective but can fluctuate in degree; repetition of spoken language can be near normal for short elements (syllables, words) but is always abnormal for long sequences (phrases, sentences). The patient's level of competency in repetition and in comprehension are closely related. Reading and writing parallel the deficit in the comprehension and production of spoken language. Naming is abnormal (often failed) but both verbal and literal paraphasias can be present; phonemic cueing does not facilitate naming. When the aphasia-producing lesion is extensive, a neologistic jargon can be observed, particularly in the early stages following onset of aphasia. In this variation, Wernicke aphasia-Type I and Wernicke aphasia-Type II are present about equally.

Obviously, all subtypes of Wernicke aphasia are variations on a continuum but differences in the clinical picture appear related to the locus of the aphasia-producing damage. It can be anticipated that the improved clinical assessment and neuroimaging techniques now available will allow considerably more precise delineation of these symptom clusters and their anatomical correlations in the future.

Summary

Three classically recognized syndromes of aphasia have been described, along with several subtypes within two of the syndromes. Although differing radically in basic clinical symptomatology, all three syndromes share one consistent language defect (impairment or even total inability to repeat spoken language) and one general anatomical feature (location of pathology in the perisylvian tissues of the language-dominant hemisphere). These three syndromes make up the most commonly recognized aphasic disorders and are supported by a great deal of corroborating anatomical and clinical data. Despite the many variations described for each, these aphasia syndromes represent the most stable material available for brain-language correlation purposes, and the dominant-hemisphere perisylvian territory can be accepted as an essential neuroanatomical substrate for basic language functions.

9

Extrasylvian (Transcortical) Aphasic Syndromes

· ·

Repetition is sometimes normal, or nearly so, in patients who are otherwise aphasic. In some aphasics repetition is considerably superior to other language functions. Aphasia without repetition disturbance almost invariably indicates pathology located outside the perisylvian cortical region. Much of the involved brain region is vascular border zone, cerebral tissue lying at the junction of the middle cerebral artery territory with the vascular beds of the anterior or posterior cerebral arteries (see Figure 9.1). The clinical varieties of aphasia with relatively good repetition can usually be correlated with the area of border zone tissue involved.

The term *transcortical aphasia* was proposed by Wernicke (1881) and Lichtheim (1885), and several varieties of aphasia gathered under this title were intensely studied by Goldstein (1917). The term was originally proposed to draw a contrast between aphasia syndromes with or without normal repetition. The word *transcortical* represented one area of a postulated model of the cortical network involved in language and ideation in which exact phonological reproduction could be accomplished by the aphasic patient but the meaning (idea) could not be extracted and/or reproduced. The hypothesis was abandoned many years ago; Goldstein, in his treatise entitled *Die Transkortikalen Aphasien* (1917), noted that the term *transcortical* was archaic and misleading. *Transcortical aphasia*, however, remains the most widely accepted designation for a distinctive group of aphasic syndromes. The syndromes are not "transcortical" in any literal sense. They are, however, almost always *extrasylvian* in location, making it reasonable to propose

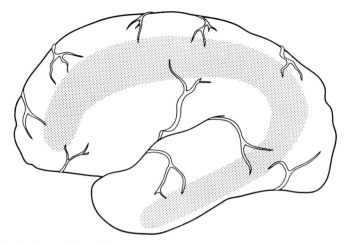

Figure 9.1. Artist's rendition of cerebral arterial border-zone (watershed) area (stippled).

that term to designate this group of aphasias. While *transcortical* may someday be dropped from the aphasia nomenclature, it remains the best-recognized term; in this chapter both terms will be used to designate the extrasylvian aphasia syndromes.

Extrasylvian (Transcortical) Motor Aphasia

A variety of labels have been applied to nonfluent aphasia with preserved repetition; these include dynamic aphasia (Luria, 1966) and anterior isolation syndrome (Benson and Geschwind, 1971), but transcortical motor aphasia (TCMA), coined by Lichtheim, remains the most widely accepted in Western literature. Goldstein (1948) hypothesized that two different problems could produce TCMA. He noted that a variation of the syndrome can occur following partial recovery from Broca aphasia at a time when repetition had recovered better than spontaneous language production. He also recognized a variation of TCMA that featured a primary difficulty in the initiation of articulation, often corrected by prompting. An extreme hesitancy in volitional articulatory initiation, almost magically corrected in the act of repetition, was the prime dysfunction characterizing the dynamic speech problem described by Luria and Tsvetkova (1967). Later, Alexander and colleagues (Alexander, Benson, and Stuss, 1989; Freedman and Alexander, 1984) distinguished a number of speech and/or language disorders that could follow left frontal pathology. Two of their subtypes presented with the TCMA symptom cluster. Damage to dorsolateral frontal structures, anterior and/or superior to the operculum, produced the classic clinical picture of TCMA described by Licht-heim (1885), Goldstein (1917), Geschwind (1965), and others. A similar language disorder, however, could also result from midline frontal damage that caused ini-tial mutism followed by reduced language formulation and eventual recovery to a TCMA symptom cluster. Differences in the speech qualities of the two disorders supported the concept of two separate types of TCMA. The nature of accompa-nying motor deficits, the locus of neuropathology and the course of language re-covery are each sufficiently different to substantiate two varieties of a single lan-guage disorder cluster, TCMA.

Both varieties of extrasylvian motor aphasia (TCMA) are characterized by nonfluent language, good comprehension, and good (essentially normal) repetition (Alexander and Benson, 1991). Articulation, prosody, and grammar are preserved but the patient's spontaneously generated verbal output shows delayed initiation, terse and poorly elaborated utterances, clipped, incomplete sentences, and verbal paraphasias. The ability to respond to yes/no questions tends to be normal, but, in contrast, responses to open-ended questions are delayed, incomplete, and show a strong tendency for repetition of the examiner's utterance (incorporation echola-lia) (Luria, 1966; Rubens, 1976).

Immediately following onset of TCMA, most patients tend to be mute (Alex-ander and Schmitt, 1980); the speechlessness is often associated with a general akinesia that improves to a right hemiakinesia (Damasio and Van Hoesen, 1983). A clinical picture of akinetic mutism (or hypophonic bradykinesia), common at the outset, is produced. Both echolalia and perseveration are common during the early recovery stage. Hemiparesis and buccofacial apraxia may occur but are not common, and limb apraxia (if observed) is mild (Alexander and Benson, 1991).

The basic language disorder in extrasylvian motor aphasia is always associ-ated with damage in the left frontal lobe but differences in the overall clinical picture are present, dependent upon the location of the damage within the left frontal lobe (see Table 9.1 for an outline of all left frontal communication disor-ders). Extrasylvian motor aphasia will be discussed as two clinically similar but separate disorders.

Extrasylvian (Transcortical) Motor Aphasia-Type I (TCMA-I)

Extrasylvian (transcortical) motor aphasia-Type I is an acquired speech/language dysfunction characterized by disordered, basically nonfluent verbal output, good comprehension, and good repetition of spoken language. This disorder has been described as dynamic aphasia (Luria, 1966, 1976a,b), as a loss of verbal initiative (Kleist, 1934a), or as transcortical motor aphasia (Benson, 1979; Benson and Geschwind, 1971; Goldstein, 1948; Gonzalez-Rothi, 1990; Hécaen and Albert, 1978; Lichtheim, 1885). It is generally recognized to result from left dorsolateral

Table 9.1. Left Frontal Communication Disorders

LANGUAGE DISORDER	NEUROANATOMICAL LOCALIZATION
Aphemia	Lower motor cortex and posterior operculum
Broca's area aphasia	Full operculum plus lower motor cortex
Transcortical motor aphasia	Dorsolateral frontal cortex
Mutism	Medial frontal cortex
Reduced formulation; impoverished discourse	Prefrontal cortex

From Alexander, Benson, and Stuss, 1989.

prefrontal damage (Alexander and Benson, 1991; Kertesz and McCabe, 1977). Table 9.2 presents the main clinical features of TCMA-I.

TCMA-I is characterized by a notable decrease (almost an absence) of spontaneous verbal output; patients with TCMA-I use as few words as possible, answer questions by reiterating many of the words and grammatical structures presented in the question (echolalia), and on occasion produce perseverative responses. Sentences tend to be started but not finished. Poor word-list generation, impoverished narrative production, reduced use of complex and precise syntax, and poor inhibition of high-association responses have been described following left prefrontal damage (Stuss and Benson, 1986). One frequently noted output feature is the attempt by the patient to use nonlanguage motor prompting to initiate speech. Patients with TCMA-I may nod their head vigorously, clap their hands, start to rise from sitting (or step out when standing), wave their hands like a conductor, or use other crude motor acts to stimulate articulatory initiation; the maneuvers are at least partially successful for many patients. Teaching a TCMA-I patient to tap with his or her hand (or just to move the hand) may facilitate verbal responsiveness. Despite the obvious difficulty initiating motor speech in TCMA-I, articulation defects are not usually observed; if present, they indicate additional (almost always deeper) pathology.

In contrast to their problems in maintaining spontaneous output, TCMA-I patients perform series speech well once the series has been initiated. If the patient fails to count on command, the first one or two numbers can be given by the examiner; the patient will repeat these and continue the series unhindered. Similarly, recitation of nursery rhymes and naming the days of the week or the months of the year are often performed successfully by these patients if initiated by the examiner. Failure at automatic speech tasks is often directly attributable to perseveration, the patient's inability to halt the continuous repetition of a single word or phrase. Open-ended phrases (e.g., red, white and _____; Mary had a

Table 9.2. Characteristics of Extrasylvian (Transcortical) Motor Aphasia-Type I

Basic Language Characteristics	
Conversational language	Sparse, echolalic
Comprehension of spoken language	Relatively normal
Repetition of spoken language	Good to fully normal
Pointing	Normal
Naming	Mildly abnormal
Reading:	
Aloud	Defective
Comprehension	Often good
Writing	Defective
Associated Neurological Signs	
Motor system	Hemiparesis may/may not be present, pathological reflexes frequently present
Articulation	Normal
Cortical sensory function	Normal
Praxis	Normal
Visual fields	Normal
Visual gnosis	Normal

little _____) are easily completed by these patients, a clinical demonstration known as the completion phenomenon (Stengel, 1947—see description in Chapter 6).

Comprehension of spoken language is usually considered good in TCMA-I patients, at least at the level of routine conversation. Many of these patients will have difficulty handling sequences of complex material, however, and some show difficulty interpreting relational words (Rothi and Heilman, 1980). Some TCMA-I patients will have difficulty controlling yes/no responses; contamination by perseveration is common and meaningless responses can be produced. Despite their apparently good ability to understand, formal demonstration of the comprehension capability of TCMA-I subjects may prove difficult.

The inability of TCMA-I patients to initiate a response may be further complicated by significant apathy, a decrease of drive sufficient to suggest behavioral withdrawal. These patients seem distant and are often difficult to engage in social conversation. They show little interest in using language, even to express their primary desires. One TCMA-I patient, when asked "Why don't you answer my questions?" responded (slowly), "I listen and I understand but it is as if you were talking to somebody else, not to me" (Ardila, personal observation). Luria (1973) proposed that in dynamic aphasia the patient's behavior was not controlled by language and that the dissociation between language and overt behavior represents an executive control disorder disrupting language at the pragmatic level. TCMA-I patients have difficulty following commands. Although they appear to understand the examiner's verbally presented commands, they often fail to respond; again, it can be interpreted that the patient's actions are no longer under the control of language.

Good repetition of spoken language is the most striking feature of the TCMA-I syndrome. The ability of these aphasic patients to repeat is unexpectedly good in dramatic contrast to their nonfluent spontaneous output. Although TCMA-I patients often echo a word or phrase, they are usually not fully echolalic; this is not the mandatory repetition seen in more posterior extrasylvian aphasia syndromes. When asked to repeat grammatically incorrect statements (e.g., "The boys is here") TCMA-I patients produce a grammatically correct response and they will reject (refuse to repeat) nonsense syllables and grammatically incorrect statements. Most often the repetition is an echoing of the examiner's statement preceding an attempt to respond.

The ability to name on confrontation is often limited in TCMA-I patients, with their delays in initiating the answer similar to those noted in their spontaneous conversation. Both contextual and phonemic cues can be helpful. Three error types are found in confrontation naming in these patients: (1) *perseveration:* the patient continues giving a past answer for a new stimulus; (2) *fragmentation:* the patient responds to a single feature of the stimulus, not to the whole stimulus (e.g., a green butterfly is called grass); (3) *extravagant paraphasias:* instead of the target name, the patient presents a free-association answer that becomes an extravagant deviation.

The generation of word lists in a given category is invariably poor in TCMA-I patients; not only do they have problems producing words belonging to a specific category but they commonly have difficulty maintaining the category (e.g., when asked to name fruits, the patient's response might be "pear, apple, tomato, potato, salad, hamburger").

The TCMA-I patient's reading ability, both aloud and for comprehension, is always better than his writing, just as spoken language comprehension is better than his expression of spoken language. Reading aloud tends to be slow and difficult to maintain, but reading comprehension is at normal levels except for syntactically complex material.

The patient's ability to write is almost always defective, often seriously. The tendency is so marked that the term "agraphia without alexia" is an appropriate description. The patient's written output features large, clumsily produced letters, poor spelling, and a hypereconomy of output—characteristics which are also noted in Broca aphasia patients. Sentences are incomplete and the patients with TCMA-I must be continuously stimulated to continue writing.

The associated neurological findings in transcortical motor aphasia-Type I are variable. Hemiparesis is uncommon but may be present transiently; more frequent is the patient's residual tendency to ignore use of the right limbs (inintention). Pathological reflexes (Hoffmann, Babinski, etc.) involving the dominant limb are often present. Neither sensory loss nor visual-field loss is characteristic although either may be seen, dependent on the size and locus of the lesion. Both conjugate deviation of the eyes and strong unilateral inattention have been recorded in the initial stages in some cases of TCMA-I.

Over a variable number of weeks, the patient's responsive language improves as spontaneous language becomes less sparse and less delayed. Language recovery is usually limited, however; TCMA-I has proved particularly difficult to treat (Alexander and Schmitt, 1980; Gonzalez-Rothi, 1990). TCMA-I has long been related to damage anterior and superior to Broca's area (Brodmann areas 45, 46, and/or part of area 9)—the posterior (dorsolateral) left prefrontal lobe. The clinical characteristics resemble the fundamental language processing features seen with left prefrontal damage (i.e., general adynamia and apathy, inability to program, tendency to perseverate).

Extrasylvian (Transcortical) Motor Aphasia-Type II (TCMA-II)

Extrasylvian (transcortical) motor aphasia-Type II is also characterized by a nonfluent output but good comprehension and repetition of spoken language. The syndrome most obviously differs from TCMA-I in the associated neurological findings and the locus of brain pathology. This type of motor aphasia has been called transcortical motor aphasia (Damasio and Kassel, 1978; Kertesz, 1979, 1985), the syndrome of the anterior cerebral artery (Alexander and Schmitt, 1980; Benson, 1979a; Rubens, 1975, 1976), mild transcortical motor aphasia (Freedman, Alexander, and Naeser, 1984), and supplementary motor area aphasia (Alexander and Benson, 1991; Ardila and Lopez, 1984).

In a review of the anatomical and clinical aspects of anterior cerebral artery occlusion, Critchley (1930) noted that aphasia was only an occasional finding; the language disturbance was not named and was only vaguely characterized. Luria (1947/1970) in his report of a large series of brain-injured aphasics, noted that damage in the mesial premotor area produced an aphasia and suggested that the language disturbance most closely resembled the efferent motor, or Broca, type of aphasia. Mutism had already been noted to result from damage to the frontal midline motor structures (supplementary motor area) by Schwab (1926) and Foerster (1936); Penfield and Boldrey (1937) observed that electrical stimulation to this area produced an arrest of speech. Following these observations, the supplementary motor area has been accorded a real, but poorly defined, role in language production.

The supplementary motor area is known to receive considerable input from the basal ganglia (Alexander, DeLong, and Strick, 1986; Cummings and Benson, 1990); a relationship between the language deficit in TCMA-II and the bradykinesia seen in basal ganglia disorder can be suspected. The supplementary motor area also receives afferents from anterior thalamus, dopaminergic mesencephalic nuclei, and the hypothalamus and has efferents to the caudate and dorsolateral frontal convexity (Brinkman, 1984; Damasio, Van Hoesen, and Damasio, 1980; Pandya and Vignolo, 1971). Pathways from the supplementary motor area to the dorsolateral frontal convexity are poorly defined but apparently extend via the anterolateral periventricular white matter and anterior-superior periventricular white matter (Alexander and Benson, 1991; Alexander, Benson, and Stuss, 1989; Freedman, Alexander, and Naeser, 1984). The supplementary motor area and the adjacent cingulate gyrus appear to play roles in limbic (motivation) and motor (initiation) tasks (Smith, Bourbonnais, and Blanchette, 1981). The initial mutism of TCMA-II patients, followed by delayed and impoverished responses during recovery phases, may be understood on the basis of disturbance to a key motor activation center (Freedman, Alexander, and Naeser, 1984). The clinical characteristics of the aphasia produced by supplementary motor aphasia damage were analyzed and categorized by Rubens (1975, 1976) who also noted that the most frequent etiology was occlusion of the left anterior cerebral artery; however, it is known that both tumor and trauma can produce similar clinical features (Damasio and Van Hoesen, 1983).

In TCMA-II patients the language disturbance following occlusion of the left anterior cerebral artery has an initial period of mutism (two to ten days). Patients then show disordered speech and language characterized by delayed articulatory initation and disturbed clarity of speech (primarily hypophonia), in contrast to their nearly normal output in repetition and their essentially normal comprehension and naming. They show neither echolalia nor the forced-completion phenomenon (Rubens, 1975, 1976). Reading aloud may be near-normal but reading comprehension is usually limited to matching of object to picture (Rubens, 1975). Inability of TCMA-II subjects to read letter-by-letter has been described in the Spanish writing system (Ardila and Lopez, 1984). Writing is slow, labored, and incomplete and shows occasional paragraphia.

The associated neurological findings in cases of midline premotor involvement (TCMA-II) are notable and often diagnostic. Profound weakness, hyperreflexia, contralateral extensor toe signs and sensory loss involve the lower extremity but there is only a mild weakness of the right shoulder and basically normal arm, hand, and face strength—a motor pattern termed crural paralysis. There may be no other neurologic involvement, but if midline frontal damage is extensive the patient may show incontinence, a right grasp reflex, alien hand syndrome, abulia, and/or gegenhalten (Adams and Victor, 1989; Stuss and Benson, 1986). The above findings make up the classic neurological findings of infarction involving the anterior cerebral artery territory (Fisher, 1975). Most TCMA-II patients show considerable recovery of language over a period of several months. Table 9.3 presents the clinical characteristics of the aphasia and associated neurological signs that follow damage to the supplementary motor area.

Damasio and Van Hoesen (1983) pointed out that small lesions in the left supplementary motor area may produce only brief mutism with rapid recovery and that once verbal output has returned, no aphasic symptomatology is present. If the lesion extends into more anterior and inferior medial frontal regions, however, numerous neurobehavioral disorders are observed; these include personality changes, motor slowness, unconcern and memory deficits (Freedman, Alexander, and Naeser, 1984; Alexander, Benson, and Stuss, 1989; Damasio and Van Hoesen, 1983). The degree of motor language defect and the degree of associated neurological problems can vary considerably but tend to be related.

A good argument can be made that extrasylvian motor aphasia, particularly TCMA-II, is a pure motor disorder that does not involve basic language function

Table 9.3. Characteristics of Extrasylvian (Transcortical) Motor Aphasia-
Type II

Basic Language Characteristics	
Conversational language	Sparse, effortful
Comprehension of spoken language	Normal
Repetition of spoken language	Good to normal
Pointing	Normal
Naming	Normal, occasional literal paraphasia
Reading	
Aloud	Defective
Comprehension	Often good
Writing	Slow with paragraphias
Associated Neurological Signs	
Motor system	Lower extremity paresis
Articulation	Mild dysarthria
Cortical sensory function	Lower extremity sensory loss
Praxis	Normal
Visual fields	Normal
Visual gnosis	Normal

and that, therefore, the extrasylvian motor verbal output disorder does not deserve inclusion as a type of aphasia. Broader views of language, however, particularly those included as metalinguistic or pragmatic language functions, would easily incorporate the extrasylvian motor disorders as language dysfunctions. Although the problem of definition remains unsettled, common usage for over a century warrants inclusion of the extrasylvian motor disorders among the aphasias.

Extrasylvian (Transcortical) Sensory Aphasia (TCSA)

Transcortical sensory aphasia was first described by Wernicke (1881) and then by Lichtheim (1885); they proposed that this syndrome represented a disconnection of the sensory (auditory) language area from a "concept area." Both investigators were initially fascinated by the phenomenon of echolalia. In fact, in many of the early papers on transcortical sensory aphasia, echolalia is the only language deficit discussed, as though it represented a specific aphasia syndrome. In his monumental study of transcortical aphasia, Goldstein (1917) clearly described the features of transcortical sensory aphasia but devoted most of his attention to repetition and echolalia. The clinical features of extrasylvian (transcortical) sensory aphasia (TCSA) listed in Table 9.4 are distinct and worthy of careful attention since the syndrome is easily (and frequently) misinterpreted as an acute psychiatric breakdown.

Conversational speech in transcortical sensory aphasia is unquestionably fluent, often featuring paraphasia (primarily neologistic and semantic substitutions) and an emptiness (lack of specific names) in content. Preserved ability to repeat is unexpected in this context. The tendency for TCSA patients to repeat is often a true echolalia. Almost routinely, these patients will incorporate words and phrases uttered by the examiner into their ongoing output while apparently failing to understand the meaning of the words. The echolalia often appears mandatory as the patient seems unable to avoid repeating the examiner's words. Unlike the echolalia seen in transcortical motor aphasia patients, TCSA patients will echo incorrect syntactical structures, nonsense words, and even foreign phrases. The total output of TCSA tends to be verbose, often almost uninhibited. Once started, TCSA patients can count, recite the days of the week and months of the year, and show a very strong completion phenomenon for poems and statements. Although their series speech, when initiated by the examiner, is good, the patients cannot perform these tasks on command.

Comprehension of spoken language is severely disturbed in TCSA patients, often to the point of total noncomprehension, and stands in stark contrast to the ease with which they reiterate the examiner's statements. Many TCSA patients

Table 9.4. Characteristics of Extrasylvian (Transcortical) Sensory
Aphasia

Basic Language Characteristics	
Conversational language	Fluent, paraphasic, echolalic
Comprehension of spoken language	Defective
Repetition of spoken language	Good to excellent
Pointing	Defective
Naming	Defective
Reading:	
Aloud	May be preserved
Comprehension	Defective
Writing	Defective
Associated Neurological Signs	
Motor system	Often normal
Articulation	Normal
Cortical sensory function	Often disordered
Praxis	Difficult to test
Visual fields	Normal or defective
Visual gnosis	Difficult to test

fail all tests of comprehension of spoken language including pointing, obeying motor commands, and answering yes/no questions. Obviously, gradations can be seen in the severity of comprehension disturbance. Partial degrees of auditory language comprehension can make TCSA even more difficult to recognize and may lead to misinterpretation of the disorder as a psychogenic problem.

Repetition of spoken language ranges from good to excellent in TCSA patients. Their span level for auditory material may be low and their ability to repeat may be limited, but in many cases the span is remarkably good. The patient tends to repeat accurately what the examiner has said and, as noted, may repeat nonsense syllables, "Jabberwocky," foreign phrases, and grammatically incorrect utterances verbatim as long as the language's sound structures resemble the patient's primary language. In TCSA patients, phonology is preserved but semantic interpretation is lost.

Naming is seriously defective in TCSA patients. Characteristically, these patients neither name an object nor identify it when the name is presented by the examiner. At times these patients will offer incorrect names but are more likely to present a phrase or sentence to describe the object and its function but most of the output is not intelligible.

Although not true in all cases, the patient's ability to read out loud may be preserved despite severe TCSA. Reading comprehension, on the other hand, is seriously defective, producing another paradox: some patients with TCSA can read aloud with accuracy but cannot understand what they have just said (and read), just as they fail to comprehend spoken language which they can repeat flawlessly. Often, however, paralexic substitutions contaminate their attempts at reading aloud, compromising the output. Writing is routinely defective in TCSA and, in general, resembles the disturbance of written output seen in Wernicke aphasia patients.

Extrasylvian sensory aphasia patients usually have no associated motor deficits although a history of right hemiparesis at the onset of the aphasia is common. Sensory abnormality is often present; it may be mild, restricted to a mild cortical sensory abnormality, or a more pervasive hemisensory loss. Unilateral inattention is common. Some disorder of the visual fields is frequent, either an inferior quadrantopia or a complete hemianopia. As many TCSA patients have no obvious elementary neurologic deficit, the potential for misdiagnosis is considerable.

As could be anticipated, patients with extrasylvian sensory aphasia who produce a plethora of real words freely intermingled with paraphasias and who have excellent repetition but almost no ability to understand can be misdiagnosed as psychotic. They are out of contact with reality, at least at the verbal level. This is particularly true if they show no evidence of basic neurologic deficit. Many such patients have been, and probably many still are, maintained in mental hospitals; many have been given a diagnosis of schizophrenia because of their garbled, paraphasic output (schizophrenic word salad) and because they are not in contact verbally.

In recent years some aphasiologists have proposed that two types of extrasylvian sensory aphasia can be distinguished. The postulated distinctions will be referred to in this volume as extrasylvian sensory aphasia-Type I and extrasylvian sensory aphasia-Type II.

Extrasylvian (Transcortical) Sensory Aphasia-Type I (TCSA-I)

The symptom cluster of TCSA-I resembles the language features described as amnesic aphasia (Hécaen and Albert, 1978; Luria, 1976a,b) and the first subtype of transcortical sensory aphasia described by Kertesz (1982, 1983).

Extrasylvian (transcortical) sensory aphasia-Type I (TCSA-I) is characterized by fluent spontaneous language, poor comprehension, and preserved repetition. Conversational language tends to be contaminated by semantic paraphasias and, particularly in the early stages, neologistic substitutions. Echolalia is common, with the patient incorporating words and sentences uttered by the examiner into his or her response. Comprehension of spoken language tends to be severely defective and naming is strongly impaired. TCSA-I patients can neither name an object on confrontation nor point to the object when the name is offered; phonemic prompting rarely helps them retrieve the appropriate word. Reading aloud may be preserved but reading comprehension is defective. Writing is defective to a variable degree.

In TCSA-I patients the presence of semantic paraphasias (correct words belonging to the language stock but inappropriate for the object in question) and the occasional helpfulness of phonemic prompting during naming tests suggests that the word itself may not be lost to the patient but it cannot be retrieved in confrontation naming tasks. For these patients a visually presented object does not trigger the appropriate word response and, conversely, a spoken word does not evoke a visual image. The patient is unable to retrieve meanings for words he can easily repeat (e.g., "draw a dog," "point to the door"). TCSA-I patients are often able to produce adequate copies of two- and three-dimensional drawings in a manner similar to their ability to repeat words spoken by the examiner. They fail, however, to match spoken or written words to visual stimuli; for these patients the visual percept is disconnected from their lexical repertoire. Other evidence suggesting a visual agnosia may be found in TCSA-I (Tsvetkova, 1979) and right visual-field impairment (and right visual attention disorder) may be present.

The brain damage associated with TCSA-I is usually located at the junction of the temporal, parietal, and occipital lobes (roughly, the lower angular gyrus and upper portion of Brodmann area 37). Damage in this area has been reported to cause increased verbal paraphasia and semantic jargon (Kertesz, 1983; Kertesz, Sheppard, and MacKenzie, 1982). Kertesz and colleagues suggested that TCSA-I can evolve into a relatively severe form of anomic aphasia; even with good recovery TCSA-I patients usually suffer a residual anomia of significant degree. The basic word-finding defect in TCSA-I is identical to the word selection anomia suggested by Benson (1988a) (see Chapter 14) but tends to be severe and is accompanied by considerable comprehension problems.

Extrasylvian (Transcortical) Sensory Aphasia-Type II (TCSA-II)

Extrasylvian (transcortical) sensory aphasia-Type II (TCSA-II) has the language features described by Kertesz (1982, 1983) as his second type of transcortical sensory aphasia and resembles, but only partially, the semantic aphasia described by Head (1926) and others (Ardila, Lopez, and Solano, 1989; Brown, 1972; Luria, 1966, 1976a,b; Wepman and Jones, 1964) and the semantic anomia described by Benson (1979a, 1988a).

Damage to the parietal-lobe angular gyrus is said to produce a verbal amnesic deficit characterized by fluent output with few semantic paraphasias, variable ability to comprehend spoken language, and excellent ability to repeat words and phrases coupled with a notable deficiency in word finding (Goldstein, 1948; Héc-aen and Albert, 1978; Kleist, 1934a); patients with TCSA-II produce an "empty speech" due to the absence of significant words and a remarkable number of circumlocutions (Benson and Geschwind, 1985). Both reading and writing tend to be seriously impaired in the syndrome and some or all components of the Gerstmann syndrome (right/left disorientation, finger agnosia, acalculia, and agraphia) will be present. Although some word-finding difficulties are present in almost every type of aphasia (Goodglass and Geschwind, 1976), word-finding difficulties are particularly evident in TCSA-II. Gloning and colleagues (1969) reported that 60% of the patients to which they gave a diagnosis of "anomic apha-sia" had pathology that involved the dominant-hemisphere parietal lobe.

Another name for TCSA-II is "semantic aphasia," a term widely used in the past but somewhat neglected in recent aphasia literature (Ardila, Lopez, and So-lano, 1989; Hier et al., 1980; Luria, 1964b). Two proponents of the term, Head and Luria, stressed the impairment of language comprehension in this disorder. Head (1926) defined semantic aphasia as an inability to recognize, simultaneously, the elements within a sentence. Luria (1966, 1976a,b) was more exact; he pro-posed that patients with semantic aphasia had comprehension problems in the following types of language constructs: (1) sentences that include a system of successive subordinate clauses, particularly forms that include the conjunction "which" or "that" or prepositions and conjunctions such as "despite"; (2) revers-ible combinations, particularly of the temporal and spatial type (e.g., "the circle underneath the square"); (3) phrases with a double negative (e.g., "I am not used to not obeying the norms"); (4) comparative sentences (e.g., "the dog is bigger than the bird"); (5) passive constructions (e.g., "the earth is illuminated by the sun"); (6) constructions with transitive verbs (e.g., "the boy slapped the girl"); (7) constructions with attributive relations (e.g., "the father's brother," "the brother's father"). It was Luria's contention that the comprehension impairment of seman-tic aphasia was not merely a problem in understanding words tinged with spatial meaning but that the disorder also included a defect in the comprehension of logical grammatical structures. Semantic aphasia as defined by Luria includes the primary characteristics of TCSA-II but incorporates a great deal of additional linguistic breakdown.

Patients with TCSA-II have difficulty integrating the elements of a sentence into a whole and fail to grasp the meaning of relationships. They almost always show some impairment in auditory comprehension and in naming; comprehen-sion of complex commands, particularly if they include elements of a spatial na-ture, is seriously impaired. Although conversational language may be adequate for social purposes in these patients, their lexicon is notably limited.

Damage involving the dominant angular gyrus has been associated with the Gerstmann syndrome by a number of investigators (Benson, 1979a; Gerstmann,

1931, 1940; Strub and Geschwind, 1974). Levine and Calvanio (1978) stressed the visuospatially oriented language disturbance of the Gerstmann syndrome components—right/left disorientation, finger agnosia, acalculia, and agraphia. A similar explanation, visuospatial language disturbance, has been proposed to explain semantic aphasia (Luria, 1966, 1976a). TCSA-II, semantic aphasia, and the Gerstmann syndrome usually coexist (Ardila, Lopez, and Solano, 1989) but may vary depending on the severity of the brain damage.

Based on clinical findings, Coslett and colleagues (1987) distinguished two types of transcortical sensory aphasia but made no attempt to relate the two with specific brain damage sites. Conversely, Kertesz and colleagues (Kertesz, Sheppard, and MacKenzie, 1982; Rubens and Kertesz, 1983) suggested two loci of damage for transcortical sensory aphasia (temporal-occipital and parietal-occipital) but did not outline well-defined clinical features to distinguish the two. Based on these observations, other studies in the literature, and our own clinical experience, it appears reasonably certain that left posterior parietal damage is associated with right-left disorientation, finger agnosia, agraphia, acalculia, anomia, and some degree of visuospatial language disturbance. If damage extends anteriorly toward the temporal lobe, the findings of alexia with agraphia and a broader, more profound comprehension disturbance will be observed. If damage involves both of these areas plus the anterior-lateral occipital lobe, a clinical picture of classic extrasylvian (transcortical) sensory aphasia occurs. Variations in the clinical expressions of cases of extrasylvian sensory aphasia, based on both the mix of language-behavior features and their severity, are readily demonstrated. The variations appear to have relatively specific neuroanatomical correlations even though the clinical picture is often mixed. The overall description presented in Table 9.4 remains appropriate but considerable variation based on lesion location can be anticipated.

Mixed Extrasylvian (Transcortical) Aphasia (MTCA)

Many pathological states that cause a significant decrease of cerebrovascular perfusion (hypoxia, anoxia, chronic hypoperfusion, carbon monoxide poisoning, acute carotid occlusion, acute hypotension [shock], cardiac arrest, and others) can produce ischemic infarction that mildly or robustly involves the cerebral border zone, the area between two major vascular territories (often termed the watershed area). If the infarction includes the border zone areas (i.e., between the middle cerebral artery territory and that of both the anterior cerebral and the posterior cerebral artery territories), a combined or mixed extrasylvian (transcortical) aphasia (MTCA) can occur. Several names have been suggested for the resulting syndrome. One, isolation of the speech area (Geschwind, Quadfasel, and Segarra,

1968; Goldstein, 1917, 1948), emphasizes the unique clinical picture. The second, mixed transcortical aphasia, recognizes the combination of the features of both the extrasylvian motor and the extrasylvian sensory aphasia syndromes (Benson, 1979a). Among the clinical characteristics of MTCA outlined in Table 9.5, the most dramatic is the preservation of an ability to repeat spoken language despite severe impairment of all other language functions. The mixed extrasylvian picture has all the characteristics of a global aphasia except for the preservation of the ability to repeat.

Although only a few well-demarcated and relatively pure cases of MTCA have been reported (Benson, 1979a; Bogousslavsky, Regli, and Assal, 1988; Geschwind, Quadfasel, and Segarra, 1968; Kertesz and McCabe, 1977; Whitaker, 1976), the syndrome awakens considerable interest. Patients with a mixed extrasylvian aphasia have little or no spontaneous language; their verbal output consists, almost entirely, of what has just been spoken by others (echolalia). The patient may, however, embellish the output, particularly showing elements of the completion phenomenon. Thus, when prompted with the beginning of a common phrase, the MTCA patient may repeat what has been said and then continue the

Table 9.5. Characteristics of Mixed Extrasylvian (Transcortical)
          Aphasia

Basic Language Characteristics	
Conversational language	Nonfluent with echolalia
Comprehension of spoken language	Severely defective
Repetition of spoken language	Relatively good
Pointing	Defective
Naming	Defective
Reading:	
Aloud	Defective
Comprehension	Defective
Writing	Defective
Associated Neurological Signs	
Motor system	Variable paresis, pathological reflexes common
Articulation	Normal
Cortical sensory function	Often disordered
Praxis	Difficult to test
Visual fields	Usually defective
Visual gnosis	Difficult to test

phrase to completion. The patient's articulation may be surprisingly clear and series speech is comparatively good once the task is started. If the series is initiated by the examiner, the MTCA patients can often continue counting, reciting the days or months, or reciting nursery rhymes or poems. If interrupted during the recitation, however, MTCA patients cannot continue. Their verbal output appears automatic, involuntary, and without understanding. Their recitations resemble those of someone reading aloud a passage written in a language that he does not comprehend.

Most reported cases of MTCA show severely limited comprehension competency and when some degree of comprehension can be demonstrated it is only transiently present. The ability to repeat spoken language, although dramatically preserved in these patients compared to other language features, remains limited and is often below normal. The length of a phrase repeated successfully is often limited to three or four words. These patients may or may not correct grammatically improper phrases when they repeat; they will repeat nonsense syllables and foreign words quite accurately up to a short span.

Patients with MTCA show a severe disturbance in confrontation naming, sometimes producing neologisms or semantic paraphasia but more often giving no response at all (Whitaker, 1976a). In one reported case, however, a subject with an aphasic syndrome otherwise clinically compatible with mixed transcortical aphasia could name many common objects (Heilman, Tucker, and Valenstein, 1976). In MTCA the ability to read out loud, the ability to comprehend written language and the ability to write are severely (usually totally) impaired. MTCA is a global aphasia, except for the preservation of the ability of the patient to repeat what the examiner has said.

The basic neurological findings in cases of MTCA can vary considerably. Some patients with MTCA show bilateral upper motor neuron paralysis, a severe spastic quadriparesis (Geschwind, Quadfasel, and Segarra, 1968), indicating bihemispheric damage. Other reported cases have had unilateral (right) hemiplegia and sensory loss. A visual-field defect, usually a right hemianopia, is present in some cases. Some individuals with MTCA, however, have few basic neurologic difficulties, showing only weakness that is most marked in the shoulder and hip musculature and variable degrees of cortical sensory loss. Most often, MTCA is found in patients with severe brain damage and a whole host of additional neurologic and neurobehavioral disorders are present. Because of the multiple sites of damage and the variety of associated neurological signs, the language syndrome of MTCA may be difficult to diagnose.

Most cases of MTCA reported in the literature have shown little tendency for recovery. Kertesz and McCabe (1977) reported two cases of "isolation syndrome" that improved only slightly, and Benson (1979a) mentioned three cases, all of whom improved only to a minimal degree. The number of reported cases is far too small, however, to allow a specific prognosis for recovery for any individual case.

Two thoroughly examined cases of MTCA (Geschwind, Quadfasel, and Segarra, 1968; Goldstein, 1948) have been considered classic. Both patients came to autopsy and had a brain lesion demonstrated neuropathologically. Both were cases of prolonged cerebral hypoxia based on suicide attempts with cooking gas. Extensive neuronal damage was present in the arterial border-zone area bilaterally, contrasting with a relative preservation of neurons in the perisylvian territory. Bogousslavsky, Regli, and Assal (1988) described four patients with impaired naming ability, semantic paraphasias, echolalia, impaired comprehension, and good repetition. Reading aloud and for comprehension were severely limited and the patients could not write spontaneously. Writing to dictation was preserved, however. These are the language findings of MTCA. All of the patients had left internal carotid artery occlusion producing ipsilateral anterior cerebral artery territory infarction plus infarction involving the cortical area at the junction of the middle and posterior cerebral artery territories; the latter lesions spared, but also isolated, the perisylvian language area.

With the advent of modern imaging techniques, neuroanatomical correlations can now be made in the living patient with MTCA. The older (now obsolete) radioisotope brain scans were particularly useful, demonstrating a characteristic crescent-shaped area of increased isotope uptake in the infarcted border-zone area (Kertesz, Lesk, and McCabe, 1977). Although far more difficult to interpret, the patterns of neural alterations indicative of border zone infarction can be seen on both CT and MRI (Damasio and Damasio, 1989).

Anomic Aphasia

An aphasia that features a defect in word finding that far exceeds any other language problem has been called amnestic aphasia (Broca, 1865), anomic aphasia (Benson, 1979a; Goodglass and Kaplan, 1972; Kertesz, 1979), amnesic aphasia (Goldstein, 1924; Weisenburg and McBride, 1935/1964), and nominal aphasia (Brain, 1961; Head, 1926). Among the fully or almost fully normal functions in patients with anomic aphasia is the ability to repeat spoken language; anomic aphasia, therefore, shows the defining characteristic of the extrasylvian aphasias. A variable characteristic in anomic aphasia is comprehension of spoken language. Comprehension is fully normal in many cases of anomic aphasia but in others some deficiencies will be noted. Based on the fluent output and excellent repetition but variable competency at comprehension of spoken language, Benson

Table 9.6. Characteristics of Anomic Aphasia

Basic Language Characteristics	
Conversational language	Fluent, empty
Comprehension of spoken language	Good to excellent
Repetition of spoken language	Good to excellent
Pointing to named object	Good to excellent
Naming	Defective
Reading:	
Aloud	Good to excellent
Comprehension	Good to excellent
Writing	Good to excellent
Associated Neurological Signs	
Motor system	Usually normal
Articulation	Normal
Cortical sensory function	Normal, or mild disorder
Praxis	Normal
Visual fields	Usually normal
Visual gnosis	Usually normal

(1979a) suggested that anomic aphasia and transcortical sensory aphasia represented a continuum, the crucial differentiating factor being the degree of ability to comprehend spoken language.

Although anomic aphasia is said by some investigators (Brown, 1972; Kertesz, 1985) to be the most common aphasia syndrome, it is well recognized that anomic aphasia cannot be reliably localized (Benson and Geschwind, 1971; Gloning, Gloning, and Hoff, 1963) and that damage in many different brain sites can cause significant word-finding difficulties (Kertesz, 1985). Although clinically defining characteristics can be listed (see Table 9.6), there is ample reason to doubt that anomic aphasia represents a true syndrome. Significant word-finding problems can occur following right-hemisphere damage and anomia represents a prominent diagnostic feature of several dementia syndromes. The ability to produce a name for a given stimulus (word finding) appears to be a consequence of the interaction of widely separated brain areas. Results of naming tests will vary dependent upon the sensory stimulus (visual, auditory, somesthetic, olfactory, gustatory) presented to the patients and their ability to form appropriate multimodal associations. Many different neuroanatomical sites and association networks apparently operate together to produce a name. Whether the language disorder known as anomic aphasia can be considered a separate entity is debatable. A reasonable clinical syndrome can be demonstrated in cases called anomic aphasia, but the marked variations in the locus of lesions producing the symptom cluster casts doubt about the reliability of anomic aphasia as a clinical entity and even stronger concern about the reality of anomic aphasia for psycholinguistic and neurolinguistic research. Chapter 14 will deal with the topic of naming in greater detail.

10

Subcortical Speech and Language Syndromes

· ·

The aphasic syndromes outlined in Chapters 8 and 9 have been discussed in the literature for over a century. Each syndrome represents a well-established clinical entity but, as every clinician realizes, many real-world aphasic disturbances cannot be clearly classified within one of the established symptom clusters. One long-standing explanation for nonclassic aphasia cases simply rejected language localization schemes (Schuell, Jenkins, and Jimenez-Pabon, 1964; Wepman and Jones, 1964); another recognized that brain pathology produces many disorders in addition to language impairment and attempted to explain variations in language disorder symptom complexes through the nonlanguage effects of the associated lesions (Brown, 1968).

At least since the days of Wernicke, investigators who are sophisticated in neuroanatomical localization have accepted that aphasia can represent the product of damage to neural networks made up of both cortical and subcortical structures; but only in recent years has it been realized that language impairment could result from noncortical pathology—an entirely subcortical aphasia. Technological advances, particularly the use of CT and MR imaging have permitted far better delineation of subcortical pathology than was previously available. The previously hypothesized effects of subcortical damage on language have been rethought, and aphasic syndromes resulting from subcortical damage alone have been proposed (Crosson, 1985; Wallesch, 1985).

When stereotactic surgery was used to treat patients with Parkinson's disease, portions of the basal ganglia or thalamus were purposefully destroyed. This produced changes in verbal output in some patients that led to increasingly sophisticated studies of both speech and language (Riklan and Cooper, 1975; Samra et al., 1969) but left doubt whether these brain structures played a role in language. The first reports of CT-demarcated cases of pure subcortical language disturbance involved patients with acute intracerebral hemorrhage (Alexander and LoVerme, 1980; Cappa and Vignolo, 1979). In later studies, focal infarctions that involved subcortical structures were demonstrated as a source of aphasia (Damasio et al., 1982; Graff-Radford et al., 1985; Naeser et al., 1982). Almost without exception, language problems following subcortical damage occurred only when certain left-hemisphere gray-matter structures (e.g., thalamus, striatum, claustrum) were involved. Most often the initial language problems included altered speech, often beginning with total mutism followed by hypophonic, slow, sparse output and poorly differentiated, amelodic articulation. At least superficially, these output qualities resembled the verbal output disorder that may accompany Parkinson's disease or the thalamotomy procedure used to treat the disorder in the 1950s and 1960s (Bell, 1968; Riklan and Levita, 1970). Language defects associated with purely subcortical damage tend to be less specific than those associated with cortical damage, but some features of subcortical aphasia (such as paraphasia-laden conversational speech contrasted with comparatively paraphasia-free repetition) appear to be unique.

Whether true aphasia results from isolated subcortical brain damage remains or unsettled question (Wallesch and Papagno, 1985). Some subcortical language findings are considered, by some investigators, to be a consequence of the mass effect caused by intracerebral hemorrhage and edema with a subsequent decrease in cortical blood perfusion (Luria, 1977; Skyhøj-Olsen, Bruhn, and Oberg, 1986). Language disorders accompanying lesions in these cases do not necessarily indicate that the involved subcortical structure has a specific language function. Symptoms characteristic of cortical damage distant from the site of subcortical involvement are common, suggesting that a secondary impairment of dominant-hemisphere language cortex exists; this interpretation is supported, at least in part, by isotopic brain-imaging studies (Metter et al., 1988; Skyhøj-Olsen, Bruhn, and Oberg, 1986). Whether the language syndromes caused by subcortical pathology represent hypoperfusion produced by the mass lesion effect or whether they represent a deactivation based on subcortical-cortical disconnection or reflect actual damage to subcortical structures involved in language function remains unsettled. Only certain loci of subcortical pathology are associated with language dysfunction; as such, they deserve consideration, either as evidence of independent subcortical functions essential for language or as the site of subcortical areas that are frequently damaged by lesions that produce the cortical aphasic syndromes.

One problem in the current aphasia literature that hampers the discussion of subcortical aphasia stems from use of the terms *deep* and *subcortical*. In contemporary linguistic literature, *deep* and *surface* have been used to differentiate the characteristics of language formulation, a connotation that has no structural correlation. Outside the linguistic literature, the term *deep* often tends to be interpreted anatomically; language impairments described as deep thus carry the implication of subcortical pathology. *Deep* is also open to neuroanatomical misinterpretation, however, particularly with respect to the role of the insula in language. The insula is located at the core of the perisylvian language area, and a role for this structure in language function has long been under consideration (Wernicke, 1874). The exact role of the insula in language, if any, remains clouded, however (Ardila, Benson, and Flynn, unpublished data). Although located deep within the brain, the insula is not subcortical. It is true cortex and its location can be correctly described as both deep and cortical.

Modern neuroimaging techniques allow relatively precise localization of the subcortical lesions associated with speech and language disorders. Two neuroanatomical areas are most frequently discussed—the striato-capsular region and the thalamus (Alexander and LoVerme, 1980; Alexander, Naeser, and Palumbo, 1987; Alexander and Benson, 1991; Brown, 1975b; Cappa et al., 1983; Crosson, 1985; Damasio et al., 1982; Naeser et al., 1982; Tanridag and Kirshner, 1985; Wallesch et al., 1983). Several relatively characteristic language features occur following subcortical brain damage. In keeping with the clinical style of the present volume, however, the features will be discussed as symptom clusters, not as general clinical-anatomical correlates. Table 10.1 outlines the major syndromes to be discussed.

The Aphasia of Marie's Quadrilateral Space

Interest in the language disorders resulting from subcortical damage was spurred when Marie (1906a,b,c) challenged the traditional discussions of aphasia. Marie

Table 10.1. Aphasia with Subcortical
Involvement

Aphasia of Marie's quadrilateral space
Striato-capsular aphasia
Thalamic aphasia
Aphasia associated with white-matter disease

described subcortical lesions that affected speech and possibly language and, with his student Moutier (1908), demonstrated that a specific subcortical region they called the quadrilateral space was critical to verbal motor output. The disorder they described is a reality (Souques, 1928), but whether damage to the quadrilateral space produces aphasia remains a source of argument. Marie contended that the aphasia described by Broca was not a true aphasia. He proposed, rather, that individuals with the Broca aphasia syndrome had pathology involving an area deep to the insula (including the external capsule, claustrum, and variable amounts of insula and putamen), subsequently known as Marie's quadrilateral space (see Figure 10.1). Damage to this area produced a severe breakdown of verbal output (speech disorder) that they called *anarthria*. Marie and Moutier proposed that the only true aphasia was Wernicke's aphasia and that pathology in the quadrilateral space did not, by itself, alter language function. They contended that if a patient with the Broca aphasia syndrome was found to be aphasic, as demonstrated by language comprehension problems, the pathology must have extended sufficiently posterior to involve Wernicke's area or connections between this region and the thalamus. Marie's suggestion, although diametrically opposed to prevailing views, was plausible; heated debate followed. Only since the demon-

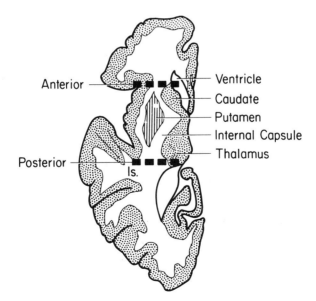

Figure 10.1. Artist's rendition of Marie's quadrilateral space indicating the subcortical tissues (between the two heavy barred lines) where Marie and others postulated that a lesion would produce anarthria but not aphasia. (From Benson, 1979a).

stration of linguistically unique comprehension and expression problems based on disordered syntactical language in patients with Broca's aphasia has Marie's contention been discredited (Alexander, Benson, and Stuss, 1989; Caramazza, Berndt, and Basilli, 1986; Samuels and Benson, 1979; Zurif, Caramazza, and Myerson, 1972). Marie's postulate of a single aphasia was of considerable influence in the genesis of aphasiology. Basic to this postulate, his contention that a destructive lesion restricted to the quadrilateral space produced anarthria but did not produce a language dysfunction remains debatable.

Although he introduced the term *anarthria*, Marie did not characterize the verbal-output impairment produced by isolated damage to the quadrilateral space. Many aphasic patients with pathology involving the quadrilateral space show speech and/or language characteristics unlike either Broca or Wernicke aphasia. Damage limited to the quadrilateral space (almost always based on hemorrhage) produces an acute mutism with a dense hemiplegia (Schiff et al., 1983). With recovery, these patients show a sparse, soft (hypophonic), poorly articulated verbal output. They may or may not show agrammatism, paraphasia, disordered comprehension, poor repetition, anomia, alexia, agraphia, or apraxia. These findings are probably dependent on whether neighboring structures are involved. Recovery, often slow, depends on the course of the basic disease process and the extent of structural damage. Even following good recovery from the basic pathology, the final verbal output attained by these patients is often unsatisfactory, with some combination of speech, language, and motor impairments remaining. Lesions in the quadrilateral space do produce serious verbal-output problems, but whether these deserve categorization as aphasia appears dependent on the involvement of neighboring structures.

Striato-Capsular Aphasia

Patients with lesions involving the striato-capsular region show obvious articulatory defects. Whether language impairment can occur if the striato-capsular lesion extends into the paraventricular white matter remains controversial.

After the introduction of CT imaging, many cases of acute basal ganglia damage associated with verbal-output disorders were reported (Alexander, Naeser, and Palumbo, 1987; Damasio et al., 1982; Hier et al., 1977; Naeser et al., 1982; Puel et al., 1986) and the verbal disturbances were catalogued. In general, patients with striato-capsular language disorders show fluent but hesitant output, good comprehension, and good repetition (Basso, Della Salla, and Farabola, 1987; Cappa et al., 1983; Damasio et al., 1982; Naeser et al., 1982). Their language output appears fluent and although routinely truncated, it is not overtly agrammatic; speech mechanics are generally impaired, with the defects in articulation and prosody resembling those observed in Broca aphasia and in recovering aphemia. In patients with striato-capsular aphasia, comprehension is sufficiently intact for casual conversation but breaks down when complex syntax or multistep, serial items are presented. Word-finding problems are often present and semantic paraphasia may be noted (Alexander and Benson, 1991; Damasio et al., 1982). Writing competency is variable but may be relatively spared.

Other behavioral disorders associated with striato-capsular aphasia tend to vary considerably. Hemiparesis and hemisensory loss are commonly present in these patients but are not mandatory. Buccofacial (oral) apraxia is frequently observed but ideomotor apraxia of the limbs tends to be absent or mild. If the lesion extends sufficiently posterior to involve deep parietal white matter, however, substantial limb apraxia may be found (Alexander, Naeser, and Palumbo, 1987; Basso, Della Salla, and Farabola, 1987).

Most of the reported deficits in verbal output in patients with striato-capsular aphasia are not distinctly linguistic. In addition to their prominent motor speech problems, most other abnormalities observed in these patients can be classed as cognitive defects. Similar cognitive problems have been recorded in patients with vascular (Fisher, 1978) or degenerative disorders of the striatum (Huber, Shuttleworth, and Freidenberg, 1989) or with dorsolateral frontal injury without evident aphasia (Nadeau, 1988).

Whether damage to basal ganglia structures or to surrounding white-matter pathways is the source of subcortical verbal-output disorder remains unsettled (Damasio et al., 1982) but most observers agree that lesions deep in the left hemisphere produce more verbal-output problems than do similarly located lesions in the right hemisphere (Wallesch et al., 1983). Some investigators hypothesize that damage to the descending dominant-hemisphere cortical-bulbar pathways underlies the disturbed speech fluency (Schiff et al., 1983). Inasmuch as the verbal output of patients with striato-capsular damage resembles the hypophonic verbal output of patients with Parkinson's disease, involvement of striatal circuitry is often implicated. Some of the other language defects seen in patients with striato-capsular aphasia (with the exception of agraphia) are traditionally attributed to damage to connections between dorsolateral frontal cortex and striatum, to damage of the striatum itself (Alexander and Benson, 1991), or to posterior extension of damage to include the temporal isthmus (Alexander, Naeser, and Palumbo, 1987). Many attempts have been made to correlate basal ganglia pathology with speech and language defects (Cappa et al., 1983; Damasio et al., 1982; Graff-Radford et al., 1985; Puel et al., 1986; Wallesch et al., 1983). As an example, Alexander and colleagues (1987) proposed six types of verbal output impairment, dependent upon the specific neuroanatomical locus of striato-capsular damage:

Type 1. Lesions limited to the putamen and head of the caudate nucleus either produce no language disturbance or only mild word-finding difficulties; if the putamen is extensively involved, hypophonia is observed. Lesions restricted to the putamen and the head of the caudate nucleus produce dysarthria but no aphasia.

Type 2. Involvement limited to the anterior limb of the internal capsule produces neither speech nor language disturbance. Similarly, lesions restricted to the paraventricular white matter produce no language or speech disturbance except for a mild alteration of prosody.

Type 3. Involvement of the anterior superior paraventricular white matter causes reduced verbal output but no overt language abnormalities; the reduction in language production is conjectured to indicate partial disconnection of the supplementary motor area from Broca's area. Extensive damage of paraventricular and periventricular white-matter structures produces a persistent nonfluent aphasia with agrammatism, presumably based on undercutting of many deep frontal pathways (limbic, association, callosal, and efferent) (Alexander, Benson, and Stuss, 1989). Generally speaking, the degree of extension of the lesion into both middle and anterior paraventricular white-matter regions determines the severity and permanency of nonfluency (Alexander and Benson, 1991). Extensive anterior extension obviates verbal production (except for stereotypies), whereas a smaller lesion will allow some recovery of single words and short phrases; lacunes in the nearby descending bulbar motor pathways may produce some dysarthria.

Type 4. Discrete injury involving the striatum, postero-medial anterior limb of the internal capsule and the anterior-superior paraventricular white matter is the smallest striato-capsular lesion capable of producing language abnormality (e.g., word-finding difficulties, occasional phonemic paraphasias and mild disturbances in comprehension) in addition to a marked dysarthria.

Type 5. Lesions of the putamen which extend posteriorly across the temporal isthmus cause a fluent aphasia with neologistic verbal output and impaired comprehension. Impaired comprehension of single words, simple sentences, and/or commands may be observed in these cases.

Type 6. When damage is primarily lateral to the putamen (insular cortex, external capsule, claustrum, and extreme capsule), the resultant language disturbance is characterized by phonemic paraphasias that increase during the patient's attempts to repeat (thus resembling conduction aphasia). The occurrence of phonemic paraphasias following striato-capsular damage is dependent on lateral extension of the lesion into the white matter of the parietal lobe deep to the fissure of Rolando or the extreme capsule.

The observations by Alexander and colleagues demonstrate that considerable variation in speech and language impairment can follow striato-capsular (subcortical) pathology. Some of the resulting disorders resemble nonfluent, agrammatic aphasia while others produce a fluent paraphasic output. Pure striato-capsular damage most often produces only hypophonia and dysprosody along with variable degrees of cognitive slowness and impairment. Slowness of mental processing, forgetfulness, apathy, and dilapidated cognitive functions of the type noted with striato-capsular damage are the characteristic clinical disturbances described in subcortical dementia (Albert, Feldman, and Willis, 1974; Benson, 1983; McHugh and Folstein, 1975).

Language impairment (aphasia) based entirely on subcortical disturbance requires extensive damage to the striatum, to the posterior medial portion of the anterior limb of the anterior capsule, and to anterior superior periventricular white matter. Such extensive damage presumably undercuts many cortical-cortical pathways that participate in language processing. The types of striato-capsular aphasia proposed by Alexander and colleagues (1987) are most often accompanied by cortical extensions; the resulting symptom clusters can be defined more accurately as cortical-subcortical aphasia. For instance, the clinical features of Type 3 (involvement of the anterior superior periventricular white matter) resemble those of transcortical (extrasylvian) motor aphasia syndrome (Types I and II) with subcortical extension. Type 5 (damage to the putamen with posterior extension across the temporal isthmus) appears to be a fluent Wernicke-type aphasia with subcortical extension. Type 6 (damage to the insular cortex, external capsule, claustrum, and extreme capsule) produces the symptom cluster of conduction aphasia. Type 1 (lesions limited to the putamen and the head of the caudate nucleus) produces a pure dysarthria of the type often associated with Broca aphasia. Finally, Type 2 (limited involvement of the anterior limb of the internal capsule) produces a speech disorder that resembles aphemia based on inferior frontal gyrus damage (Schiff et al., 1983).

In summary, in addition to the evident speech impairments, true language disorders can be observed in patients with striato-capsular damage; however, extension that involves the cortex is usually present in these cases. Extensive subcortical damage is required to produce a pure (noncortical) striato-capsular aphasia.

Thalamic Aphasia

The role, if any, played by the dominant-hemisphere thalamus in language and aphasia has been debated for many years. At one time, an entire mechanism of aphasia, primarily based on pathology involving the thalamic pulvinar, was proposed. In this proposal, variations in the language symptom clusters implied involvement of neighboring sensory and/or motor regions (Brown, 1968), with the thalamus assumed to play a crucial role in language formulation. Scattered reports documenting thalamic involvement in individuals with distinct language disturbance supported the postulation that the thalamus played a significant role in language function (Ciemins, 1970; Samarel et al., 1976; Van Buren, 1975; Van Buren and Burke, 1969). Other reports, however, demonstrated that the thalamus could be damaged without production of aphasia. For instance, follow-up studies of the thousands of patients who underwent thalamic destruction for treatment of Parkinson's disease failed to demonstrate any consistent alteration of language (Brown, 1974; Riklan and Levita, 1970; Van Buren, 1975). Although aphasia following pure thalamic destruction has been considered rare (Crosson et al., 1986), the impossibility of proving a negative and the occasional report of some verbal output disturbance following a thalamic destruction procedure used to treat Parkinson's disease kept the controversy alive (Bell, 1968; Riklan and Cooper, 1975).

With the introduction of CT, several cases of thalamic hemorrhage with language disorder were reported (Alexander and LoVerme, 1980; Cappa and Vignolo, 1979; McFarling et al., 1982; Mohr, 1983). Not only was hemorrhage demonstrated; infarctions of the thalamus could also be associated with aphasia. Most reported cases of thalamic aphasia have been based on CT or MRI findings of focal pathology (Bogousslavsky, Regli, and Uske, 1988; Gorelick et al., 1984; Graff-Radford et al., 1985). There are few neuropathological confirmations but Crosson and colleagues (1986) have reported cases in which aphasia followed an ischemic thalamic infarct demonstrated by CT and later confirmed by neuropathological study.

Hemorrhage, the most common thalamic pathology associated with aphasia, usually produces an acute, catastrophic clinical picture with hemiplegia, hemisensory loss, right visual-field defect and alteration of the level of consciousness, often to the state of coma. The initial language abnormality is mutism (or near mutism) which typically improves to a verbose, paraphasic, but hypophonic jargon output. Anomia is often severe, almost to the point of a total failure to name on confrontation. Although thalamic aphasia resembles other fluent paraphasic aphasias with serious anomia, patients with thalamic aphasia show relatively good comprehension and their verbal output when they attempt to repeat is far better than their conversational speech. Paraphasia disappears, or decreases dramatically, during repetition. The verbal output of the case reported by Crosson and colleagues (1986) showed only relatively mild anomia and paraphasia when the patient discussed familiar topics but deteriorated to a jargon output when discussing unfamiliar material. Mohr, Watters, and Duncan (1975) interpreted similar fluctuations in the patient's verbal output as alterations of alertness. Reading and writing are usually disturbed to a significant degree in thalamic aphasia patients, although not to the degree of severity seen when cortical damage produces fluent aphasia plus alexia and agraphia.

The language disorders that follow thalamic hemorrhage tend to be transient (Benson, 1979a; Crosson, 1985). Recovery usually begins within days or weeks after the cerebrovascular accident and, except in cases complicated by widespread damage, the course is usually one of consistent language improvement over a period of a few weeks or months. Recovery from paresis in these cases tends to be even more rapid but some degree of hemisensory abnormality almost always remains. Clinically, the combination of logorrheic, paraphasic output, comparatively good comprehension, and unexpectedly good repetition suggests posterior subcortical (thalamic) aphasia.

Although the prognosis for an aphasia due to thalamic hemorrhage is generally good, the same is not true for the underlying brain pathology. Thalamic hemorrhage produces a serious brain disorder; many patients never recover sufficiently to allow aphasia evaluation. The mortality rate in cases of thalamic hemorrhage remains high, and many patients who survive left thalamic hemorrhage have severe residual cognitive deficits including language dysfunction. Because of the poor prognosis of the disorder, study of the clinical course remains clouded and the role of the left thalamus in language remains controversial.

Thalamic aphasia does not produce the pattern of any cortical aphasic syndrome (Alexander and LoVerme, 1980) and a unique aphasia syndrome based on thalamic damage can be postulated: (1) reduction in spontaneous verbal output, (2) word-finding difficulties, (3) verbal paraphasias, (4) preserved repetition competency, (5) defective comprehension (Basso, Della Sala, and Farabola, 1987; Cappa and Vignolo, 1979). A similarity to transcortical (extrasylvian) sensory aphasia has been noted. Support for a distinct thalamic aphasia syndrome stems from several sources, the most robust being direct clinical-pathological observations of thalamic damage associated with aphasia; additional support comes from demonstration of aphasic elements (paraphasia and anomia) following electrical stimulation of the left thalamus (Fedio and Van Buren, 1975; Ojemann, 1975, 1976; Ojemann and Ward, 1971).

Other investigators, however, have found no evidence of aphasia despite severe thalamic damage and note that even when aphasia is present, it is often not permanent (Cappa et al., 1986; Mohr, 1983; Wallesch et al., 1983). It has been postulated that the aphasia that follows thalamic hemorrhage is a variant of transcortical (extrasylvian) sensory aphasia based on ischemia in the posterior cortical border zone (watershed) vascular territory secondary to acutely increased intracranial pressure (Benson, 1979a). Another proposal considers the language disturbance that follows thalamic damage to be based on cortical deactivation secondary to thalamo-cortical disconnection. With cerebral blood flow studies, thalamic damage has been shown to produce cortical hypometabolism when there is no demonstrable structural damage (Metter et al., 1981, 1984, 1988). Functional disturbance based on reduced blood flow and/or metabolism in cortical areas which appear undamaged on CT or MR images may be responsible for language symptoms in cases of thalamic damage.

Alexander and Benson (1991) categorized the language disorder syndromes that can be noted following thalamic damage into three types—medial, anterior, and lateral. Data concerning a fourth type—posterior—were too uncertain to warrant inclusion.

1. Lesions in the left paramedial thalamic area, involving dorsomedial and centromedianum nuclei plus the medial intramedullary lamina, produce deficits in attention and memory (Bogousslavsky, Regli, and Uske, 1988; Graff-Radford et al., 1985; Motomura, Yamadori, and Mitani, 1986). Accompanying language deficits are restricted to anomia and language-related impairments attributable to inattention. Neurological examination can be normal in these cases but paramedian mesencephalic damage may be associated with oculomotor abnormalities.

2. Lesions in the left anterolateral thalamus produce more-distinctive language impairments (Alexander, Hiltbrunner, and Fischer, 1989; Gorelick et al., 1984; McFarling, Rothi, and Heilman, 1982). When damage involves the anterior, ventral-anterior, dorsolateral, ventrolateral, and anterior dorsomedial nuclei and/or the anterior medial intramedullary region, the language impairment profile resembles the extrasylvian sensory or mixed extrasylvian aphasia syndromes. Language output in anterior thalamic aphasia is grammatically correct but terse, with a tendency for echolalia; repetition is good but comprehension is impaired. Alexia, agraphia, and anomia are usually severe. Neurological examination is normal, with the exception of right hypokinesia, decreased mimetic facial activity, and hypophonia.

3. Lesions involving the left lateral thalamus without penetration to deeper thalamic structures can be associated with language disorder, but often only a mild anomia is observed. If there is extension of the lateral thalamic lesion to involve the globus pallidus, the posterior limb of the internal capsule, and/or the reticular thalamic nucleus, a more significant aphasia, resembling that following anterolateral thalamic damage, can occur; hemiparesis, hemisensory loss, and/or visual-field deficits may result. In addition, lesions in the lateral thalamus invariably damage pathways to or from the thalamus and can be associated with distant cortical hypofunction.

Based on current clinical evidence, it is reasonable to believe that damage to the left thalamus could produce aphasia and that a left thalamic aphasia syndrome or syndromes could be anticipated. Supporting evidence for a purely thalamic source for aphasia is weak, however, and remains under scrutiny. What is firmly established is that left thalamic damage from hemorrhage or ischemia is often associated with language abnormality, sometimes with distinctive features, and deserves recognition.

Aphasia Associated with White-Matter Disease

One reason aphasia was long considered a strictly cortical abnormality by so many neurologists was the virtual absence of aphasia in CNS disorders featuring significant white-matter destruction. The most striking example is multiple sclerosis (MS), a relatively common neurologic disorder in which demyelination destroys white-matter tracts but rarely involves cortex (Kurtzke, 1970). Although aphasia has been reported in sporadic cases of MS, it is notably uncommon.

Olmos-Lau, Ginsberg, and Geller (1977) reported a case of motor aphasia in a young woman with a clinical diagnosis of MS; her aphasia was characterized by reduced spontaneous speech, word-finding difficulties, and marked oral facial apraxia; written language and auditory comprehension were intact. These language symptoms did not correspond to any of the then-accepted aphasia syndromes but did resemble the findings in the disorder now called subcortical dementia (Cummings and Benson, 1984). Two large studies (Heaton et al., 1985; Jambor, 1969) concluded that MS patients perform many language tests at slightly, but not significantly, lower levels than normal control subjects; word fluency, naming, and reading competency are reduced, but auditory comprehension is unimpaired (Rao, 1986). Again, the pattern described corresponds to the clinical picture of subcortical dementia, a total symptom cluster that includes some findings present in the traditional aphasia syndromes.

Estimates of the frequency of aphasia in MS range narrowly, from absolute zero to very rare (Heaton et al., 1985). In contrast, speech disturbances are common in MS, although not universal (Farmikides and Boone, 1960). A study of speech quality in over one hundred patients with a clinical diagnosis of MS studied at the Mayo Clinic showed that fewer than 50% had clinically significant speech disturbance (Darley, Aronson, and Brown, 1975). Four speech abnormalities predominated in the Mayo series: (1) nasal voice, (2) weak phonation, (3) variability of pitch, (4) slow rate of output. The scanning speech emphasized by Charcot (1877) and widely accepted as a diagnostic characteristic of MS is decidedly uncommon, occurring only in the late stages of the disorder in selected patients.

The true language disorders observed in MS tend to have one of two clinical pictures. One rare syndrome features an acute onset with prominent motor language disturbance and right hemiplegia; the disorder is usually transient and resembles an acute vascular accident until later exacerbations point to the correct diagnosis (Adams and Victor, 1989). In a second variant, an apparent anomia appears in the course of a progressive dementia that includes a prominent amnesia. In the former case and most of the latter cases, a severe speech abnormality obscures the presence (or absence) of aphasia.

In the rare cases of MS with an acute onset of aphasia along with the right hemiplegia, involvement of cortical structures in the inflammatory reaction surrounding the MS plaque can be conjectured. In the more chronic variation, the dementing process is usually advanced and the degree of language disability mirrors the degree of mental impairment. Thus, not only is aphasia rare in MS, but it appears doubtful that it ever occurs on the basis of pure white-matter pathology.

Another subcortical white-matter disorder, progressive multifocal leukoencephalopathy (PML), has been reported to cause aphasia. Buchwald (1978) described one patient with PML who complained of only two symptoms—headache and severe anomia. The anomia was manifested by emptiness in conversational speech, confrontation naming failures and occasional verbal paraphasic substitutions. Repetition and comprehension were only mildly abnormal. The course was one of rapid deterioration; the patient sank into stupor and died. Postmortem examination suggested that the original lesion, the one thought to have produced the anomia, involved the white matter deep in the posterior aspects of the left temporal lobe. PML is now considered a viral encephalopathy occurring primarily in individuals with an immunodeficiency disorder that affects deep white matter. PML rarely presents with a primary language disorder.

It is evident that when aphasia is associated with white-matter pathology, extensive damage is present and most often involves the left hemisphere paraventricular and periventricular pathways (Alexander, Naeser, and Palumbo, 1987). Aphasia is rarely present when pathology affects white matter only. When a distinct aphasia disorder is present in pure white-matter disease, the onset of the pathology is usually acute and the area of surrounding tissue involvement is extensive; it can be suspected that the aphasia in such cases can be attributed to secondary cortical involvement.

Summary

Aphasia, defined as an acquired impairment of language based on brain damage, does occur with subcortical brain pathology, particularly when it involves both subcortical nuclei and adjacent white-matter pathways in the left hemisphere. In most instances of subcortical pathology, the language disorder is mild in comparison to motor speech problems and/or cognitive dysfunction. A characteristic symptom cluster and course (initial mutism developing into a hypophonic, hesitant, paraphasic output that improves considerably with repetition) is sufficient to warrant a diagnosis of subcortical aphasia. The transient nature of the disorder, with complete recovery in most cases, poses a serious question as to whether the subcortical damage itself causes the language impairment. Subcortical aphasia is both real as a clinical syndrome and a paradox since subcortical pathology does not permanently impair language function.

11

Alexia

· ·

Alexia refers to an acquired disturbance in reading, adequately defined as loss or impairment of the ability to comprehend written or printed language caused by brain damage.

One key consideration in defining alexia concerns the concept of loss. As defined above, alexia is limited to situations in which the ability to read was present and then was lost after brain damage; it is an acquired illiteracy. Many contemporary aphasiologists use the term *alexia* to designate all acquired reading impairments, but others reserve it for a total loss of reading ability, applying *dyslexia* to the more common condition of partially impaired reading comprehension. While this distinction is rational, it is a source of confusion as *dyslexia* is used by many investigators (pediatricians, psychologists, educators) to designate a form of abnormal language development, an inherent inability to acquire reading skills (Critchley, 1985). Dyslexia was formally defined in 1968 by a committee of the World Federation of Neurology as "a disorder manifested by difficulty in learning to read despite conventional instruction, adequate intelligence, and sociocultural opportunity. It is dependent on fundamental cognitive disabilities which are frequently of constitutional origin." Thus defined, dyslexia is very different from alexia, and the difference goes far beyond a mere matter of derivations from the Greek. Both the clinical phenomenology and the linguistic impairments that characterize the two disorders are totally different (Duffy and Geschwind, 1985). Many contemporary investigators attempt to side-step the problem by using the terms "developmental dyslexia" and "acquired dyslexia". In the present volume the established custom of referring to all acquired reading impairments as alexia will be retained.

Another crucial distinction inherent in the definition of alexia is the significant variable—the subject's ability to comprehend written material. The ability to read out loud represents a separate function. Thus, a subject's inability to read out loud even though he can comprehend written language is not to be called alexia. On the other hand, when a person can read out loud accurately but cannot comprehend the material, the term alexia is correct.

Several other terms often used in discussion of alexia deserve mention. *Literal alexia* refers to a comparative inability to read (name) individual letters of the alphabet; in the older terminology this problem was termed *letter-blindness*. *Verbal alexia* refers to an inability to read words (aloud and for comprehension), despite comparative retention of letter recognition, and has been called *word-blindness*. *Hemialexia* indicates an inability to attend to (and therefore comprehend) one-half of a word or line of printed language. *Paralexia* designates a substitution in written language while reading aloud that is comparable to paraphasia in freely spoken language.

Historical Background

Alexia has been recognized for millennia but only in the twentieth century did literacy become sufficiently widespread that alexia represented a significant medical problem. Reports of alexia precede the time of Christ and many cases were recorded before Broca (Benton, 1964). Invariably, however, the reading disturbance was included as part of a more widespread physical and language disorder. Even the surging interest in aphasia during the late nineteenth century stimulated only limited interest in alexia.

A major impetus to the understanding of alexia stemmed from two case reports published by Dejerine in 1891 and 1892. In the 1891 paper Dejerine described a patient who had suffered a cerebrovascular accident that produced mild right-sided weakness, some degree of right-sided visual-field defect, and mild difficulty in naming and spoken language comprehension, but a complete loss of the ability to read. The patient could write nothing but his signature. Over time, the paresis and the aphasia cleared but the alexia and agraphia remained basically unchanged until his death several years later. Postmortem examination of the brain demonstrated an old, scarred infarct in the left parietal lobe involving three-quarters of the angular gyrus cortex and extending deep to the lateral ventricle. Destruction of most of the dominant angular gyrus had produced an acquired illiteracy.

One year later Dejerine (1892) reported a patient who awoke to note an inability to read but no other language disturbance. The only basic neurologic finding of significance was a right hemianopia. A left posterior cerebral artery terri-

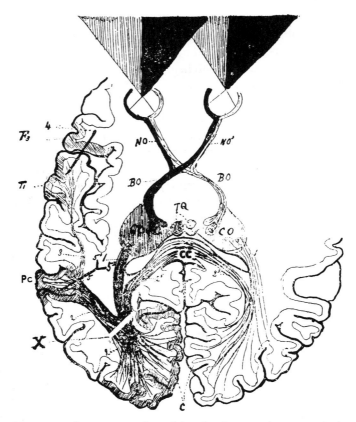

Figure II.I. Diagrammatic representation of the visual processing network showing lesions (brain damage) at both *cc* and *x* producing an occipital alexia (alexia without agraphia). (From Dejerine, 1892; reprinted in Geschwind, 1962).

tory infarction was presumed. Unlike the case described in 1891, this patient, while unable to read except for a few individual letters, could write adequately. Although he was not able to comprehend written language symbols, he had no difficulty producing copies of them. Four years later a second cerebrovascular accident led to death. Postmortem examination revealed two different infarcts. One was a large softening that involved the left angular gyrus and was obviously of recent origin; the other was an old gliotic infarct that involved the medial and inferior aspects of the left occipital lobe and the splenium of the corpus callosum. The recent infarct had led to the patient's demise but the old infarct was the source of the alexia without agraphia. Dejerine conjectured that the visual pathways leading to the visual cortex of the dominant-hemisphere occipital area had been destroyed in this patient, causing the right visual-field defect. The callosal lesion had separated the intact right-hemisphere visual area from the equally intact left-hemisphere language area (see Figure 11.1). Thus, the patient had suffered no language defect (even writing skills) but was unable to comprehend written language symbols that he was able to visualize sufficiently to copy.

Dejerine's papers excited many investigators and in the next decade a number of case reports were published supporting the clinical and neuropathological pattern of alexia he had described (Bastian, 1898; Hinshelwood, 1900; Wylie, 1894). In that period two distinct alexia syndromes were recognized—*alexia with agraphia* (a syndrome based on dominant-parietal-lobe damage), and *alexia without agraphia* (a syndrome in which pathology damaged the dominant occipital lobe and the splenium of the corpus callosum). Many patients with significant reading comprehension disorders, however, did not appear to have pathology involving either of these sites. A third, clinically distinct alexia syndrome—*frontal alexia* (associated with pathology in the frontal language areas)—was established (Benson, 1977; Dejerine and Mirallie, 1895; Henderson, 1984), and a number of other variations of alexia have been proposed in recent years (see Table 11.1).

The following discussion will focus on the first three syndromes of acquired reading impairment. Over the years many different terms have been used to delineate these variations of reading disorder. In this chapter the three major alexia

Table 11.1. Classification of Alexia

Parietal-temporal alexia (central alexia)

Occipital alexia (posterior alexia)

Frontal alexia (anterior alexia)

Other reading disorders
  Spatial alexia
  Hemispatial alexia
  Aphasic alexia
  Hemialexia

Linguistic models of alexia
  Central Alexias
    Phonological alexia
    Surface alexia
    Deep alexia
  Peripheral alexias
    Letter-by-letter reading
    Neglect alexia
    Attentional alexia

syndromes will be categorized according to the general location of brain pathology—parietal-temporal, occipital, frontal—but we recognize that many other terms are currently used (see Table 11.2).

Testing for Alexia

Reading ability is usually assessed at the time oral language ability is tested; certain tasks should be included routinely. Table 11.3 lists an extensive number of tests of reading abilities for use in selected cases of alexia and for discussion here. In most patients, however, abbreviated testing will be sufficient. Reading aloud and reading comprehension should always be tested separately and writing ability may be tested at the same time as reading.

Recognition of individual letters is frequently the initial task to be assessed. Reading letters, syllables, words, and sentences aloud represents progressively more complex levels of reading competency. Different types of written material can be presented (e.g., uppercase, lowercase, and cursive letters) and words of different levels of familiarity for the patient should be used. Reading of highly logographic, almost automatically comprehended words (such as the patient's

Table II.2. Nomenclature—The Three Alexias

PARIETAL-TEMPORAL ALEXIA	OCCIPITAL ALEXIA	FRONTAL ALEXIA
Alexia with agraphia	Alexia without agraphia	
Aphasic alexia	Agnosic alexia	
Central alexia	Posterior alexia	Anterior alexia
Semantic alexia	Associative alexia	Syntactic alexia
Subangular alexia	Splenio-occipital alexia	
Angular alexia	Postangular alexia	Preangular alexia
Total (literal plus verbal) alexia	Verbal alexia	Literal alexia
Cortical alexia	Optic alexia	
Letter-blindness and word-blindness	Word-blindness	Letter-blindness
Surface alexia	Visual alexia	
Acquired illiteracy	Pure alexia	Third alexia

Adapted from Benson, 1985a.

Table II.3. Assessment of Reading

Reading aloud and recognition (identification) of:
  letters
  syllables
  words
  logotomes
  sentences
  paragraph reading

Logographic (symbol) reading

Ability to match different types of writing (e.g., script, block letters)

Reading comprehension
  matching written words with objects
  carrying out written commands
  paragraph comprehension

Spelling
  spelling of words out loud
  comprehension of orally spelled words

Comprehension (reading) of other symbolic systems
  traffic signals
  musical notation
  chemical symbols

---

name, the name of his country, etc.) may be preserved in an otherwise totally alexic patient. The patient's ability to match words written in different forms (e.g., script or block letters) can be informative; patients with parietal-temporal alexia find it almost impossible to perform this task.

Words with different frequency of use should be offered: it is desirable to include logotomes (zero frequency), low-frequency, and high-frequency words. The patient's ability to read concrete and highly imageable words versus abstract and poorly imageable words should be compared. In different alexia types the subject's ability to read different phrase elements (e.g., nouns, verbs, adjectives, and grammatical connectors) may be individually disordered; these elements should be assessed separately.

Reading comprehension is tested by noting the patient's ability to match words with objects or to follow written commands. More complex levels of difficulty can be sampled by the silent reading of paragraphs following which the patient is asked to answer specific questions or to report on what he has just read.

The ability to spell aloud and to recognize spelled words can be difficult for patients with brain pathology and the disorder can be correlated with some specific types of alexia (see below). In bilingual (and polyglot) patients, reading should be tested in both (or several) languages, as their reading ability in the different languages may be dissociated (Luria, 1964a).

The ability to read in other symbolic systems (e.g., musical notation, traffic signals, chemical symbols, computer language) is rarely tested but may be indicated in individual cases. Recognition of ideographic logotypes (e.g., "Coca-Cola") represents an additional written language comprehension task that may be lost (or preserved) in brain-damaged patients.

The testing techniques presented in Table 11.3 can distinguish a number of varieties of alexia. Based on the clinical differences, distinct syndromes of alexia can be outlined.

Three Major Syndromes of Alexia

Parietal-Temporal Alexia

The original alexia syndrome reported by Dejerine (1891), most often called *alexia with agraphia,* has been described many times in the literature. Other terms used for this symptom cluster include parietal-temporal alexia, central alexia, angular alexia, letter-blindness, and semantic alexia. The symptom picture in parietal-temporal alexia is striking and relatively precise (see Table 11.4) but the associated clinical findings vary considerably, depending on the amount and location of cerebral pathology.

The characterizing features of parietal-temporal alexia are the impairments of reading and writing—alexia and agraphia. The loss of these functions may be total but is more often partial. In patients with parietal-temporal alexia, the ability to read out loud and to comprehend written language are both disturbed and cues are of little help. Their ability to read both letters and words is impaired, and as a rule they have difficulty in comprehension of numbers and of musical notations. Patients with parietal-temporal alexia will fail to recognize a word when it is spelled aloud and will often state that they cannot understand a word that is spelled aloud because of an inability to read.

For patients with parietal-temporal alexia the writing disturbance is usually equal to the severity of the alexia. These patients often produce real letters and even combinations of letters that resemble words, however; the letter combinations are often nonwords that fail to carry meaning. Their ability to copy written and printed words is far superior to their ability to write them spontaneously or to dictation; in general, they fail to transpose cursive to printed forms and vice versa. The patient with parietal-temporal alexia is truly illiterate for written and printed language symbols.

Number reading is usually disordered in parietal-temporal alexia, and most

Table II.4. Differential Features of the Three Alexias

	PARIETAL-TEMPORAL ALEXIA	OCCIPITAL ALEXIA	FRONTAL ALEXIA
Written Language			
Reading	Total alexia	Primarily verbal alexia	Primarily literal alexia
Writing	Severe agraphia except copying	Mild or no agraphia	Severe agraphia including copying
Copying	Slavish	Slavish	Poor, clumsy, omissions
Letter Naming	Anomia for letters	Normal	Anomia for letters
Comprehension of spelled words	Failed	Good	Poor
Spelling out loud	Failed	Good	Poor
Associated Clinical Findings			
Language	Fluent, paraphasic aphasia	Normal or mild anomia	Nonfluent aphasia
Motor	Mild, (usually transient) paresis	Normal	Hemiplegia
Sensory	Often hemi-sensory sensory loss	Normal	Usually mild sensory loss
Visual Field	May or may not have visual-field defect	Right homonymous hemianopia	Normal
Gerstmann Syndrome	Frequent	Absent	Absent

Adapted from Benson, 1985a.

patients also have acalculia. Although the disorder appears to be based on an inability to encode or decode number language, anarithmetria (an inability to perform computations) may also be present (see Chapter 14). Reading of other symbolic systems such as musical notations, chemical formulae, and others is likely to be impaired. Parietal-temporal alexia tends to affect all systems of notation about equally.

Associated neurologic and neurobehavioral findings may or may not be present in patients with parietal-temporal alexia. Right upper-extremity paresis is often present initially but usually disappears in a short time. Right-sided sensory loss is common and is more likely to remain as a permanent residual. A right visual-field defect (often an inferior quadrantanopia) may be present, indicating involvement of the geniculo-calcarine pathways, but many cases of parietal-temporal alexia with no visual field defect have been recorded. Patients with parietal-temporal alexia may show a variety of aphasic findings, including paraphasic verbal output, defective comprehension of spoken language, inability to repeat, and almost always some degree of anomia. Only rarely is all evidence of aphasia absent. The Gerstmann syndrome (see Chapter 17) and constructional disturbance are often present but are not consistently noted nor necessary for the diagnosis of parietal-temporal alexia. Parietal-temporal alexia may occur without any associated clinical findings, particularly in its chronic state.

The neuroanatomical location of the causative pathology in the parietal-temporal alexia syndrome is often clearly demonstrated, demarcated not only by the alexia syndrome but also by the associated neurologic defects. Numerous confirmations by site of trauma, CT, MRI, isotope brain scan, surgical exploration, and autopsy have been presented. Even brain trauma localized only by the site of focal skull defects has demonstrated the parietal-temporal locus for the acquired alexia and agraphia syndrome (see Figure 11.2) (Luria, 1947/1970).

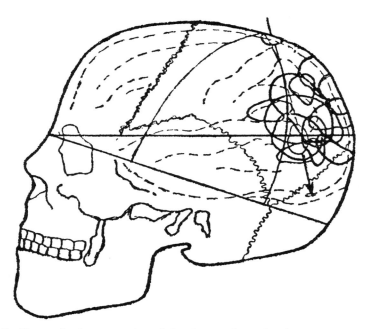

Figure 11.2. Composite demonstration of the sites on the scalp of wounds that caused parietal-temporal alexia (alexia with agraphia) in brain injured soldiers. (From Luria, 1947/1970).

The clinical course of parietal-temporal alexia depends on the underlying etiology and the size of the lesion. Rapid recovery of some or all reading skills can occur; more often recovery is partial, permitting limited reading comprehension, and remains in this state. Both the degree of the reading problem and the degree of recovery will be strongly influenced by the patient's premorbid literacy level and the importance of reading in the lifestyle of the patient. Many individuals have never been regular readers and are not greatly disturbed by acquired illiteracy. Unfortunately, some patients who have a strong desire for resumption of literacy maintain both the alexia and the agraphia indefinitely.

A variety of disease processes can produce parietal-temporal alexia. The most common is cerebrovascular disease, particularly occlusion of the angular branch of the middle cerebral artery. Arteriovenous malformation or infiltrating glioma may be the cause. Trauma, gunshot wound, abscess, or metastatic tumor are other possible etiologies. In all instances, it is the location of the lesion, not the disease type that determines the language symptomatology.

One cluster of findings frequently noted in clinical practice includes parietal-temporal alexia, the Gerstmann syndrome and extrasylvian sensory aphasia. This group of findings has been called the *angular gyrus syndrome* and, almost without exception, indicates a dominant-hemisphere inferior parietal location for the causative pathology.

Despite location of the primary pathology in the posterior vascular border zone, parietal-temporal alexia is not commonly reported as the primary finding following carotid occlusion, probably because the alexia is accompanied and obscured by additional language and cognitive defects.

In 1891 Dejerine reported that the syndrome of alexia with agraphia followed dominant-hemisphere angular gyrus damage. Many subsequent reports support this localization (Alajouanine, Lhermitte, and Ribaucourt-Ducarne, 1960; Benson and Geschwind, 1969; Greenblatt, 1983; Nielsen and Raney, 1938; Wolpert, 1930). The number of cases of alexia with agraphia with pathology involving the parietal-temporal junction area recorded in the literature is large, whereas reports of other brain damage sites in cases with this syndrome are rare.

Occipital Alexia

Alexia based on occipital pathology, a disorder termed "alexia without agraphia" by Dejerine (1892), is spectacular but not common. The syndrome has been given many different names including pure alexia, pure word-blindness, agnosic alexia, occipital alexia, posterior alexia, and optic aphasia, as well as alexia without agraphia.

Occipital alexia is a relatively specific syndrome and, based on the dramatic findings, is easily recognized by clinicians. The definitive clinical findings include a serious disturbance of reading contrasted with a much better preservation of writing competency. The patient with occipital alexia actually finds himself unable to read what he has just finished writing. Most patients with occipital alexia, however, do recognize (understand) some common written words such as the name of their city and state, their own name, and the acronym U.S.A. or similarly common language symbols; they fail, however, to read most other words. Most patients with occipital alexia eventually regain their ability to read aloud (i.e., to name) many or all individual letters of the alphabet. Letter naming is performed slowly and insecurely at first, but with practice the skill at spelling aloud improves and from oral spelling the words can be deciphered. This process has been called *verbal alexia* (Benson, Brown, and Tomlinson, 1971) with only mild literal alexia. Obviously, the process of reading individual letters aloud in order to recognize the word is slow and open to error, particularly on long words dependent on a suffix for exact meaning (e.g., "refrigerator" read as "refrigeration," "medical" read as "medicine," etc.)—in which the incorrect suffix suggests a word-length effect (Henderson et al., 1985). Morphological paralexia, the misreading of final morphemes (Payne and Cooper, 1985) is a common characteristic of occipital alexia; these patients are routinely much better at reading the initial than the ending morphemes of a word.

When a word is spelled aloud by the examiner, the patient with occipital alexia immediately recognizes it, a sharp contrast to patients with parietal-temporal alexia, who fail this task. Testing of recognition of spelled words is a simple and relatively specific way to differentiate occipital alexia from parietal-temporal alexia. With improvement, the "reading" of patients with occipital alexia becomes speedier; no longer is it necessary for them to spell out loud but their "reading" is still accomplished by identifying individual letters and combining them to form words.

Patients with occipital alexia can identify individual letters outlined on the palm or when the shapes of the letters are palpated from embossed blocks; they will decipher words presented in this manner at about the same speed as normal subjects. In addition, they can match letters formed with different writing forms (e.g., cursive to block letters) and can even switch the form of letter they write. Patients with occipital alexia have not lost the ability to perceive the language aspects of written language; rather, the delivery of adequately perceived stimuli containing written language symbols to the cortical language area for interpretation is impaired in these patients.

Patients with occipital alexia can usually write without difficulty. However, letter omissions and/or substitutions may occur. They may also show errors in the reading of individual letters (literal paralexia), particularly with lower frequency or complexly constructed letters such as *W*, *R*, or *M* (Dejerine's patient described the letters *A*, *P*, and *Z* as a sawhorse, a loop, and a snake) (Dejerine, 1892). At one stage of recovery, these patients can actually write personal letters or long descriptive paragraphs but can neither read nor remember what they have just written. Additional difficulties such as a tendency to slant their writing upwards (Martin, 1954) and a tendency for the writing to deteriorate over the years (Adler, 1950), based on the absence of visual monitoring, can occur. Patients with occipital alexia have more difficulty copying written material than in writing words to dictation; again, this is a sharp contrast to the performance of patients with parietal-temporal alexia. The difficulties in copying words and sentences contrasted with much better spontaneous writing represents a distinguishing feature of occipital alexia.

Patients with occipital alexia can spell out loud excellently, another feature that differentiates them from patients with parietal-temporal alexia. Also, although patients with occipital alexia cannot read words, they perform relatively well at the matching of words (Grossi et al., 1984).

Right homonymous hemianopia is present in most patients with occipital alexia, although individual cases without hemianopia have been described (Ajax, 1967; Goldstein, Joynt, and Goldblatt, 1971). Nonright-handers may show occipital alexia with a left visual-field defect (Erkulvrawratr, 1978; Pillon, Bakchine, and Lhermitte, 1987). Some investigators base variations in occipital alexia on the presence or absence of hemianopia (Greenblatt, 1983) but others note variations which are not related to visual-field defect (Damasio and Damasio, 1983). Most cases without hemianopia are based on tumor, either a meningioma compressing the dominant-hemisphere medial occipital region or a glioma infiltrating this region. Most reported cases of occipital alexia, however, are caused by vascular infarction and unilateral visual-field defect is present. Not only do these patients often have a blind right hemifield, but they often exhibit decreased smooth pursuit when moving the eyes from left to right (the direction essential for reading in Western languages). A residual lateral-gaze paresis may represent a core deficit in occipital alexia (Luria, 1966).

Although most language functions are normal or near normal, many patients with occipital alexia show difficulty in naming tasks. Most prominent is a disturbed ability to name colors (Geschwind and Fusillo, 1966). If the testing process is reversed (e.g., the patient is asked to point to a color named by the examiner), the problem is just as severe. These same patients have no difficulty using color names in conversation or in presenting a color name to answer a question (e.g., "What is the color of a banana?"); if appropriately tested, they can sort colors easily and accurately. Only in the process of visual-verbal association (i.e., naming a color or pointing to a named color) do they fail. This two-way defect has been considered a true agnosia for colors (Benson, 1988a; Geschwind and Fusillo, 1966; Kinsbourne and Warrington, 1964). Not all patients with occipital alexia have color-naming disturbance (Greenblatt, 1973, 1983). In one large series of patients with occipital pathology (Gloning, Gloning, and Hoff, 1963), "color-naming disturbance" was present in just over 70% of the cases of "pure" alexia. Damasio and Damasio (1986) noted that some patients with occipital alexia show a hemiachromatopia in addition to their reading defect.

Other clinical findings are less dramatic and consistent than the color-naming disturbance in patients with occipital alexia. Anomia for objects, less severe than the color-naming disturbance but still appreciable, may be noted. Difficulty in number reading, particularly with multiple digits, may be seen, and anarithmetia (inability to compute) may be present. The ability to read musical notations is lost in some but not all cases. Most people are illiterate for music notation, however, making this an insecure finding. In patients with occipital alexia, there is no paralysis, no sensory deficit or any other basic neurological deficit except the right homonymous hemianopia. And, except for anomia, there is no aphasia in cases of occipital alexia.

Because of the separate, somewhat distant neuroanatomical locus of pathology (the dominant-hemisphere posterior cerebral artery territory) in cases of occipital alexia (Henderson, 1986), many techniques have successfully demonstrated the site of the lesion. A number of cases of occipital alexia have been correlated with neuropathological findings (Benson and Geschwind, 1969); other successful localizing techniques include the CT scan, MRI, isotope brain scan, EEG, and even cerebral angiography.

The clinical course of occipital alexia varies but a slow, persistent improvement is common; although incomplete, reading ability usually improves to a useful level. Reading therapy, using elementary reading materials and large-print newspapers and books coupled with many hours of practice and considerable encouragement, is often successful. The patient's reading ability, however, rarely returns to the level of pleasure.

Both the lesion site and the typical pathology tend to be consistent in occipital alexia. The neuroanatomical defect described by Dejerine (1892) (see Figure 11.1), with variations, can be demonstrated in most cases (occlusion of the dominant-hemisphere posterior cerebral artery). Occipital alexia can also occur with either intracerebral or extracerebral tumor or arteriovenous malformation (Ajax, 1967; Greenblatt, 1976). In these cases most tissue destruction involves the medial and inferior occipital region, particularly the fusiform and lingual gyri, and damages the posterior segment of the geniculo-calcarine pathway. In addition, at least partial destruction of the splenium of the corpus callosum is present. In the few reported cases of occipital alexia without splenial damage, pathology has involved the deep white matter immediately adjacent to the splenium (Greenblatt, 1973). Damasio and Damasio (1983, 1986) proposed subtypes of pure alexia with or without hemianopia, color anomia, and/or hemiachromatopia. Neither color anomia nor visual-field deficit is requisite for a diagnosis of occipital alexia, although both are usually present. Alexia without agraphia has also been reported in left-handed individuals following a right occipital lesion (Pillon, 1985).

Greenblatt (1973, 1976, 1977) described an entity closely related to occipital alexia in which the patient suffered alexia but neither agraphia nor hemianopia. He termed the disorder *subangular alexia*, because the case he reported had structural pathology that involved the white matter deep in the dominant parietal cortex, undercutting the angular gyrus. The presence of alexia without other language impairment suggests that the "subangular" lesion acted to disconnect the intact dominant-hemisphere angular gyrus from visual stimuli arising from both the right and left hemispheres but did not interfere with angular gyrus function or primary geniculo-calcarine transmission. Subangular alexia can be considered a separate alexia syndrome including segments of parietal-temporal alexia and of occipital alexia; clinically, however, subangular alexia most closely resembles occipital alexia. Detailed descriptions of differences in the symptom pictures of parietal-temporal alexia and occipital alexia, coupled with postulated neuroanatomical correlates (see Figure 11.3), have been presented by Greenblatt (1977, 1983).

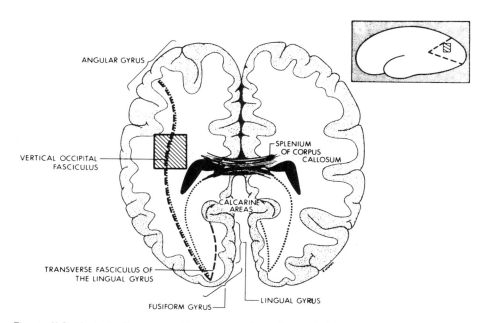

Figure II.3. Artist's diagrammatic representation of postulated visual processing network and the area of brain damage involved (shaded square) that will produce subangular alexia. (From Greenblatt, 1977).

Frontal Alexia

The third syndrome of alexia has a somewhat more controversial history. For years investigators had noted that many patients with Broca aphasia had either lost the ability to read or found the task difficult and unpleasant. According to the accepted theories of written language processing, alexia was not expected with a frontal lesion. In 1891 Freud used the relatively common co-occurrence of Broca aphasia and alexia as a strong argument against the prevailing localization theories. In most cases of Broca aphasia with alexia reported in the nineteenth century, poor premorbid reading ability was accepted as the probable explanation. With the spread of literacy in the twentieth century, however, this explanation became untenable but alexia remained a common finding in patients who had Broca aphasia based on frontal pathology. In a review of sixty-one cases of Broca aphasia evaluated at the Boston VA Hospital, fifty-one were found to have a significant degree of reading comprehension disorder (Benson, 1977).

A number of features of frontal alexia are sufficiently distinctive to allow clinical differentiation from the other two major syndromes of alexia (see Table 11.4). Most patients with frontal alexia do understand some written material but this is usually limited to individual words. Patients may decipher a newspaper headline but will fail (or refuse to try) to comprehend the sentences that make up the article. If they can read a word aloud they will understand it. The words that can be recognized are almost exclusively substantives, words that have individual meaning. If the gist of a sentence depends upon only one or two substantive words, patients may correctly interpret the meaning of the entire sentence. If, however, relational words such as adjectives, prepositional phrases, and the like are significant for sentence meaning, then patients with frontal alexia may misinterpret the sentence. Thus, both "The Yankees did score" and "The Yankees did not score" may be interpreted as having the same meaning; the negative of the second sentence is not appreciated by patients with frontal alexia.

The difficulty that patients with frontal alexia have comprehending written material closely resembles the auditory comprehension disturbance demonstrated in patients with Broca aphasia (Samuels and Benson, 1979; Zurif, Caramazza, and Myerson, 1972). Even though patients with frontal alexia are able to understand some words, they insist that they cannot read and consistently avoid reading. In direct contrast to patients with occipital alexia, patients with frontal alexia will read some words but fail when asked to read (or even name) the individual letters of a word (literal alexia) (Benson, Brown, and Tomlinson, 1971). They also commit more morphological errors in reading (Payne and Cooper, 1985). Although they may recognize some words spelled aloud (usually substantive words), they fail to comprehend most.

A severe agraphia almost always accompanies frontal alexia. Their writing, most often performed with the left hand because of right motor paresis, is crude, with poorly formed letters, faulty spelling, and agrammatic sentences. Although these patients can copy written language, motor problems cause them to have more difficulty in this task than patients with the other major syndromes of alexia. Even in copying, there is a tendency for patients with frontal alexia to omit letters.

The associated clinical findings in frontal alexia are distinct and unquestionably helpful in confirming the diagnosis (see Table 11.4). Broca aphasia is present in most cases. Numerous observations suggest that patients with extrasylvian motor aphasia, even though severely nonfluent, comprehend written material adequately, a sharp contrast with the frontal alexia seen in most cases of Broca aphasia (Alexander and Benson, 1991; Gonzalez-Rothi, 1990; Hécaen and Albert, 1978). The verbal output of patients with frontal alexia is usually limited but their comprehension of spoken language is relatively good, appearing better than their comprehension of written language. Right hemiplegia is usually present in patients with frontal alexia. A sizable number show some degree of sensory loss and a few patients will have a visual-field defect (Benson, 1977). Frontal alexia tends to remain severe, often the most disabling residual impairment of Broca aphasia. On the other hand, some patients with clinically defined Broca aphasia show no alexia whatsoever; alexia, although common and frequently severe, is not a characterizing feature of Broca aphasia.

The neuroanatomical locus of pathology in frontal alexia can be demonstrated by the techniques that localize frontal aphasic lesions (see Chapter 8). Definitive autopsy studies (Neilsen, 1938) and neuroimaging techniques clearly establish the site of lesions which cause frontal alexia. The pathology involves the posterior portion of the inferior frontal gyrus with extension into the tissues of the anterior insula (Greenblatt, 1983). Whether the reading disturbance seen in frontal alexia can occur with involvement of other anterior sites remains controversial (Rothi, McFarling, and Heilman, 1982). The etiology in cases of frontal alexia is the same as that causing Broca aphasia; cerebrovascular problems predominate.

The difficulty with reading noted in many patients with Broca aphasia is a real alexia. Although such patients can decipher some written words and some can comprehend many written words, the degree of impairment is significant. Frontal alexia is not, however, the full-scale illiteracy seen in parietal-temporal alexia and differs from occipital alexia in many features. Frontal alexia deserves recognition as a unique and relatively common clinical syndrome.

Other Types of Reading Impairment

Spatial (Visuospatial) Alexia

As an acquired language function, alexia is strongly related to left-hemisphere pathology, and reading comprehension (the decoding of written language) has been shown to be a strongly lateralized function (Benson, 1982, 1985a). Reading is not only a linguistic task, however, and disturbances in reading after right-brain damage are sufficiently significant to warrant discussion as a variety of alexia (Ardila and Rosselli, 1988a; Benson and Geschwind, 1969; Gloning et al., 1955; Hécaen and Albert, 1978).

Reading demands rigorous spatial discrimination and disorder of this function based on right-hemisphere damage may be sufficient to impair reading comprehension. Recognition of a symbolic system (letters) presented in space is crucial to written language comprehension. Letters in a word are separated by spaces, and word separations are indicated by larger intervening spaces. If spatial separation is not properly maintained, words will appear fragmented, incorrectly joined and difficult to decipher.

In Western languages written material is presented from left to right, demanding that left hemispace be explored initially. After a line has been visualized, the reader must return to the left extreme in order to read the next line; if this sequential act cannot be performed accurately, the same line may be revisualized or a line skipped. Reading comprehension becomes difficult, almost impossible, when spatial control cannot be maintained. Spatial alexia, then, refers to impairments in reading based on disordered visuospatial control.

Following right-hemisphere damage, a patient's spatial discrimination may be so impaired that problems in sentence reading may resemble those seen in left-hemisphere-damaged patients (Ardila and Rosselli, 1994). There are distinctions, however. Spatial alexia involves sequences of written material (words, sentences, and texts) and is not evident when only letters or even individual words are to be interpreted. Ardila and colleagues (1989) found that all patients with right retrorolandic hemispheric damage made errors in text reading.

Hécaen (1972) found spatial alexia in 23.4% of 146 right-hemisphere-damaged patients. He characterized spatial alexia by (a) inability to fix the gaze on the word or text and to move in an orderly fashion from one line to another; (b) neglect of the left side of the text. Ardila and Rosselli (1994), in a sample of twenty-one right-hemisphere-damaged patients, observed that although hemi-spatial neglect was the most evident reading error, several other reading errors are also present. Substitutions, additions, and omissions of letters and words at the left margin were frequent; occasionally additions, omissions, and/or substitutions of letters and words to the right (or in the middle) of words or sentences were observed. Some word substitutions noted in these patients appeared to be interpreted as semantic paralexias. Punctuation marks were misused by these patients; for instance, when reading a text they would not stop with a period. Their oral reading was monotonous and difficult to comprehend. An inability to follow lines is frequent in this population. While reading a line they might move to the upper or lower one (e.g., skipping a line or reading it twice; after reading one line the patient would not know where to continue reading). Grouping (reading two words as one) and splitting (reading one word as two different words) were rare.

Most patients with spatial alexia present one or several associated disorders such as hemiparesis, left visual-field defect, left hemispatial neglect, constructional apraxia, spatial agraphia, or spatial acalculia.

Hemispatial Alexia

Another problem in spatial arrangement that can interfere with a patient's comprehension of written language has been termed hemispatial alexia. Unilateral neglect may be demonstrated in patients with hemispatial alexia by testing their ability to read individual words out loud. These patients will read either the initial or the final morpheme(s) of a word while omitting the other segment (e.g., "basketball" will be read as "basket" or as "ball") (Kinsbourne and Warrington, 1962b). Patients with right-hemispatial neglect tend to guess the missing segment of the word, producing a confabulation. For example, these patients may correctly read the initial part of the word (or sentence) but will guess the remainder (e.g., "national" for "nationwide"). Right-brain-damaged patients tend to substitute the left side of a word; this is best demonstrated when they are presented with logotomes, which they often read as meaningful words (e.g., "nall" is read as "wall"). Almost 80% of patients with right retrorolandic damage and 50% of those with right prerolandic lesions make confabulatory errors in attempts to read logotomes (Ardila et al., 1989c). Letter omission and/or letter addition may also produce disordered written-word comprehension in patients with hemispatial alexia. Their omissions and additions often lead to their producing literal paralexias (e.g., "threaten" becomes "threat"; "ahead" becomes "head").

In addition to the spatial orientation difficulties in their reading, patients with hemispatial alexia almost always show evidence of spatial hemi-inattention demonstrated by disturbances in writing (spatial agraphia), calculation (spatial acalculia), and construction; some may also have topographagnosia, environmental agnosia, and/or prosopagnosia.

Hemispatial alexia is most commonly observed in patients suffering right retrorolandic lesions (Ardila and Rosselli, 1994; Hécaen and Albert, 1978) but can just as readily occur following left-hemisphere damage, particularly retrorolandic; with left-hemisphere damage, however, hemispatial alexia is almost always masked by other acquired reading problems.

Aphasic Alexia

Aphasic patients present characteristic reading difficulties that can be attributed directly to their basic language impairment. Thus, in conduction aphasia reading comprehension is better than reading out loud, just as auditory comprehension is superior to repetition of spoken language. When reading aloud, patients with conduction aphasia produce literal paralexias, parallel to the literal paraphasias in their spoken language. In addition, their oral reading of high-frequency words and meaningful phrases and sentences may be better than their reading of low-frequency words or semantically complex written material. Conduction aphasia patients are consistently unsuccessful when attempting to read logotomes. Their errors in reading out loud may be substitutions (e.g., "pal" for "par"), additions, or omissions of letters, but even more frequently they will refuse to attempt the task.

Patients with extrasylvian motor aphasia-Type I may show "frontal deficits" when reading. Thus, they can misread a phrase due to perseveration (e.g., "The boy went boy") and they tend to make meaningful words out of meaningless letter combinations (Luria, 1966). They will read logotomes as real words (e.g., "contimout" might be read as "commission").

By definition, patients with Wernicke aphasia have a problem understanding written language. In some reported cases of Wernicke aphasia, however, the patient was totally unable to comprehend written language even though no significant extension of pathology into the parietal or the occipital lobe was demonstrated (Nielsen, 1939). Patients with cortical damage restricted to the dominant-hemisphere temporal lobe may produce substitutions, omissions, and additions of letters and even neologistic reading. Occasionally, the patient may show letter-by-letter reading aloud (e.g., "table" is read as "t-a-b-l-e") without comprehension; an inability to interpret meaning for the word despite ability to name the letters is suggested. Comprehension of written language is often severely impaired and even word-picture matching tends to be difficult for the patient with Wernicke aphasia. Only if the Wernicke aphasia disorder primarily involves phonemic discrimination (word-deafness) may the reading disturbance be insignificant.

Pure word-deafness, the relatively rare condition that features severe auditory comprehension deficit without alexia, usually has a dominant hemisphere posterior superior temporal-lobe locus of pathology. If the damage extends upward toward the parietal lobe, parietal-temporal alexia results; if the damage extends posteriorly, the patient may show a variation of occipital alexia.

Most extrasylvian sensory aphasias are associated with reading difficulty and some, but not all, anomic aphasia patients have difficulty interpreting the meaning of a written word; the severity of the comprehension defect tends to correlate with the degree of naming deficit. Extrasylvian sensory aphasia is almost routinely associated with a parietal-temporal alexia (Benson, 1985) but the severity of the alexia can vary. If the underlying damage involves the posterior parietal and/or parietal-temporal regions, the reading defect is evident. With damage to the more temporal-occipital region, the patient's reading tends to be better preserved, but if the temporal damage extends farther posteriorly, some degree of occipital or subangular alexia may be present.

Hemialexia

In a few cases reported in the literature, the splenium of the corpus callosum was purposefully severed by neurosurgeons to approach a pinealoma or other retro-mesencephalic tumor or to separate the hemispheres to help control epilepsy. In some of these reports the patients showed no disturbance of reading (Akelaitis, 1941, 1943, 1944); in others, however, the patient could not understand written material visualized in their left visual field but could correctly read material presented to their right visual field (left hemisphere), a condition termed hemialexia (Gazzaniga and Sperry, 1967; Maspes, 1948; Trescher and Ford, 1937). This condition differs from hemispatial alexia in that both visual fields are intact in hemialexia; only the fibers connecting right visual processing areas from the left language processing areas are damaged. Hemialexia is rare and has only been reported in patients following neurosurgical section of the posterior corpus callosum; in theory, however, hemialexia could occur with any pathology that destroys the splenium of the corpus callosum.

Linguistic Models of Alexia

Significant variability in reading disturbances is evident and the classical, neuro-anatomically based distinctions appear insufficient to explain the degree of variability. Parietal-temporal alexia, in particular, presents considerable variability in patterns of linguistic disturbances (Alajouanine, Lhermitte, and Ribaucourt-Ducarne, 1960); subtypes of reading disorders can be distinguished.

During the 1970s and 1980s new approaches to the analysis of alexia were developed. Experimental and cognitive psychologists analyzed alexic disorders from linguistic and cognitive-psychology perspectives, and neuropsychologists analyzed the disorders from a brain-behavior approach (Beauvois and Derouesne, 1979, 1981; Caramazza et al., 1985; Coltheart, 1980b, Coltheart et al., 1983; Marshall and Newcombe, 1973; Patterson, 1978; Patterson and Kay, 1982; Shallice and Warrington, 1980; Shallice, Warrington and McCarthy, 1983). Interest shifted from the anatomical correlates of acquired reading disturbances to the functional mechanisms underlying alexias (Coslett, Gonzalez-Rothi, and Heilman, 1985; Friedman, 1988; Friedman and Albert, 1985).

In 1966 Marshall and Newcombe reported a patient who was unable to read pronounceable nonwords but could read words of an open class (nouns, adjectives, verbs) and, to a lesser degree, closed-class words (grammatical connectors).

This patient presented a significant number of semantic, morphological, and formal verbal paralexias. The disorder was initially termed "literal alexia" (Hécaen, 1972) and later "deep dyslexia" (Marshall and Newcombe, 1973). The introduction of the concept of *deep dyslexia* initiated a new, linguistically oriented epoch in the study of acquired reading and writing disorders.

Normal Reading

The cognitive and linguistic approaches to the study of alexia demanded development of models for normal reading. Several cognitive models of normal reading were presented (Coltheart, 1980a; Friedman, 1988; Marcel, 1980; Morton and Patterson, 1980; Roeltgen, 1985). In general, most of these models proposed that after initial letter identification, reading proceeds along two linguistically distinct routes:

1. The direct route: the written word is associated with a visual word in the lexicon memory. Thus, the string of letters is matched to an abstract representation of the orthographic composition of the word from which the meaning of the written word can be retrieved.
2. The indirect route: the written word is transformed into a spoken word following a graphophonemic set of rules, and the meaning of the word is attained through its phonological mediation, as when an individual understands spoken speech (Marcel, 1980; Friedman and Albert, 1985).

If one or the other of these two reading systems is altered, different error patterns will be observed (Marshall and Newcombe, 1973; Morton and Patterson, 1980; Patterson, 1978; Shallice and Warrington, 1980). In some instances both reading systems can be disrupted simultaneously. Research was focused around the types of errors (paralexias) observed in alexic patients (see Table 11.5), and on the linguistic properties of the words that influenced word-reading competency.

Figure 11.4 presents a basic model of the neurolinguistic aspects of reading, stressing the two reading routes—direct and indirect. Graphophonemic reading systems (e.g., Spanish) rely almost entirely on the indirect route, whereas ideographic or logographic systems (e.g., Chinese) primarily use the direct route. English written language has been described as a compromise between the graphophonemic and logographic reading principles (Sampson, 1985); comprehension of written words is partially achieved following specific grapheme-phoneme correspondence principles and partially following a visual *gestalt* recognition without analysis into individual letters. In written English, considerable homophonic heterography is observed (e.g., morning/mourning; blue/blew) and the direct route must be used frequently.

The ultimate goal of the linguistic approach was to identify components of

Table II.5. General Classification of Paralexias and Paragraphias

TYPE OF ERROR	EXAMPLE
Literal Paralexia and Paragraphia	
Omission	HAND → HAD
Addition	BOY → BOYS
Displacement	MEAT → TEAM
Substitution	RED → NET
Verbal Paralexia and Paragraphia	
Formal verbal paralexia and paragraphia (phonological relation)	PEAR → DARE
Morphemic verbal paralexia and paragraphia	
Lexical (or derivational) paralexia and paragraphia	KINDNESS → SADNESS
Morphologic (or flexional) paralexia and paragraphia	FREQUENCY → FREQUENT
Semantic verbal paralexia and paragraphia (semantic relation)	
Same semantic field	LAWYER → ATTORNEY
Antonym	BIG → SMALL
Superordinate	DOG → ANIMAL
Proximity	CIGARETTES → MATCHES
Unrelated verbal paralexia and paragraphia	PEOPLE *MEET* AT THE PARK → PEOPLE *TOMORROW* AT THE PARK
Syntagmatic paralexia and paragraphia	THE BOY WALKS → THE MAN GOES
Other Types of Paralexia and Paragraphia	
Neglect paralexia	
Omission	SAND → AND
Substitution	WINE → PINE
Neglect paragraphia	FURNITURE → TURE
Spelling paralexia	TABLE → T,A,B,L,E
Visual paralexia	MILD → SLID
Graphemic paragraphia	PHONE → FONE
Regularization paralexia and paragraphia	CAS → CAN
Decomposition paralexia and paragraphia	THERAPIST → THE RAPIST
Grouping paralexia and paragraphia	A HEAD → AHEAD
Neologisms	TABLE → NARTRAN

From Lecours (unpublished doctoral dissertation).

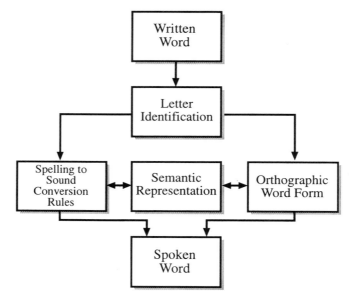

Figure II.4. Basic neurolinguistic representation of reading process. (From Caplan, 1993).

the normal reading system that are disturbed in alexia syndromes and to provide clinical data to support models of normal reading (Friedman, 1988). Initially, occipital alexia was ignored and most linguistic discussions centered around parietal-temporal (aphasic) alexia. Eventually, a further distinction between a central (parietal-temporal) alexia and a peripheral (occipital) alexia was introduced (Riddoch, 1990; Shallice and Warrington, 1980). Table 11.6 presents a comparison between classic, anatomically based alexia syndromes and psycholinguistically based alexia syndromes.

Table II.6. Comparative Classification of Alexias

ANATOMICALLY BASED CLASSIFICATION	LINGUISTICALLY BASED CLASSIFICATION
Parietal-temporal (central) alexia	Surface alexia
Frontal (anterior) alexia	Phonological alexia
Global alexia	Deep alexia
Occipital (posterior) alexia	Letter-by-letter reading
Spatial alexia	—
Hemispatial alexia	Neglect alexia
Literal alexia	Attentional alexia

Central Alexias (Dyslexia)

In central alexia (or dyslexia, as used by English investigators), the patient can perceive a word correctly, but has difficulty recognizing (identifying) it with either semantic or phonological processing (Shallice and Warrington, 1980). Three different types of central alexia—phonological, surface, and deep—were distinguished. Each features a specific pattern of reading errors (paralexias).

Phonological Alexia

Phonological alexia is characterized by inability to read legitimate (pronounceable) pseudowords despite relatively well preserved ability to read real words. In theory, patients with phonological alexia are presumed to read known words because these words are stored in a lexical memory bank. Pseudowords are not present in the lexicon and, in consequence, cannot be read. Reading pseudowords requires the use of the nonlexical (or graphophonemic) route. This dissociation implies that the nonlexical (phonological or "indirect") route is impaired and the subject must rely exclusively on the lexical (direct) route. Patients with this problem also suffer an inability to use the spelling-to-sound correspondence (graphophonemic) rules of the written language (Beauvois and Derouesne, 1981; Friedman, 1988; Shallice and Warrington, 1980) although the lexical matching route in preserved.

In phonological alexia, linguistic frequency plays a crucial role; high-frequency words are more likely to be read correctly than low-frequency words. Pseudowords (with a frequency of zero) are usually impossible to read (Derouesne and Beauvois, 1985; Patterson and Kay, 1982).

Disagreement has existed with regard to the relative difficulty of reading different grammatical classes of real words. Patterson (1982) reported that in phonological alexia, errors in reading real words occurred with closed-class (grammatical, connectors) words whereas open-class words were read correctly. This finding would indicate that reading was mediated through semantics, considering that connectors and bound morphemes have little semantic value. This difference in the ability to read words belonging to different grammatical categories has not been fully confirmed by other investigators (e.g., Funell, 1983).

Patients with phonological alexia will produce visual paralexias; that is, they will misread real words as other words that are visually similar to the target words. The similarity refers not just to the visual form but to the orthographic composition; the target word and the paralexic error have many letters in common (e.g., mild → slid) (Friedman and Albert, 1985). Shallice and Warrington (1977) found that at least half of the letters of the words interchanged by these patients were the same. Friedman (1988) considered this reading error to be an "orthographic paralexia" rather than "visual paralexia."

A significant effect, called *pseudohomophony*, has been observed in phonological alexia. Patients with this disorder read pseudowords better if the pseudowords are homophonous with a real word (e.g., rair) (Beauvois and Derouesne, 1979). Patterson (1982) posited this to be the result of a deliberate strategy: the patient attempts to obtain a reconstruction of the phonological form by applying a lexical strategy. Derouesne and Beauvois (1985) reported that pseudohomophony was observed only when the patient was instructed to try to find a word that sounded similar to the pseudoword.

The degree of associated aphasia and agraphia in patients with phonological alexia are not consistent. Aphasia is not severe, and different aphasia types may be present. The aphasia may be either fluent or nonfluent (Friedman, 1988). Phonological alexia has been reported in cases of right-hemisphere pathology (Derouesne and Beauvois, 1985; Patterson, 1982). Phonological alexia has been associated with impaired spelling (Shallice and Warrington, 1980), and anomia (Rapcsak, Gonzalez-Rothi, and Heilman, 1987). Agraphia is present, but usually not severe (Friedman and Albert, 1985).

Surface Alexia

Surface alexia represents an acquired disorder characterized by the superior reading of regular words and legitimate pseudowords in comparison to irregular words (Patterson and Morton, 1985). The graphophonemic reading system is available to patients with surface alexia, although they do make some errors when using the grapheme-to-phoneme conversion system (Behrman and Bub, 1992). Marshall and Newcombe (1973) described two patients, unable to read irregular words but capable of reading legitimate pseudowords, and proposed that the grapheme-to-phoneme correspondences used in regular words were preserved in these patients, whereas the lexical reading of irregular words was impaired (Coltheart et al., 1983; Deloche, Andreewsky, and Desi, 1982; Kay and Lesser, 1986; Shallice, Warrington, and McCarthy, 1983; Shallice and Warrington, 1980).

In surface alexia the inadequate application of grapheme-phoneme conversion rules produces specific types of paralexias (Deloche, Andreewsky, and Desi, 1982; Marcel, 1980; Shallice and Warrington, 1980). The patient seems to rely exclusively on grapheme-phoneme decoding and tends to present numerous "regularization errors" (Coltheart et al., 1983) in which irregular words are read following standard graphophonemic rules. Unambiguous words are read successfully by these patients but words with ambiguous or irregular orthography are misread.

In languages like English, the dichotomy of "regular" versus "irregular" words is not simple (Shallice, Warrington, and McCarthy, 1983). Some irregular words are more irregular than others. Patients with surface alexia read mildly irregular words better than very irregular words. Furthermore, their ability to read a word correctly may depend on its frequency—frequently used words tend to be read more accurately than regular but low-frequency words.

Friedman (1988) summarized thirteen published reports of cases of surface alexia and noted the following characteristics:

1. Some patients produced predominately regularization errors; others produced only a few such errors.
2. Frequency effects, grammatical category effects, and length effects are reported in only a few cases.
3. The agraphia associated with surface alexia resembles lexical agraphia; the patient's writing errors mirror their reading errors, with regular words more likely to be written correctly than irregular words.
4. All but two reported cases were in fluent aphasics (anomia, Wernicke, conduction, or transcortical sensory aphasia).
5. Almost all patients had a left temporal or temporoparietal lesion; the others had widespread cortical atrophy that included the left temporoparietal region.

Deep Alexia

If both the lexical (direct) reading route and the phonological (indirect) route are impaired, only limited residual reading ability will remain. In patients with deep alexia both the lexical route and phonological route appear impaired (Jones, 1985) and the patient's reading deficit is severe.

Deep alexia has been studied intensely and several relatively consistent distinguishing characteristics have been outlined:

1. The most striking feature of deep alexia is the occurrence of semantic paralexias in oral reading (Coltheart, 1980a). Semantic paralexias refer to reading errors related to the meaning of the target word (e.g., hand → foot; building → house). Varieties of semantic paralexias have been distinguished: (a) the paralexic error may be a synonym of the target word (e.g., lawyer → attorney); (b) it may be an antonym (e.g., big → small); (c) it may be an associate of the target word (e.g., cigarettes → matches); or (d) it may be a superordinate word (e.g., dog → animal) (Friedman, 1988).
2. Success in reading single words is affected by: (a) the grammatical category: function words (grammatical particles) are particularly difficult to read, and nouns are easier to read than adjectives or verbs. This reading pattern is similar to that observed in alexia associated with Broca aphasia (anterior alexia); some investigators consider deep alexia to be associated with a Broca's aphasia (Coltheart, Patterson, and Marshall, 1980; Kaplan and Goodglass, 1981); (b) concrete nouns are read better than abstract

nouns. Paralexic errors are more frequent with abstract than with concrete words.

3. The patient cannot make use of the grapheme-phoneme rules of conversion and, as a consequence, cannot read pseudowords (Coltheart, 1980a).
4. Visual and derivational (i.e., verbal morphological) paralexias are always present.
5. Deep alexia is always associated with aphasia and agraphia (Friedman and Albert, 1985).

Different explanations have been proposed for the production of semantic paralexias: (1) It has been noted that the semantic system is imprecise. Following presentation of some written words, several semantically distinct words can be activated; the correct selection requires the use of phonological mechanisms that are not available to patients with deep alexia (Marshall and Newcombe, 1973; Newcombe and Marshall, 1980; Saffran and Marin, 1977). (2) Some semantic paralexias are not clearly related to the target word (they correspond to verbally unrelated paralexias, not to semantic paralexias); in consequence, a semantic deficit compounds the phonological deficit (Morton and Patterson, 1980). (3) Some investigators argue that deep alexia, particularly the presence of semantic paralexias, reflects the reading capability of the intact right hemisphere (e.g., Benson and Geschwind, 1969; Coltheart, 1980b, 1983b). (4) Deep alexia in general, and semantic paralexia in particular, have been interpreted as a stage in the recovery from total alexia (Benson, 1985a).

Peripheral Alexias (Dyslexias)

In the peripheral alexias the reading impairment corresponds more exactly to a perceptual disturbance; the patient has difficulty attaining a satisfactory visual word form (Riddoch, 1990; Shallice and Warrington, 1980). There is impairment of the prelexical reading processes. Three patterns of defects have been grouped under peripheral alexia.

Letter-by-Letter Reading
The disorder characterized by letter-by-letter reading corresponds to the literal alexia seen in patients with occipital alexia. Although the syndrome characterized by letter-by-letter reading was described a century ago by Dejerine (1892), cognitive neuropsychologists have contributed new theoretical models for this reading disorder (Bub, Black, and Howell, 1989; Coslett and Saffran, 1989; Friedman and Alexander, 1984; Kay and Hanley, 1991; Patterson and Kay, 1982; Price and Humphreys, 1992; Rapp and Caramazza, 1990; Reuter-Lorenz and Brunn, 1990; Shallice and Saffran, 1986).

A lexicality effect is sometimes present in letter-by-letter reading. Reading is better for words and pseudowords than for letter strings (Rapp and Caramazza, 1990). Word length is significant; increased latencies are noted in reading as the length of the word increases (Kay and Hanley, 1991).

Investigations of letter-by-letter reading have been focused on attempts to explain the reading impairment. Farah and Wallace (1991) have summarized the three different hypotheses that have been put forth to explain this reading deficit.

The classic explanation for letter-by-letter reading (occipital alexia) is the disconnection hypothesis (Benson, 1979a, 1985; Geschwind, 1965). This hypothesis proposed that for reading comprehension, visual information in the occipital lobe must be connected, via white-matter pathways, to the brain language areas of the posterior left-hemisphere cortex. The angular gyrus plays a critical role in the multimodal associations that link visual patterns of printed words to both sounds and meanings. Letter-by-letter reading results from functional separation of the visual cortex from the left angular gyrus. Farah and Wallace (1991) point out that although this hypothesis is consistent with a disorder producing letter-by-letter reading, it does not explain all of the characteristic features.

A second hypothesis proposed that letter-by-letter reading results from an extended impairment in visual perception (visual agnosia) including, but not limited to, the perception of printed words, and that alexia will be evident in this context. Patients would thus be suffering a form of simultanagnosia (Kinsbourne and Warrington, 1962b; Luria, 1966). Letter-by-letter reading is the most evident manifestation of a perceptual disorder that is not limited to verbal material. Levine and Calvanio (1978) termed this disorder "alexia-simultanagnosia" and demonstrated that the patient's inability to simultaneously recognize several stimuli is not restricted to the naming of letters or words. Friedman and Alexander (1984) proposed that letter-by-letter reading represents a manifestation of a deficit in the speed of visual identification which is not specific to orthographic material. Several investigators (Bub, Black, and Howell, 1989; Kay and Hanley, 1991; Reuter-Lorenz and Brunn, 1990) have shown that individuals with "pure" alexia have difficulty in letter-matching tasks (in which pairs of letters must be judged "same" or "different" as quickly as possible).

A third hypothesis was proposed by Farah and Wallace (1991): letter-by-letter reading occurs following disruption of reading-specific processes. Warrington and Shallice (1980) proposed that for normal reading individual letters must be grouped into recognizable higher-order units, corresponding to words. Letter-by-letter reading represents a disorder in the "word form system" (Shallice and Saffran, 1986). Word recognition is failed by patients with this disorder because the word form needed to match with the string of perceived letters is not available to them. Warrington and Shallice emphasize that these alexics have adequate visual perception of letters. They also emphasize that these patients recognize script better than printed words and suggest that their recognition of words in script relies more on overall word form than does their recognition of printed words (written-word limits are imprecise in script). Patterson and Kay (1982) modified this reading-specific process impairment hypothesis by proposing that the patient's word form system is intact but that input from the letter recognition system is limited to a single letter at a time. Letter-by-letter identification is thus essential for reading.

All three hypotheses are based on plausible explanations and each has gained some support. The letter-by-letter reading strategy is a real phenomenon that has exerted a strong influence on both clinical diagnosis and academic models.

Neglect Alexia

As noted earlier, reading defects may result from right-hemisphere damage that produces a left hemispatial neglect (Bisiach and Vallar, 1988; De Renzi, 1985; Friedland and Weinstein, 1977; Heilman, Watson, and Valenstein, 1985c; Kolb and Whishaw, 1990; Weinstein and Friedland, 1977). Benson (1979a) used the term *unilateral paralexia* to describe a condition in which the patient fails to read (neglects) one side of a word or sentence. At times these patients substitute ("confabulate") the neglected portion of the visualized word (Friedland and Weinstein, 1977). This reading disorder is best known as hemispatial alexia or neglect alexia, a disorder that produces considerable difficulty in the comprehension of written material. Kinsbourne and Warrington (1962a) reported six right-handed patients with right-hemisphere damage causing neglect alexia. The neglect-type errors were associated with the tendency for these patients to replace the initial letters of words with others (e.g., "basketball" read aloud as "baseball").

A number of reported studies (usually single-case studies) have been devoted to the analysis of neglect alexia (Behrmann et al., 1990; Bruhn and Farah, 1991; Ellis, Flude, and Young, 1987; Hillis and Caramazza, 1990; Patterson and Wilson, 1992; Warrington, 1991; Young, Newcombe, and Ellis, 1991). The disorder is most frequently associated with right-hemisphere pathology, particularly parietal-lobe lesions (Riddoch, 1990; Riddoch et al., 1990), but some cases of right neglect alexia (associated with left-hemisphere damage) have been reported (Ardila, 1983; Hillis and Caramazza, 1990; Warrington, 1991; Warrington and Zangwill, 1957).

Neglect can fractionate into a number of discrete syndromes, each observable in isolation (Bisiach et al., 1986; Laplane and Degos, 1983). Thus, a patient can present severe motor neglect, but normal sensation and strength, and absence of neglect in drawing or line bisection. Unilateral neglect in reading can be observed in patients without a generalized neglect (Baxter and Warrington, 1983; Riddoch et al., 1990). Furthermore, neglect alexia may also fractionate; different forms of written material (text, words, single letters) may be differentially affected in patients with neglect alexia (Riddoch, 1990) and isolated neglect for numbers has been observed in some cases (Cohen and Dehaene, 1991). In some patients, single-word reading may be impaired, while the reading of text remains intact (Costello and Warrington, 1987; Patterson and Wilson, 1992).

Reading can be affected by the lexical quality of the material. Reading of words is superior to reading of nonwords, and wordlike nonwords are better read than unpronounceable letter combinations. Word length can also influence the type of errors observed in neglect alexia. Warrington (1991) noted that substitution errors predominated with three- and four-letter words whereas omission errors were observed with longer words. Inverted or mirror-image presentations make little difference to the reading difficulties in these patients; they continue to misread letters on the neglected side (Riddoch et al., 1990). Vertical presentation of words, however, can improve most instances of neglect alexia (Kinsbourne and Warrington, 1962b; Young, Newcombe, and Ellis, 1991), but some patients also find vertical reading difficult.

Attentional Alexia

Shallice and Warrington (1977) reported two patients with deep left parietal tumors in which word reading was preserved but the naming of the constituent letters was failed. The patients could, however, name individual letters in isolation. Both patients presented right homonymous hemianopia and aphasia. Their impairment was not specific for letters but included all stimuli in which more than one item of the same category was simultaneously present in the visual field (numbers and even pictorial material). Shallice and Warrington proposed that the lesions involved the area at which visual input is selected for visual analysis. They further proposed that category-specific transmission routes exist and that when only one item of a specific category is present, the transmission route connecting the different classificatory stages of perception is not overloaded. From this they proposed that word recognition involves a transmission route that is different from letter recognition; the perceptual classification unit could process combinations of letters but not words.

Inability to read letters within a word despite preserved ability to read words was first described toward the end of the last century (Hinshelwood, 1900) and most often has been known as "literal alexia" (Hécaen, 1972). It is a prominent characteristic of frontal alexia (Benson, Brown, and Tomlinson, 1971).

Alexia in Oriental Languages

All discussion thus far in this chapter has concerned alexia in English or related Indo-European languages. The possibility that acquired disturbances of written language might be considerably different in the Oriental languages, particularly those that utilize ideographic characters, was raised many years ago (Assayama, 1914; Benson and Geschwind, 1969; Lyman, Kwan, and Chao, 1938; Panse and Shimoyama, 1955) and the literature now contains considerable case material that defines this difference. The most convincing evidence comes from Japan (Sasanuma and Fujimura, 1971; Yamadori, 1975) where essentially isolated alexias of Kana (the phonetic, syllabic written form) and Kanji (the nonphonetic, ideographic written characters) have been demonstrated. Some investigators initially suspected that the right hemisphere might be of particular significance for the reading of Kanji characters (Halta, 1977; Sasanuma, 1975) but this postulation has not been confirmed. Although the number of cases in the literature showing a clear separation of Kana reading disorder from Kanji reading disorder remains limited, it is now apparent that patients with more posterior (parietal-occipital) dominant-hemisphere lesions sustain greater impairment in understanding Kanji (Yamadori, 1980) whereas patients with more anterior (temporal-parietal) pathology have the most difficulty reading the Kana script (Iwata, 1986; Yamadori, 1975).

An intriguing distinction between the impairment in reading of the two different types of Japanese script had been suggested, again based on limited case data. Iwata (1986) proposed that a dominant-hemisphere parietal-temporal lesion would impair Kana (phonetic) but not Kanji (ideographic) reading. In contrast, a dominant temporal-occipital lesion would do the opposite. Iwata's case demonstrations suggest that the stronger visual aspects of the Kanji characters and the stronger auditory aspects of the Kana characters are subserved by dedicated corti-

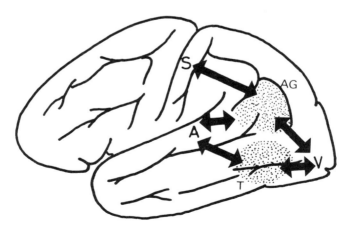

Figure II.5. Diagrammatic representation of left-hemisphere areas crucial to the reading of Japanese characters: (V) visual area; (T) Brodmann area 37, temporal-occipital junction area; (A) auditory cortex; (AG) angular gyrus; (S) somesthetic cortex. (From Iwata, 1986).

cal areas (and/or dedicated pathways) (see Figure 11.5). Iwata's results, however, are based on a few selected cases and have been criticized (Sugishita et al., 1992). Although the Japanese use of two separate written language systems in combination is unusual, almost unique, it would be reasonable to believe that the system diagrammed in Figure 11.5 may be present in all literate humans. It can be proposed that both the auditory (phonetic) and the visual imagery aspects of reading are simultaneously active but that separate anatomical networks subserve these two types of written language processing. Thus, most reading (for comprehension) includes simultaneous activity in both (auditory and visual) spheres.

Summary

Alexia, the acquired impairment of the comprehension of written language, is a complex entity intimately associated with the processing of spoken language but unique in anatomical, linguistic, and behavioral ways. The classic alexia categorizations—alexia with agraphia (parietal-temporal) and alexia without agraphia (occipital)—have been augmented by a third symptom cluster (frontal alexia); each syndrome has distinguishing language-processing characteristics, distinct symptom clusters, and different neuroanatomical loci. Nonlanguage factors such as visual neglect and visuospatial discrimination disorders can influence written language comprehension. In addition, the relatively rigid format of written language lends itself to formal linguistic analysis, and a rich corpus of linguistic models has been developed. Disordered processing of written language provides many avenues for fruitful investigation.

12

Agraphia

· ·

Agraphia may be defined simply as a loss or impairment of the ability to produce written language caused by brain damage. There is nothing simple about agraphia, however. In fact, the complexities of written language disorder have made useful clinical correlations difficult. Almost without exception, aphasic patients show some degree of agraphia. Not only does agraphia accompany many brain disturbances other than aphasia, but writing competency varies immensely between normal individuals. Writing is, at best, a tenuous accomplishment for many humans and almost any brain abnormality can significantly disrupt a poorly established writing skill.

Written language mirrors the complexities of spoken language and its loss. The distinct varieties of aphasia can be reflected by equally distinct agraphic disorders, but many other elements, some language-related but others independent of language, influence writing. Written language demands a precise output that must be presented in a specific spatial orientation; visuospatial orientation and constructional competency are important for written language. Abnormalities of visuospatial discrimination, of spatial orientation, or of constructional ability, all common in brain damage, can produce nonaphasic varieties of agraphia. In addition, motor and, to a lesser degree, sensory abnormalities can adversely affect the patient's written language production. Ataxia, rigidity, spasticity, chorea, myoclonus, and either central or peripheral sensory loss involving the dominant limb will alter the quality of graphic output.

Paralysis is a common cause of abnormal written language and the problem is so obvious that motor disability tends to be overemphasized. Many aphasic patients are paralyzed in the favored upper extremity, so that writing must be attempted with the nondominant hand. Agraphic writing is often attributed to the forced use of the nonfavored hand, but this is a false conception. Right-handed individuals forced to write with the left hand because of right upper-extremity injury rapidly learn to produce an acceptable written language; both the linguistic and the motor quality of their left-handed writing is considerably better than the written output of the aphasic patient with right hemiparesis. Not only is the language aspect preserved in the non-brain-injured patient forced to write with the nondominant hand, but these individuals have no motor apraxia complicating their cross-hemisphere motor activities. A combination of language disorder and motor disturbance affects the written output of many aphasic patients.

Writing is a complex brain activity that demands knowledge of language codes (phonemes, words), ability to convert phonemes into graphemes, knowledge of a graphemic system (alphabet), highly skilled motor ability, and precise spatial ability to distribute and separate letters. With so many potential disturbances to complicate the production of written language, it is not surprising that agraphia has proved difficult to analyze. Distinct varieties of writing disturbances can be observed in clinical practice but combinations are the rule.

Historical Background

Ogle (1867) introduced the term *agraphia* to designate acquired impairment in writing resulting from brain damage. Exner (1881) proposed the existence of a "writing center" located at the foot of the second frontal gyrus immediately above Broca's area and just anterior to the primary motor cortex controlling the hand. Dejerine (1891) described the syndrome of acquired illiteracy (alexia with agraphia) and Gerstmann (1931) proposed that agraphia combined with acalculia, right/left disorientation and finger agnosia could indicate a single, focal injury to the dominant left parietal lobe.

Several classifications of agraphia have been proposed. Goldstein (1948) suggested that writing consisted of linguistic and praxic components, and distinguished two types of agraphia—apractoamnesic agraphia and aphasoamnesic agraphia. Luria (1966, 1976a,b) subdivided agraphia into five types—three paralleling major aphasic disorders (sensory agraphia, afferent motor agraphia, and sequential or kinetic motor agraphia) plus two types related to visuospatial deficits. Hécaen and Albert (1978) proposed four varieties of agraphia—pure, apractic, spatial, and aphasic. Roeltgen (1985) proposed linguistically oriented classifications of agraphia—phonological, lexical, and deep.

Using a pragmatic approach, we will divide the agraphias into two primary types—aphasic and mechanical (see Table 12.1). Aphasic agraphia is based on

Table 12.1. Classification of the Agraphias

Aphasic Agraphias

Agraphia in Broca aphasia

Agraphia in Wernicke aphasia

Agraphia in conduction aphasia

Agraphia in other aphasias

Mechanical Agraphias

Motor agraphia
   Paretic agraphia
   Dyskinetic agraphia
   Hypokinetic agraphia
   Hyperkinetic agraphia
   Dystonic agraphia

Pure Agraphia

Apractic agraphia

Spatial agraphia

Other Writing Disturbances

Hemiagraphia

Prefrontal writing disturbances

Agraphia in confusional states

Hypergraphia

Psychogenic agraphia

---

linguistic impairment; nonaphasic disturbances in writing include both motor and spatial impairments. Agraphia based on apraxia is often classed as a motor disorder but may represent a symbolic deficit and deserves separate discussion. Pure agraphia has proved to be a controversial designation; some investigators regard it as a frontal agraphia (Dubois, Hécaen, and Marcie, 1969), others equate it with apractic agraphia (Auerbach and Alexander, 1981).

Strictly speaking, some writing disturbances should not be considered agraphia. Thus, the inability to produce written language with the left hand following callosal disconnection (hemiagraphia), the lack of writing based on inertia (akinesia), the perseveration seen in some general cognitive disorders (confusional states), excessive writing (hypergraphia), and the pseudoagraphia seen in some psychiatric disorders have explanations that are not based on disorder of either language or the motor system for writing.

Testing for Agraphia

Tests of writing ability are included in most aphasia test batteries and, with appropriate tests, the different aspects of a patient's graphic skill can be analyzed (see Table 12.2).

Automatic writing skills are easily tested but the results demand critical interpretation. The subject's own signature is the most overlearned writing capability and is often performed well by aphasic subjects who cannot write any other words or even letters upon command. Other automatic writing such as address, hometown, state, country, numbers, letters of the alphabet, or days of the week are considerably less overlearned, and many aphasic subjects are unable to write them on request. The aphasic patient's performance on automatic writing tests is generally superior to performance of other written functions; therefore, testing of auto-

Table 12.2. Evaluation of Writing

Automatic writing
  Signature
  Address
  Days of the week

Writing to copy
  Letters
  Logotomes
  Words
  Sentences

Writing to dictation
  Letters
  Logotomes
  Words (high-frequency and low-frequency, high-image and low-image, grammatical forms)
  Sentences

Narrative writing

Changing writing form (script, block letters, etc.)

Spelling words (aloud, with block letters)

Arranging the letters of a word

Writing in other symbol systems
  Shorthand
  Musical notation
  Chemical formulas
  Computer languages

---

matic skills can be useful as an initial step. First, it helps to establish the set for the more difficult writing requests that follow; second, it demonstrates the patient's best possible mechanical production, particularly valuable when he is forced to write with the nondominant limb because of hemiparesis.

A second step in testing graphic competency is to request the subject to copy letters, words, logotomes, and sentences written by the examiner or presented on a card. Copying can be performed without comprehension, although both analysis and comprehension accompany most attempts to copy. Normal subjects easily copy nonsense words and foreign language words even if they do not understand them; some aphasic patients can also copy written text without difficulty. Although the test of copying is not sufficient to demonstrate agraphia, it will show spatial disturbances affecting written output.

A better test of the patient's command of written language is to dictate material to be written: letters, logotomes, high- and low-frequency words, phrases, and sentences. Words belonging to different grammatical categories (e.g., nouns, verbs, adjectives, connectors) and easily imageable words and nonimageable words should be included. Tests of writing to dictation probe both the language and the writing skills of the patient.

An even more challenging writing test is to request that the patient produce a written narrative on a designated topic: for instance, description of the weather, the patient's job, the route from one part of the city to another, or how to change a punctured tire or to prepare a meal. The patient's written description of a picture (e.g., the cookie theft picture from the BDAE [Goodglass and Kaplan, 1983]) can be used to demonstrate the patient's narrative writing competency. Testing of narrative writing evaluates both the mechanics of writing and the ability of the subject to formulate thoughts and integrate them into language. The formulation and integration of thought is a complex process and testing at this level often reveals abnormality in patients who have succeeded in the easier tests. Almost without exception, patients with aphasia will be agraphic at this level; successful completion of a narrative paragraph with appropriate use of complex grammatical features almost excludes significant language pathology.

The patient's performance at changing the form of writing (from uppercase to lowercase or from block letters to script, and vice versa) may demonstrate unanticipated deficits in writing. Thus, this task may be failed by patients who can copy adequately and even by some who can write fluently. An equivalent task, but easier to test, is to match letters or words written in different case (A to a). Similarly, spelling words aloud (and conversely, recognizing spelled words) is easily performed by some and may be informative when demonstrated in patients who are unable to the write words they know how to spell (see Chapter 11).

Some additional tests are occasionally used to probe for writing deficit.

Motor-impaired patients may be given individual block letters or a typewriter and asked to form words. A related but far more demanding test is to request that the patient find a word (or words) that can be formed with a selected group of letter blocks (anagrams). The Cloze Test (Taylor, 1953) can be used to challenge normal subjects but has proved too difficult for most patients with aphasia. In this test, the subject is asked to provide an appropriate word for a blank space in a sentence (e.g., The car _____ through the city streets).

Routine evaluation of aphasic patients challenges only language and number writing. Other writing systems (e.g., shorthand, typewriting, chemical-formula writing, musical notation, computer languages, etc.) are rarely tested, as only a minority of people are literate in these symbolic systems. Competency in these systems may be of interest in patients who have had the ability to use them. Only on rare occasions has agraphia for alternative writing systems been reported (Boyle and Canter, 1987) or, the opposite, retained skills in the face of significant agraphia (Regard, Landis, and Hess, 1985). Needless to say, in bilingual (or polyglot) patients, each written language must be evaluated separately. In general, agraphia in one language will be mirrored in the patient's other language.

Varieties of Agraphia

Aphasic Agraphias

One aspect of writing impairment is based on disordered language function; aphasia is an important component of agraphia. As could be anticipated, variations in the linguistic malfunction noted in varieties of aphasia will be reflected in aphasic agraphia.

Agraphia in Broca Aphasia

Patients with Broca aphasia show a relatively characteristic written language impairment, and correlations between their oral and written language deficits are evident (see Table 12.3): writing is sparse, effortful, clumsy, abbreviated, and agrammatic. Literal paragraphias, anticipations (anterograde assimilations, e.g., "table" becomes "bable"), perseverations (retrograde assimilations, e.g., "table" becomes "tatle"), and letter omissions, particularly in syllabic clusters (e.g., "table" becomes "tabe"), are noted. Mechanically, the letters tend to be large, poorly formed, and messy.

Broca aphasia patients often refuse to write unless coerced and then demonstrate considerable effort and strain. In most, writing must be performed with the nonpreferred hand, an additional source of difficulty. Their writing difficulties

Table 12.3. Comparison of Spoken and
Written Output in Broca Aphasia

SPOKEN OUTPUT	WRITTEN OUTPUT
Sparse output	Sparse output
Effortful	Effortful
Poor articulation	Clumsy calligraphy
Short phrase length	Abbreviated output
Dysprosody	—
Agrammatism	Agrammatism
Poor spelling	Poor spelling

cannot be related only to the clumsy performance with the nonpreferred hand, however. Spelling is often incorrect, words (particularly the grammatical connectors) are omitted, and word-ending grammatical morphemes are absent. Agrammatism is even more obvious in written than in oral language production; it can be surmised that clumsiness of the nonpreferred hand encourages a leaner, more economical written expression but it is also true that writing demands a more elaborate and exact level of language than speaking (Vygotsky, 1934/1962).

Several investigators (Brown, Leader, and Blum, 1983; Leischner, 1983) have promoted use of a special device that allows right hemiplegics to write with their paralyzed hand. Investigations with this implement suggest that the agraphic output produced by the left hand of Broca aphasia patients has a disconnection component (hemiagraphia) in addition to the aphasic component.

Many patients with nonfluent aphasia have damage that involves deeper structures, obliterating connections between the cortex and the basal ganglia and/or damaging primary motor cortex control of hand movements. Paralysis or dystonic movement disorder consequent to this damage can produce a mechanical writing disorder that complicates the aphasic component. The agraphia of Broca aphasia includes a mixture of aphasic (particularly agrammatic) agraphia, a motor paresis agraphia, disconnection (hemiagraphia), and in some cases even a movement disorder agraphia. Figure 12.1 illustrates the abnormal written language of a patient with Broca aphasia.

Agraphia in Wernicke Aphasia
Graphic language output problems in Wernicke aphasia are quite distinct from those of Broca aphasia; ease of production and the generation of well-formed, recognizable letters that are incorrectly combined are distinct features of the writ-

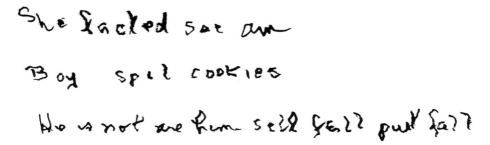

Figure 12.1. Writing sample showing combined mechanical and linguistic agraphia in a patient with Broca aphasia. (From Goodglass, 1993).

ten output of Wernicke aphasia patients. Table 12.4 compares the characteristics of the spoken and written outputs of Wernicke aphasia.

Letter substitutions are frequent (literal paragraphias) and letter combinations may be completely incomprehensible (neologisms). As in the spoken output of Wernicke aphasia, the grammatical elements of writing tend to be preserved and even overused; grammatical elements, however, can be substituted, and the sentences (as in oral language) lack precise limits (written paragrammatism); substantive words are decreased in number and frequently miswritten, with letter additions, substitutions, and omissions. The written production, although fluent and well formed, is often incomprehensible (jargon agraphia). That the mechanical aspects of writing are preserved is most evident when the patient attempts to write words and sentences (particularly spontaneously, but even to dictation). By definition, the closely related problem of pure word-deafness causes minimal or no difficulty with written language except, of course, when the patient attempts

Table 12.4. Comparison of Spoken and Written Output in
            Wernicke Aphasia

SPOKEN OUTPUT	WRITTEN OUTPUT
Normal vocal characteristics	Normal graphic characteristics
Easy output	Easy production
Good articulation	Well-formed letters
Normal phrase length	Normal sentence length
Normal prosody	—
Lack of substantive words	Lack of substantive words
Paraphasias	Paragraphias

to write to dictation (see Chapter 8). Literal paragraphias may be present, particularly early in the course of pure word-deafness, but the preserved writing competency is the factor that clearly distinguishes this disorder from Wernicke aphasia.

Comparison of Table 12.3 with Table 12.4 demonstrates not only that the writing disturbances in Broca aphasia and Wernicke aphasia resemble the spoken disturbances of the two varieties of aphasia, respectively, but that the agraphias in each variety are also distinctly different. Figure 12.2 demonstrates writing disorder in a Wernicke aphasia patient.

Agraphia in Conduction Aphasia

Agraphia also occurs in conduction aphasia but the mechanism is not as well defined as the agraphia of Broca or Wernicke aphasia. Luria (1966, 1947/1970) described a patient with afferent motor agraphia in which spontaneous writing ability was better than writing to dictation. He claimed the writing disorder paralleled the spontaneous spoken output/repetition characteristic of conduction aphasia. Articulatory-based literal paragraphia occurs in conduction aphasia patients when phonologically complex, infrequently used words are written to dictation (Luria, 1966) or when logotomes or words in a partially known foreign language are written. Letter substitutions, additions, and omissions can be sufficiently

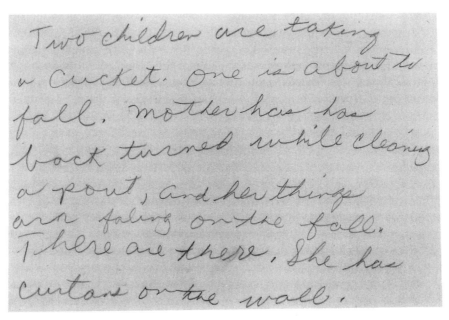

Figure 12.2. Written production of a patient with Wernicke aphasia. (From Goodglass and Kaplan, 1983).

abundant in the writing of these patients that their written words become incomprehensible (neologism). In contrast to the agraphia seen in Wernicke aphasia patients, the patient with conduction aphasia usually recognizes that he has written the word incorrectly, but cannot correct it; attempts to correct a misspelled word often produce new mistakes. As a consequence, written text by a conduction aphasia patient often shows multiple corrections and crossouts. The patient usually states that he knows the word (and may say it aloud) but cannot remember how it should be written (Ardila, Rosselli, and Pinzon, 1989).

Writing in conduction aphasia is often slow and effortful. If the patient has right hypesthesia and/or significant limb apraxia, the letters may be poorly formed but individual letters are routinely better written than words. Although the patient can perform the movements required to write individual letters and produces no scribbles or "nonletters," when spontaneously writing more complex material, the necessary letter combinations are not achieved. Word selection and grammar are basically unimpaired, another contrast to Wernicke aphasia.

One additional complexity is found in the agraphia associated with conduction aphasia. An apraxia for writing (apraxic agraphia) may complicate the aphasic agraphia. In this situation the patient will not write the letters well; instead scribbles or nonletters will be produced. The apraxic defect may be more prominent than the aphasic deficit.

Agraphia associated with conduction aphasia varies considerably in degree. In some patients, the writing deficit will be mild, evident only when they attempt to write low-frequency words to dictation. In other cases, however, agraphia may be so severe that it virtually precludes any useful written output.

Agraphia in Other Aphasias

All patients with global aphasia suffer severe agraphia. Their output may be unintelligible and is usually limited to a few perseverated letters or strokes. It is particularly difficult to induce patients with global aphasia to write. Not only does the language comprehension deficit keep them from understanding the request but most have a right hemiplegia and refuse to attempt writing with the nonpreferred hand.

In patients with mixed extrasylvian aphasia, a severe inability to write will be present although some ability to copy may be preserved (Benson and Cummings, 1985). Writing to dictation or to request is virtually impossible for these patients.

Writing impairment may be observed in both extrasylvian sensory aphasia and anomic aphasia. The inability to use nouns, noted in their spoken language, will be reflected in their writing, and verbal substitutions may appear in their spontaneous writing (verbal paragraphias). It is rare for anomic aphasia to be present without some impairment of written language output. Many patients with extrasylvian sensory aphasia fail to express their thoughts in writing but can write to dictation. The latter tends to be misspelled or otherwise inadequate, however.

The written output of extrasylvian motor aphasia varies considerably, at least partially dependent upon the anatomical site of the causative lesion. In patients with extrasylvian motor aphasia-Type I writing is often seriously compromised, in contrast to their reading comprehension, which is at near-normal levels. Their written output tends to be clumsy, sparse, incomplete, and poorly spelled. The difference between the comprehension and the production of written language has led to the term "agraphia without alexia."

Extrasylvian motor aphasia-Type II produces a different writing disturbance, characterized by marked slowness and effort leading to incomplete sentences with some substitutions (literal and/or verbal paragraphias). In this disorder reading competency is compromised as much as writing.

Anomia and agraphia are the most common residuals remaining after recovery from aphasia. Recovered Wernicke aphasics often have a fluent agraphia when their only obvious impairment of spoken language is an anomia. Most often, however, their naming difficulty is associated with some degree of impaired language comprehension and mild degrees of both alexia and agraphia (Benson, 1981, 1982).

Acquired illiteracy—alexia with agraphia—has been recognized for over a century (Dejerine, 1891). When the causative lesion is limited to the angular gyrus area, the abnormal written production usually has the characteristics of a fluent agraphia. The associated language disturbances can vary considerably, depending on lesion site and size. Alexia with agraphia is almost always accompanied by an anomic or an extrasylvian sensory aphasia.

The agraphia seen in patients with the Gerstmann syndrome consists of real letters produced with comparative ease and accuracy but arranged in an incomprehensible order. The combination of letters may be meaningless, but true words may be interspersed; omissions or reversal of letters or words are frequent. The agraphia in the Gerstmann syndrome is basically identical to the fluent agraphia associated with extrasylvian sensory aphasia (Benson and Cummings, 1985). Some investigators (Ardila, Lopez, and Solano, 1989), however, suggest that agraphia in the Gerstmann syndrome can be considered an apractic agraphia; if the lesion involves occipital- or temporal-lobe tissues, apractic components are not expected, but if the lesion extends to involve the inferior parietal gyrus an apractic element may be noted.

Mechanical Agraphias

In addition to linguistic competence, writing demands both motor and visuospatial skills. Motor disturbances can severely impair written language production; spatial deficits can produce disarrangement of the written material in space. Either can make written production difficult or even impossible. The term *mechanical agraphia* has been suggested to designate these motor and attentional disorders (Benson and Cummings, 1985).

Motor Agraphias

Motor disturbances affecting writing can arise from CNS lesions involving the basal ganglia, cerebellum, the cortical-spinal tracts, or the peripheral nerves; joints and tendons are needed for mechanical operation of the hand, and pathology affecting these structures (e.g., arthritis) can produce a mechanical agraphia. Only the writing disturbances that result from disorders of the peripheral nerves, the cortical-spinal tract, the basal ganglia, or the cerebellum will be discussed.

PARETIC AGRAPHIA. Peripheral nerve disturbances, either symmetric polyneuropathy or asymmetric nerve entrapment, may disrupt writing. In particular, radial, ulnar, and/or median nerve involvement of the dominant hand can produce a flaccid weakness making impossible many manual tasks including writing. Lower motor neuron dysfunction secondary to anterior horn cell pathology or anterior root comprehension can affect the muscles needed for writing. Upper motor (cortical-spinal) damage can produce weakness and spastic rigidity. In a typical hemiparesis the arm and fingers assume a flexed posture. Even when the paralysis is mild, dexterity, speed, and precision are significantly impaired even though gross movements may appear spared. The patient with a paretic hand tends to print rather than write in script and to produce crudely formed characters that are larger than normal.

DYSKINETIC AGRAPHIA. Functional disorders of the basal ganglia and closely related neural structures can disrupt writing without producing weakness in the involved limbs. These so-called extrapyramidal dysfunctions may be manifested by hypokinesia (as in Parkinsonism) or as a hyperkinetic disorder (e.g., chorea, athetosis, dystonia, ataxia, or tremor).

HYPOKINETIC AGRAPHIA (MICROGRAPHIA). The most prominent difficulty of handwriting in the Parkinson syndrome is diminished letter size—micrographia. Two types of micrographia have been described: in one the writing is small throughout; in the other the lettering becomes progressively smaller as the line of letters proceeds. The former type is not an extrapyramidal dysfunction and may also be produced by cortical-spinal lesion (Wilson, 1925); the latter is recognized as a common (but not fully pathognomonic) indicator of Parkinsonism. Micrographia is common in Parkinson's disease, where it may even antedate other demonstrable extrapyramidal signs (McLennan et al., 1972), and micrographia can also be seen in other disorders producing the Parkinson syndrome.

HYPERKINETIC AGRAPHIA. Hyperkinetic movements such as tremors, tics, chorea, and dystonia often involve the upper limbs and disturb writing. Of the three principal types of tremor—parkinsonian (resting), postural, and cerebellar—the latter two types disrupt the writing process most. As the parkinsonian tremor is most pronounced at rest, it interferes relatively little with the action of writing. Postural tremors occur with attempts to sustain a posture; they appear in a variety of clinical conditions including drug-induced or metabolic encephalopathies, systemic weakness, and peripheral disorders such as myalgia or arthritis, and are often idiopathic (e.g., familial or essential tremor). Postural tremors are exacerbated by fatigue and stress and are particularly likely to be manifested during writing (Marshall, 1968). Cerebellar tremors occur with limb movement (intention tremor) and can be sufficiently severe that the patient can accomplish only a few sweeping marks when attempting to write.

Choreiform movements cause an agraphia with letters that are large, crudely formed, and barely legible. Huntington's chorea often involves the proximal limb and trunk musculature in large-amplitude movements that almost preclude writing. The movements of Sydenham's chorea tend to be distal, producing smaller-amplitude but abrupt movements of the hands and fingers. Tardive dyskinesia, a potential complication of neuroleptic medications, has become a common cause of "choreic" disorder. Although the choreiform movements frequently involve the hand and fingers, writing is only mildly disturbed, as the movements can be suppressed volitionally (Benson and Cummings, 1985).

DYSTONIC AGRAPHIA. One of the more controversial motor disorders involving writing is the so-called writer's cramp, which is now categorized as a dystonic agraphia (Sheehy and Marsden, 1982). In this disorder one or several muscles of the preferred writing hand will go into a cramp when the hand posture necessary to hold a writing instrument is assumed. "Simple writer's cramp" is produced only by attempts to write but the problem is often part of a more severe dystonia involving any repetitive hand posture. In some instances the disorder is progressive, starting as the simple writer's cramp but progressing toward a broader dystonic disorder (Sheehy and Marsden, 1982).

Writer's cramp has been described for over a century and a variety of explanations have been offered. Some initial postulations suggesting focal motor disorder were discarded because of failure to demonstrate appropriate pathology; psychogenic explanations were then invoked (Bindman and Tibbetts, 1977; Crisp and Modolfsky, 1965). Attempts were made to treat writer's cramp with behavioral conditioning and/or psychotherapy (Liversedge and Sylvester, 1955; Modolfsky, 1971) but these processes did not prove effective. In recent years neurological explanations have regained prominence (Sheehy and Marsden, 1982). Many patients with writer's cramp are found to have other motor abnormalities such as abnormal posturing of the affected limb, diminished arm swing, increased limb tone, or postural tremor. Writer's cramp is first seen in adult years (onset varies from age 20–50), most often occurring in people who perform a great deal of writing. As the disorder progresses, the problem occurs earlier and earlier in the writing process until any attempt to write will cause cramping. No specific neuropathological changes have been identified but available evidence suggests that a disturbance of neurotransmitter function affecting basal ganglia activity underlies the problem and writer's cramp is now considered as a form of dystonia (Sheehy and Marsden, 1982).

Pure Agraphia

Exner (1881) proposed the existence of a writing center located at the foot of the second frontal gyrus—the premotor cortex lying immediately in front of the primary motor cortex area for the hand. Disagreement regarding the existence of a pure agraphia consequent to Exner's area damage has been extensive, primarily because so few cases correlating pure agraphia with damage to this area have been recorded. Dubois, Hécaen, and Marcie (1969) reported six cases of pure agraphia, four of which had frontal-lobe damage; additional reports (Assal, Chopins, and Zander, 1970; Penfield and Roberts, 1959) have supported a frontal localization for pure agraphia. However, pure agraphia has also been reported with lesions that involve the left superior parietal lobe (Kinsbourne and Rosenfield, 1974; Russell and Espir, 1961). Auerbach and Alexander (1981) suggested that superior parietal agraphia represents a defect of visual control of hand movements.

Anderson, Damasio, and Damasio (1990) reported a patient with a stable alexia and agraphia following a circumscribed lesion in the left premotor cortex (Brodmann area 6) above the Broca's area in the region traditionally called Exner's area. The alexia and agraphia occurred in a setting of otherwise normal cognitive and neurological function. The patient was not aphasic or hemiparetic, and visual perception, intellect, memory, oral spelling, and drawing were normal. Croisile and colleagues (1990) reported a case of pure agraphia following hematoma in the left centrum semiovale that spared parietal and frontal cortices. The patient suffered a total inability to produce graphemes in the absence of limb apraxia.

Chedru and Geschwind (1972) suggested that all cases of pure agraphia were based on some fundamental defect, most often a movement disorder or confusional state. Although agraphia may occur as an isolated defect in rare instances, it is far more common in the context of other cerebral abnormalities.

Apractic Agraphia

A strong association between apraxia and agraphia has been posited for many years (Henschen, 1922). Kleist (1934a) suggested several varieties of apractic agraphia (apraxia in the manipulation of writing implements, apraxia for written discourse, and apraxia for the correct formation of letters). Goldstein (1948) referred to an apractamnestic agraphia which he considered to be based on loss of the motor engrams (patterns) needed for writing. Hécaen and Albert (1978) defined apractic agraphia as the inability to form normal graphemes, producing inversions and distortions instead. The patient with apractic agraphia retains the ability to spell and can compose words with block letters, but spelling errors and iterations are abundant. Apractic writing difficulty involves all modalities— spontaneous writing, writing to dictation, and copying. With time, most patients recover sufficiently to write short sentences but paragraphic errors will still be observed.

Hécaen and Albert (1978) proposed two varieties of apractic agraphia. In one, the patient has neither aphasia nor alexia; in this disorder ideomotor apraxia is evident only in the left hand but agraphia is observed in the right hand. A second, considerably more common variety is found in combination with elements of dominant parietal dysfunction, including both alexia and language comprehension difficulties. They did not consider the agraphia of this parietal disorder to be aphasia dependent, however; rather, it represented a motor writing disorder, an inability to program the movement required to form letters and words. Crary and Heilman (1988) stress that "pure" agraphia can be observed without limb apraxia or other nonwriting language disturbances. Coslett and colleagues (1986) consider ideomotor limb apraxia and apractic agraphia to be dissociable entities; on this basis, apractic agraphia has been considered a pure agraphia (Auerbach and Alexander, 1981).

Spatial Agraphia

Spatial agraphia is a recognized clinical entity (Benson and Cummings, 1985; Hécaen et al., 1956) but few studies have systematically probed the writing disturbances associated with visuospatial discrimination. Hécaen and Marcie (1974) analyzed the writing disturbances present in a large sample of patients with right-hemisphere damage, noting their tendency to reiterate strokes and letters and the progressive enlargement of the left-sided margin. Reiteration was considered a perseverative phenomenon linked to spatial aspects of writing, while the increased left-hand margin appeared to represent unilateral spatial neglect. Ardila (1984b) found that 50% of patients with pre-Rolandic right-hemisphere damage and 75% of patients with post-Rolandic right-hemisphere damage demonstrated some degree of difficulty in the spatial aspects of writing.

Incorrect use of space to separate or join words seriously obscures written language (e.g., "Themanwal ksint hes treet" versus "The man walks in the street"). Misuse of space is particularly associated with right post-Rolandic lesions but can also be present with right pre-Rolandic damage. Reiteration of strokes (particularly in letters such as *m* and *n*) and reiteration of letters, particularly when a letter has to be duplicated (e.g., "bee" becomes "beee") are more frequent in right pre-Rolandic than in right post-Rolandic brain-damaged patients, suggesting perseveration rather than a spatial error. Omissions of letters or parts of letters (individual strokes) can also occur following right hemisphere damage; omissions are considerably more frequent with right post-Rolandic lesions.

Slanting of written lines toward the top or the bottom of the page has been noted in the writing of patients after right-hemisphere damage (Benson and Cummings, 1985; Marcie and Hécaen, 1979), and these patients often write sentences at an oblique angle of about 15 degrees. The left side of the paper is underused, with a progressively wider left-hand margin. If the problem is brought to their attention, these patients will return to the left margin. Unsteadiness in maintaining the left margin of written output ("cascade phenomenon") is most common following right (particularly post-Rolandic) hemisphere damage, possibly indicating unilateral inattention (Heilman and Valenstein, 1979).

Even highly automatized graphic productions such as one's signature can be impaired by spatial disorder. Left hemisphere damage probably produces similar spatial writing disorders but they are hidden by the many other linguistic and motor problems.

Spatial agraphia can co-occur with spatial alexia, spatial acalculia, left visual-field and oculomotor defects, constructional disturbance, unilateral spatial agnosia, and/or decreased topographical competency (Hécaen and Albert, 1978; Hécaen and Marcie, 1974). Thus, writing defects in right-hemisphere-damaged patients can be associated with: (a) left hemi-neglect, reflected in increased left margins; (b) constructional deficits in writing, reflected in disautomatized and altered handwriting; (c) spatial-discrimination disorder, reflected in the inability to use correctly the spaces between words, difficulty in writing in a horizontal line, and spatial disorganization of the written material; (d) a tendency for perseveration (Ardila and Rosselli, 1993a). Although similar errors follow both pre-Rolandic and post-Rolandic damage, patients with pre-Rolandic lesions show more iterative errors such as feature additions and letter additions, whereas those with post-Rolandic lesions produce abnormal groupings of elements and/or letter omissions.

Other Writing Disturbances

Hemiagraphia

A patient whose corpus callosum has been sectioned, either for control of epilepsy for tumor removal, may write in a normal manner with the right (preferred) hand but may totally fail to write with the nonpreferred hand (Bogen, 1969). Geschwind (1965) proposed that the left hemisphere, dominant for language and motor activity, is needed to produce writing with the left hand. Disconnection of the two hemispheres can isolate the right hemisphere (left hand) from language input for writing. Hemiagraphia is usually associated with other unilateral linguistic disturbances (Bogen, 1986) and has also been called disconnection agraphia or unilateral agraphia (Lebrun, 1987).

Prefrontal Writing Disturbances

Patients with prefrontal brain damage may not present a primary deficit in writing, despite having a deficit in oral production (extrasylvian motor aphasia-Type II) characterized by decreased spontaneous verbal output but preserved repetition and language comprehension. Their reading comprehension and ability to read aloud tend to be better preserved than their writing (production). As in the oral language defect, their spontaneous written output will be sparse. The patient may not finish what he has started to write and must be coaxed to continue the task. Both copying and writing to dictation are performed better than spontaneous writing.

Although perseveration can follow brain damage in many different areas (Luria, 1966; Stuss and Benson, 1986), it is often regarded as a fundamental sign of frontal-lobe damage. Perseveration may occur in writing, as in any other motor act. The perseveration in writing may involve words, parts of words, individual letters, or even parts of the letters themselves. Repeated letters in words (e.g., book) are particularly likely to elicit a perseverative response (e.g., boook); motor perseveration can often be demonstrated by having the patient draw multiple loops or other repetitive figures (see Figure 12.3).

Agraphia in Confusional States

Chedru and Geschwind (1972) observed that patients in the confusional state could speak, comprehend, and repeat spoken language and could name and read aloud but could not express their thoughts in writing. Their written output was sparse, clumsy, and contained only vague meaning. Chedru and Geschwind explained this finding by emphasizing the sensitivity of written language production to any alteration of brain function.

Hypergraphia

Hypergraphia has been recorded as one striking manifestion of an interictal personality disorder present in some patients with partial complex seizures (Bear and Fedio, 1977; Blumer and Benson, 1982; Waxman and Geschwind, 1974). In pa-

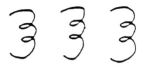

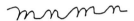

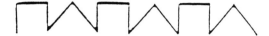

Figure 12.3. Standard tests for seeking evidence of perseveration: multiple loops, alternating *m* and *n*, alternating square and triangle.

tients with this clinical state, hypergraphia is associated with overinclusive verbal output, circumstantiality, viscosity, hyposexuality, intense interest in philosophic/ religious issues, and increased emotional responses. Patients with this disorder (now called the Geschwind syndrome [Benson, 1990]) may write long essays, stories or even novels, compose poetry, write numerous letters to their physicians, to family members, or to government officials, and frequently keep detailed logs or diaries. Hypergraphia is also observed, however, in schizophrenic patients; here it tends to be associated with bizarre topics, mixed metaphors, repeated changes in construction, rhymed effusions, odd punctuations, and verbal repetitions (Benson and Cummings, 1985; Mayer-Gross, Slater, and Roth, 1969). Hypergraphia does not appear to be a language abnormality.

Psychogenic Agraphia

Psychogenic (hysterical) paralysis tends to involve the nonpreferred hand and psychogenic (hysterical) agraphia is rarely reported. It is probable that most of the patients reported as having psychogenic (hysterical) agraphia suffered from idiopathic dystonia (writer's cramp) or a unilateral tremor (Benson and Cummings,

1985). The agraphia could, however, be based on conversion reaction or a false tremor involving the preferred hand. The fundamental importance of recognizing "hysterical" symptoms is that they often indicate major neurologic or psychiatric disorder that demands careful evaluation and management (Gould et al., 1986).

Linguistic Models of Agraphia

Linguistic models of agraphia have attracted considerable interest (Bub and Chertkow, 1988; Goodglass, 1993, Roeltgen, 1985). Different linguistic processing levels (phonological, lexical, semantic) have been proposed for correlation with written language disturbances (see Figure 12.4).

Two types of agraphia (called dysgraphia in the cognitive neuropsychology

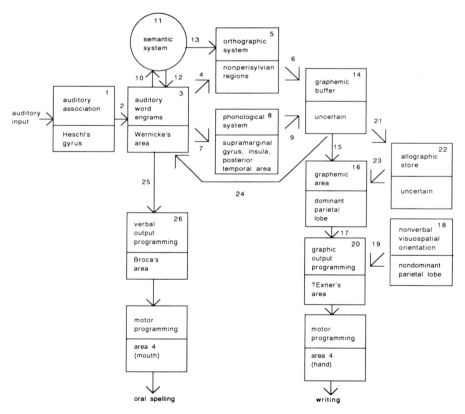

Figure 12.4. Outline of postulated neurolinguistic steps necessary to convert auditory (word) input into either oral spelling or written language. (From Roeltgen, 1993).

literature) are recognized: central agraphia and peripheral agraphia (Ellis, 1988; Ellis, Young, and Flude, 1987), paralleling the distinction between central alexia and peripheral alexia (Shallice and Warrington, 1980). Anatomically based and linguistically based agraphia syndromes are listed in Table 12.5).

Central Agraphia

Central agraphia affects one or more of the processes needed to generate spelling of familiar and unfamiliar words (and pseudowords). Central agraphia affects spelling in all output modes (handwriting, typing, oral spelling, spelling with cardboard letters, etc.). Several varieties of central agraphia can be distinguished.

Lexical (Surface) Agraphia

In some languages (such as English) two different systems are available for spelling—lexical and phonological (Beauvois and Derouesne, 1981; Hartfield and Patterson, 1983; Roeltgen, 1985; Roeltgen, Sevush, and Heilman, 1983; Shallice, 1981). The lexical system is used to spell orthographically irregular words (words that cannot be spelled by direct phonographemic methods—e.g., island) and ambiguous words (words with sounds that may be represented by multiple letters or letter clusters—e.g., phase), requiring the use of visual word images (Roeltgen and Heilman, 1984). The lexical system may also be used to spell orthographically

Table 12.5. Comparative Classification of Agraphias

ANATOMICALLY BASED CLASSIFICATION	LINGUISTICALLY BASED CLASSIFICATION
Aphasic Agraphias (classified by basic language disorder)	*Central Agraphias*
	Lexical agraphia
Agraphia in Broca aphasia (nonfluent agraphia)	Phonological agraphia
	Deep agraphia
Agraphia in Wernicke aphasia (fluent agraphia)	
Agraphia in conduction aphasia	
Mechanical Agraphias	*Peripheral Agraphias*
Motor agraphia	—
Pure agraphia	—
Spatial agraphia	Spatial (afferent) agraphia
Apractic agraphia	Apractic agraphia

regular words (e.g., editor). Dysfunction of the lexical system produces lexical (or surface) agraphia, a disorder characterized by difficulty in spelling irregular and ambiguous words but preserved ability to spell phonographically regular words.

In lexical agraphia, the patient's ability to write deteriorates as the orthographic ambiguity of the target word increases. Word frequency plays a decisive role, suggesting that the vulnerability of the whole-word orthographic units depends on the subject's premorbid competency in writing (Bub, Cancilliere, and Kertesz, 1985).

Patients with lexical agraphia tend to show a "regularization" of writing: the target word is written so that it can be phonologically correct, although orthographically incorrect (e.g., jelly → gely). Such errors indicate overuse of the phonographemic system and decreased use of visual word images. Bub and Chertkow (1988) emphasized that patients with lexical agraphia show variability in selecting an orthographic segment; at times they employ the correct principles of translation between sound and spelling but they can also fail to apply these phonographemic principles. In languages with a high homophonic heterography (e.g., French), this defect is particularly prominent. In Spanish language, with some homophonic but no homographic heterophony, lexical agraphia is uncommon and is simply called "dysorthography."

Lexical agraphia usually occurs following damage involving the left posterior angular gyrus and/or the parieto-occipital lobule (Roeltgen, 1985). Rapcsak, Arthur, and Rubens (1988), however, reported a case of lexical agraphia following damage to the left precentral gyrus. No definitive correlation of brain pathology with lexical agraphia is firmly accepted.

Phonological Agraphia
In phonological agraphia, the patient retains ability to write familiar words, both regular and irregular, but cannot spell nonwords. Even low-frequency words containing unusual spelling patterns are correctly written. In contrast, these patients cannot write legitimate pseudowords to dictation (Baxter and Warrington, 1985; Bub and Kertesz, 1982a; Hartfield, 1985). Their spelling errors are usually not phonologically correct but show some visual similarity to the target word (Roeltgen, 1983; Shallice, 1981). The existence of phonological agraphia supports the existence of a lexical writing system in addition to the graphophonemic system.

Roeltgen (1985) relates phonological agraphia to damage at the level of the supramarginal gyrus and the insula medial to it. Alexander and colleagues (1992), based on data from their own cases and some previously reported cases, propose that phonological agraphia can follow damage over a range of perisylvian cortical regions that share some role in central phonological processing.

Deep Agraphia

Deep agraphia refers to a writing disorder characterized by: (a) the inability to spell non-words and grammatical function words, (b) better spelling of high-image than of low-image nouns, and (c) semantic paragraphias (Bub and Kertesz, 1982b). Deep agraphia is often associated with phonological agraphia. The disorder follows damage to the supramarginal gyrus and insula but with extended lesions; the angular gyrus, however, is spared. It has been proposed that deep agraphia could represent a right-hemisphere writing process (Roeltgen, 1985), a hypothesis similar to that proposed for deep dyslexia (Benson, 1982).

Peripheral Agraphia

Peripheral agraphia shows defects specific to a single output mode. Most often, good oral spelling is combined with impaired handwriting (Baxter and Warrington, 1986; Papagno, 1992; Roeltgen and Heilman, 1983), although the reverse has also been reported (Kinsbourne and Warrington, 1965).

Writing requires generation of the spatial form of each letter in the correct sequence as well as skilled performance in the distribution of written materal in external space. Ellis (1988) refers to these letter distributions as allographs. An allographic code would specify the shape of a letter but not the overall dimension of the muscle system executing the response. In patients with peripheral agraphia, retrieval of the allographic code is impaired but knowledge of orthography is adequate. Their writing is thus affected by improper execution, although knowledge of the written code is preserved. Two prime varieties of peripheral agraphia are recognized.

Spatial Agraphia

Spatial agraphia, usually associated with right-hemisphere pathology, has been relatively well analyzed in the neuropsychology literature (Ardila and Rosselli, 1993a; Benson and Cummings, 1985; Ellis, Flude, and Young, 1987; Hécaen, Angelergues, and Douzenis, 1963; Hécaen and Marcie, 1974; Lebrun, 1985; Lebrun and Rubio, 1972; Simernitskaya, 1974). Lebrun (1976) discussed this writing disorder as "afferent agraphia." Spatial agraphia was described earlier with the classic agraphia syndromes.

Apractic Agraphia

Apractic agraphia produces disorder at the implementation of peripheral motor processes, the "graphic motor patterns" (Ellis, 1982). In apractic agraphia the product should be appropriate in spelling but letter malformations may be severe. Copying is usually normal. Several well-studied cases have been presented in the literature (Baxter and Warrington, 1986; Margolin and Binder, 1984; Papagno, 1992; Roeltgen and Heilman, 1983). Baxter and Warrington (1986) propose that the diagnosis of pure apractic agraphia requires a disturbance in writing but no disturbance of spelling or reading, or any other language problem, and that neither major apraxia nor visuoconstructional disturbance should be present.

Papagno (1992) described a patient with a posterior parietal ischemic lesion who had preservation of oral spelling and no impairment in oral language or any other cognitive skill except writing. In spontaneous writing as well as in written naming and writing to dictation, this patient frequently presented stroke and letter duplications or omissions and gap errors. Some letter substitutions and nonletters were also present. Both copying and transcription from uppercase to lowercase letters were impaired. Word length, imageability, frequency, and class of words were not pertinent factors. The apraxia for writing was present in the absence of any other form of apraxia.

Summary

Written language is a complicated, multifactorial function that is inadequately mastered by many individuals. Acquired defects in the production of written language can result from a wide variety of language and/or motor disturbances. The resulting disorder, agraphia, is usually based on a complicated mixture of language and motor abnormalities that makes precise analysis difficult. There are, however, distinct clinical attributes for the language and motor problems of agraphia, and at least some diagnostically useful information can be gathered from the study of agraphia.

13

Acalculia

· ·

Calculation, defined here as the operation of mathematical computation, demands a complex set of cognitive operations. Calculation originated as a form of counting but has developed into many different levels of number performance that resemble but can be distinguished from other cognitive activities (Klein and Starkey, 1987).

Global quantification, or *numerosity perception*, refers to the rough discrimination made between sets of different numbers of objects (Davis, Albert, and Barron, 1985). Global quantification does not represent a truly numerical process, however, because there is no one-to-one correspondence between the proposed number and the actual count.

Enumeration can be considered the most elementary type of numerical knowledge (Klein and Starkey, 1987). *Correspondence construction* is a form of enumeration in which the approximate number of objects in a set is identified for comparison with the number of objects in other collections. It implies but does not provide an exact one-to-one correspondence. *Counting* is a more sophisticated form of enumeration; a unique number-name is paired with each object in a collection, and the final number-name used represents the total for the entire collection. Arithmetic is an advanced numerical system that involves number permutability (e.g., adding, subtracting).

Historical Background—Calculation

Historically, human abilities in calculation almost undoubtedly developed from counting, which, as in child development, begins with the sequencing of the fingers—a correspondence construction (Hitch et al., 1987). In counting the fingers or toes, these digits are sequenced in a particular order, a basic procedure that is common to different cultures, both ancient and contemporary, throughout the world (Ardila, 1993; Cauty, 1984; Levy-Bruhl, 1910/1947). Thus, it is not surprising that mathematical disabilities and finger agnosia occur together in a clinical syndrome (Gerstmann, 1940). The word *digit* in English or *digito* in Spanish is derived from the Latin word *digitus,* which means both number and finger, and this combination is the probable reason that the decimal system has developed. Simultaneously (or at least close in time), decimal systems were devised in different countries (Sumeria, Egypt, India, and Crete) and distinct symbols were used to represent 1, 10, 100, and 1000 (Childe, 1936). There is, however, one intriguing exception. The Sumerians and later the Babylonians (about 2000 B.C.) developed both a decimal and a sexagesimal system in which a symbol represented the number 60 or any 60-multiple whereas a different symbol represented the number 10 or any 10-multiple. Sixty remains the base for most contemporary measures of time.

Computation, the ability to manipulate number language, has evolved in a spectacular fashion during the past few centuries. Sophisticated advances in calculus, geometry, physics, and mathematical logic have emerged. And from a technical point of view, the introduction of calculating machines including electronic computers has once again radically altered our competency to perform calculation tasks.

Individual variations in calculating abilities are both considerable and important. Some children fail to develop calculating capability, a developmental disability termed *developmental dyscalculia* (Shalev, Weirtman, and Amir, 1988; Slande and Russell, 1971). In contrast, *acalculia* is the acquired loss or impairment of the ability to perform calculating tasks based on brain pathology.

Because of the considerable individual variability in calculation abilities, demonstration and assessment of acalculia has always proved difficult. For example, a university professor of mathematics was forced into retirement because of a calculating impairment resulting from a right frontal tumor. However, he could still perform most mathematical tasks far better than any of the medical staff in the hospital. The staff was unable to design a test sufficiently stringent to demonstrate the patient's calculating impairment. (Ardila, personal observation).

Development of calculation skills in children provides some insight into the organization and processing of calculation capability in the brain. Human infants can recognize numerosity for small quantities (usually three to six items [Antell and Keating, 1983]), and the ability to construct correspondences emerges during the child's second year (Langer, 1986). At that age the child begins to use some number-names, developing the ability to count to three. The young child thus acquires knowledge of two basic principles of counting—a one-to-one principle (each object in a collection is paired with only one number name) and a stable-order principle (each number-name is assigned a permanent position in the list of numbers). At this age, however, they have not realized one principle of addition—that the final number-name used in a counting sequence refers to the cardinal value of the sequence (Klein and Starkey, 1987). This principle can be observed in 3-year-old children (Gelman and Meck, 1983). Number value strategies (e.g., when a new item is included the collection becomes larger and a new cardinal number-name will be given to the collection) are found in 3- to 5-year-old children but only for small quantities at first. Ability to add and subtract numerical quantities can be observed in first- or second-grade children, but more complicated mathematical manipulations (e.g., multiplying and dividing) are acquired only after a long and painstaking training period during the third to fifth school grades.

Additional factors add to the difficulty of demarcating acquired calculation disorders. A gender difference in calculation capability (males normally outperforming females) has been reported (Benbow, 1988), but the reason for this difference remains unclear. Calculating abilities strongly reflect educational and professional factors. A store cashier may perform basic arithmetic operations better than a professional engineer. As the use of pocket calculators for routine tasks increases, simple arithmetical skills are not practiced and a person's competency in these skills deteriorates. Currently, very few people are competent in using a slide rule, a commonly held skill a generation or two ago. The teaching of mathematics in school has changed considerably in the last few decades. "New mathematics," computer training, pocket calculators, and broad diversification of educational goals have all tended to decrease simple, "mental" calculating competency. Many contemporary humans are less literate in mathematical language than their parents (or even than they themselves were decades earlier).

Observations of illiterate individuals disclose that they use simple numerical concepts and easily handle money in their daily activities. Subtraction, however, is particularly difficult and tends to confuse illiterate individuals. They usually cannot multiply or divide, except by ten (e.g., 3, 30, 300, etc.) or by two, doubling and halving figures (e.g., 200, 100, 50, etc.). The ability to multiply and divide by ten or by two permits some simple arithmetic calculations. Illiterates make use of important everyday numerical facts such as dates (e.g., "Today is August 18, 1993"), time (e.g., "I work eight hours a day, from 8 A.M. to 4 P.M.; "I am 46 years old"), weight (e.g., "The cow weighs 350 kilograms"), and distance (e.g., "From my house to the park is five blocks"). Illiterates can also understand simple fractions (e.g., half, quarter, tenth). In brief, some calculation competency (counting, magnitude estimation, simple adding and subtracting) can be accomplished without knowledge of number language.

Arithmetical skills benefit from schooling, and basic calculating abilities, including counting and the four basic arithmetical operations, appear known to all literate individuals. Counting demands the concept of number as a quantity, the concept of bigger and smaller, and the concept of plurals; all three concepts are syntactic functions. Arithmetical manipulations (e.g., addition, multiplication) depend on syntactic rules plus a rigidly fixed semantic code. Basic calculation is, to a considerable degree, a language function.

The most widely used numerical system contains several particular features: (1) there are nine numerical symbols or digits; (2) 0 (zero) indicates the absence of quantity; (3) digits change in value based on their spatial position (e.g., tens, hundreds, thousands, and so on); (4) a new number always follows the preceding one; numbers are, consequently, infinite.

Historical Background—Acalculia

Most interest in acalculia (calculation disturbance caused by brain damage) has developed in the twentieth century (Kahn and Whitaker, 1991). Henschen (1926) coined the term *acalculia* and both collected and described cases of disturbances of calculation produced by focal lesions of the brain. Berger (1926) distinguished primary and secondary acalculia; primary acalculia indicated a defect in the calculating process, whereas secondary acalculia referred to a defect in a fundamental cognitive function such as memory, attention, etc. Gerstmann (1940) noted that when acalculia appeared with agraphia, right/left disorientation, and finger agnosia, the group of findings formed a clinical syndrome known since as the Gerstmann syndrome. All four components of the Gerstmann syndrome (including calculation impairment) were once explained as disorders of body schema (Schilder, 1935) occurring after dominant-parietal-lobe damage.

Advances in the study of acquired calculation disturbance came from the research of Hécaen and colleagues (Hecaen, 1962; Hécaen and Angelergues, 1961; Hécaen, Angelergues, and Houiller, 1961). Three distinct varieties of acquired calculation disorder were defined: (1) aphasic acalculia, an inability to read and write numbers; (2) spatial acalculia, an impairment of spatial positioning of digits, often accompanied by unilateral neglect; (3) anarithmetia, an inability to perform computational operations. Anarithmetia and aphasic acalculia were most often observed in cases of left pre-Rolandic damage, whereas spatial acalculia most characteristically followed right posterior hemisphere damage.

Additional varieties of acalculia have been suggested. Grewel (1960) described a frontal acalculia and denied that this problem is based on disorder of abstracting ability only; he suggested, instead, a general lowering of the patient's intellectual level plus a decreased ability to initiate mental activity. Some investigators suggest that the acalculia associated with the Gerstmann syndrome is a form of anarithmetia (Boller and Grafman, 1983, 1985) in which the patient has lost the hierarchic strata of numbers, mathematical relations cannot be integrated and mathematical signs cannot be recognized. Others, however (Benson and Denckla, 1969; Poeck and Orgass, 1966), have found an aphasic defect (verbal paraphasia) present in patients with the Gerstmann syndrome.

The distinction between aphasic acalculia and anarithmetia, although conceptually valid, may be difficult to establish and the suggested neuroanatomical topography of damage for the two entities often overlaps (Levin and Spiers, 1985). Thus, anarithmetia is often associated with aphasia, alexia, and agraphia (Poeck and Orgass, 1966).

Luria (1966, 1976a) presented a different interpretation for acalculia. He proposed that left posterior parietal or parietal-temporal-occipital lesions could produce components of spatial apraxia and spatial agnosia, semantic aphasia, and acalculia. Luria believed that the same cognitive defects were present in semantic aphasia and acalculia. Consequently, the two were necessarily associated.

Critchley (1953) and Cohn (1961) emphasized the spatial deficit in acalculia, particularly apparent in written calculations, and related the disturbance to parietal damage. Kinsbourne and Warrington (1962a) noted the simultaneous presence of computational, spatial, and symbolic errors in acalculia, and Luria (1966, 1973) further suggested that difficulties with calculation in patients with left parietal damage might be directly related to deficits in the grammatical structure (relationship) of complex numbers. Dahmen and colleagues (1982) studied calculation disorders in patients with Broca and Wernicke aphasia. Using factor analysis, they identified two main factors: numeric-symbolic, and visuospatial. They proposed that the less serious calculation defects found in patients with Broca aphasia were derived from linguistic defects, whereas the more severe calculation difficulties of Wernicke aphasia were derived from defects in visuospatial processing.

Several additional considerations in the study of acalculia deserve mention. Deloche and Seron (1982, 1984) postulated the existence of a double code (alphabetic and numerical) that was used in calculation. Using transcoding tasks designed to probe both codes, they observed lexical substitution errors (errors due to position in a series—such as 7 for 8) in the patients with Wernicke aphasia. Most calculation errors in the Wernicke aphasia patients were semantic deficits, however, based on lexical semantic errors in the reading and writing of numbers. Broca aphasia patients, in contrast, produced stack errors (e.g., 15 for 50) that were considered syntactic.

Boller and Grafman (1983, 1985) proposed that calculation defects can be explained in a variety of ways: (1) inability to appreciate the meaning of the names of the numbers; (2) visuospatial deficits that interfere with the spatial arrangement of numbers and with the mechanical aspects of the operations; (3) inability to remember mathematical facts and to use them appropriately; (4) defects in mathematical processing and/or in understanding the underlying operations. Inability to conceptualize quantities (numerateness) and to perform reverse operations (e.g., subtract, divide) were also noted. According to Boller and Grafman, angular gyrus acalculia (as in the Gerstmann syndrome) would feature the defects listed in points 2 and 4 above but could also be associated with the defects described for the first type (aphasic acalculia).

Jackson and Warrington (1986) found significant differences when they compared the arithmetic skills of patients who had suffered left-hemisphere damage with those who had right-hemisphere damage. The patients with left-hemisphere damage showed greater overall impairment and were more impaired in arithmetical language than in problem-solving.

Spiers (1987) critically reviewed neuropsychological approaches to acalculia and, from this review, proposed a classification of acalculia based on error analysis. Spiers's classification included (1) place-holding errors, (2) digit errors, (3) borrow-and-carry errors, (4) basic fact errors; (5) algorithm dysfunction, (6) symbol errors. Under each heading, from two to seven distinct types of errors could be demonstrated, suggesting that a sizable array of different problems can manifest as calculation impairment.

McCloskey and colleagues (McCloskey, Caramazzo, and Basili, 1985; McCloskey, Sokol, and Goodman, 1986; McCloskey and Caramazza, 1987; McCloskey, Aliminosa, and Sokol, 1991) proposed a general cognitive model of number processing and calculation. They separate the number-processing system (the mechanisms for comprehending and producing numbers) from the calculation system (the processing algorithms required to carry out a calculation). Facts (e.g., the multiplication tables), rules (e.g., $N \times 0 = 0$), and procedures (e.g., multiplying goes from right to left) are considered elements of the calculation system.

Even though arithmetical calculation is a complex cognitive activity demanding appropriate action of many subcomponents, the study of arithmetical impairments in brain-damaged patients produces a relatively restricted and comprehensible avenue for the study of information manipulation. Warrington (1982) was able to demonstrate a dissociation between arithmetical processing and the retrieval of computation facts. Selective deficits can be observed in the use of operational rules, in retrieving arithmetical facts and in carrying out calculation procedures (Caramazza and McCloskey, 1987; Ferro and Betelho, 1980). The analysis of patterns of impaired performance in single-case studies has enhanced the understanding of the cognitive processes used in calculation; models of both normal and abnormal processing of numbers and systems for calculation have been developed (Benson and Weir, 1972; Caramazza and McCloskey, 1987; Ferro and Botelho, 1980; McCloskey and Caramazza, 1987; Singer and Low, 1933; Warrington, 1982).

Table 13.1 presents a simplified classification of acalculia based on distinc-

Table 13.1. Types of Acalculia

Anarithmetia

Aphasic acalculia
  in Broca aphasia
  in Wernicke aphasia
  in conduction aphasia
  in extrasylvian aphasias

Alexic acalculia
  in parietal-temporal alexia
  in occipital alexia

Agraphic acalculia

Frontal acalculia

Spatial acalculia

tions between acalculia derived from a language deficit and acalculia related to other neuropsychological breakdowns; overlap exists. For instance, anarithmetia and aphasic acalculia often coexist; spatial deficits may be present in cases of anarithmetia; spatial acalculia resulting from right-hemisphere damage may be associated with an alexia that further interferes with calculating ability. Despite the absence of specificity, the proposed classification describes and contains the principal clinical syndromes of acalculia. A review of the standard tests of calculating ability is advisable before discussion of the individual types of acalculia listed in Table 13.1.

Tests of Calculating Competency

No single well-standardized test effectively assesses calculation defects; a variety of tasks must be included. The traditional technique—simply presenting problems and grading on the correctness of the subject's response—fails to demonstrate many problems and interpretation may be seriously misleading.

Counting forward and backward (1 to 20, 20 to 1) is an initial number language task (Seron and Deloche, 1987). Naming the number of fingers exposed by the examiner can be used to demonstrate number-word finding. Assessment of calculation competency should include written as well as mental tasks; the two operations may be dissociated. Testing of the subject's ability to read and to write numbers (single and multiple digits) can disclose both alexia and agraphia for numbers and may disclose spatial difficulties. Assessing the subject's competency at recognizing relations such as bigger/smaller (e.g., which number is bigger) not only demonstrates difficulty in recognizing numbers but probes the appreciation of quantity.

Basic arithmetical operations (addition, subtraction, multiplication, and division) should be performed both orally (e.g., "How much is $12 + 15$?") and in written form. Different levels of difficulty should be included (e.g., one, two, three or more digits). In oral testing, patients may be asked to perform successive operations (100 minus 7; and minus 7, and so on); instead of the standard 7, the numbers 3, 13, 17, etc. may be used to alter the level of difficulty. In written calculations, the ability to recognize arithmetical signs ($+$, $-$, $\times$, $:$, $=$, $/$) can be assessed. Some investigators have observed patients with isolated difficulty in the reading of arithmetical signs (Ferro and Botelho, 1980) and it is well to ask the patient to read the arithmetical signs and to explain their use. Patients may read the signs simply as "x" rather than "multiplied by" or "dash" rather than "minus," or provide a similarly concrete response, thus failing to recognize their mathematical context.

Transcoding tasks have been proposed as a means to assess calculation skills (Deloche and Seron, 1984). The patient is presented with a series of numbers of different levels of difficulty (3, 8, 37, 276, 1003) and asked to write them with the number-name (transcoding from numerical to verbal code), or vice versa. Both tasks challenge the subject's number language competency.

The alignment of numbers in columns (position in relation to other numbers) represents an essential element for the appreciation of the value of numbers. A simple test of this function requests that a list of dictated numbers be positioned for summing. Inability to align numbers to represent appropriate place-value is immediately evident, a significant factor in spatial acalculia (Cohn, 1961).

If the examiner presents the mathematical problems orally, the patient's ability to handle serial quantities and to use problem-solving techniques can be evaluated. Luria (1973) routinely used the problem: "There are eighteen books placed on two shelves; one shelf has double the number of the other; how many books are on each shelf?" When difficulties were observed, he asked the patient to repeat the problem. If the patient's response was incorrect, the problem was repeated until the basic idea was comprehended.

The subject's ability to recognize temporal variables may be informative. The patient can be asked questions about how long ago something happened (e.g., "How long have you been married?") or asked to appreciate the passage of time (e.g., "How long have we been talking?"), in addition to the usual questions concerning temporal orientation (e.g., "What year is it?," "When were you born?"). Arithmetical calculations using time (e.g., "How much time is there between 2:45 and 4:20?") probes use of 12-base arithmetic; this can prove difficult for some normal subjects, however, and is sensitive to educational level. Similarly, numerical appreciation of quantity is often difficult for normal subjects (e.g., "How much do you think an egg weighs?," "How long would a person take to walk a block at a normal speed?").

As a screening test, a few computation problems can be presented and if the patient is successful with the more difficult problems, acalculia is not a significant problem. If, however, the patient has difficulty, it is well to backtrack to probe a variety of arithmetical language and computational functions. Many distinct problems can interfere with calculation competency and, at least in some instances, variations of the disorder provide pertinent localizing information.

Types of Acalculia

Anarithmetia

Anarithmetia can be considered the basic disorder of computation. Among the disorders included in the category anarithmetia are the loss of mathematical concepts, inability to understand quantities, inability to use syntactic rules in calculation (e.g., "carry over"), and/or confusion of arithmetical signs causing defective performance of basic arithmetical operations. Some or all of these processes may be impaired.

In their seminal study of patients with acalculia, Hécaen, Angelergues, and Houiller (1961) found a considerable overlap between anarithmetia and impaired written number competency (alexia and agraphia for numbers). In addition, of their sample of seventy-two patients with anarithmetia, 62% were aphasic, 61% had visual constructive deficit, 54% had a demonstrable visual-field defect, 50% had some degree of general cognitive deterioration, 39% had verbal alexia, 37% had sensory impairment, 37% had directional confusion, and 33% had ocular motor disturbances. Although their sample was etiologically heterogenous, anarithmetia has been related to even more deficits.

Rosselli and Ardila (1989) analyzed acalculia in patients with left posterior parietal damage. Sign confusion was observed in 75% of the patients and all made errors in transcoding tasks, in successive operations, and in solving mathematical problems. Decomposition errors (e.g., 1223 was written as 12   23) and inversions (23 changed to 32) were noted in almost half of the subjects. In addition, order errors (7 changed to 8) and hierarchy errors (15 written as 50) were present in transcoding. All subjects had similar problems in language-oriented tasks.

Anarithmetia isolated from other linguistic deficits is sufficiently unusual as to be almost nonexistent, and only a few single-case reports of relatively pure anarithmetia have been published. Benson and Weir (1972) presented a well-educated patient who, following a focal left parietal lesion, was able to read numbers accurately, recognized arithmetical signs, could write numbers, and maintained his rote arithmetical knowledge (e.g., multiplication tables) but was unable to carry over. Ferro and Botelho (1980) described a patient who was unable to perform simple arithmetical operations based on inability to distinguish arithmetical signs. Takayama and colleagues (1994) described two subjects who had lost the ability to perform computation following small, focal embolic lesions involving the left posterior parietal cortex. The locus of pathology in cases with anarithmetia is generally regarded as the dominant angular gyrus, based on evidence gathered by Henschen (1922, 1926) and supported by Gerstmann (1940) and Benson (1994).

Luria (1973) correlated posterior parietal acalculia with a subject's inability to deal with complex grammatical relations, spatial concepts and/or numerical features. It has been suggested that most patients showing the acalculia of the Gerstmann syndrome also suffer at least some degree of extrasylvian sensory aphasia (Ardila, Lopez, and Solano, 1989). Acalculia, including loss of numerical concepts, routinely develops in patients with Alzheimer's disease, but always in conjunction with many additional cognitive deficits.

Aphasic Acalculia

Based on language impairment, difficulties in calculation can be demonstrated in all types of aphasia, and aphasic calculation deficits can usually be correlated with the basic language impairment that characterizes the aphasia syndrome.

Acalculia in Broca Aphasia

Dahmen and colleagues (1982) observed that Broca aphasia patients presented calculation disorders of a numeric-symbolic type derived from their linguistic impairment. Deloche and Seron (1982) stressed that in Broca aphasia the errors are stack errors (e.g., 15 read as 50) and are, therefore, syntactic. Rosselli and Ardila (1989) observed that all patients with Broca aphasia made errors in counting backwards and in successive operations (e.g., 100, 93, 86, . . . ; 1, 4, 7, . . .). Both hierarchy (reading) and order (writing) errors were demonstrated. Inversion errors were occasionally observed in number reading, and omission of grammatical function words was observed when the patients were given transcoding tasks. Carrying procedures were difficult and often confused.

The grammar and syntax of calculation are particularly impaired in patients with Broca aphasia and the production and maintenance of sequences is difficult. Just as disorder in the sequences of language is one characteristic of Broca aphasia, number sequences are similarly impaired. Although number language is difficult and often anomalous, the most fundamental calculating problem of Broca aphasia is a disorder of relationship (syntax).

Acalculia in Wernicke Aphasia

There is less accord on the cause of acalculia in Wernicke aphasia patients. Deloche and Seron (1984), in their study of calculation disorders in aphasics, found that Wernicke aphasia patients produced semantic errors in the reading and writing of numbers. Dahmen and colleagues (1982), on the other hand, suggested that calculation deficits in Wernicke aphasia can be correlated with a defect in visuospatial processing. Luria (1973) emphasized that calculation mistakes in acoustic-amnesic aphasia reflect verbal memory impairment, particularly notable in mathematical problem solving when the patient must retain multiple segments of the problem.

When the Wernicke aphasia patient is asked to recall numerical facts (e.g., "How many days are there in one year?"), paraphasic errors become evident. They show lexical errors in a variety of tasks. When writing numbers to dictation, Wernicke aphasia patients can produce completely irrelevant sequences (e.g., if "257" is dictated, the patient may say "820" but write "193"), suggesting impairment of both decoding and encoding of written numbers. In reading and writing numbers these patients may show decomposition errors (e.g., 463 is written "46 3"). Oral and written operations, successive operations and mathematical problem solving appear equally difficult for these patients. Number-language comprehension deficits, lexical access impairments, disordered visual-spatial processing, and defects in verbal memory may interfere with calculation tasks in Wernicke aphasia patients.

Acalculia in Conduction Aphasia

Calculation disturbance is frequently overlooked in patients with conduction aphasia but both oral and written mathematical operations tend to be disordered. Sequencing operations and mathematical problem solving tasks are impaired and even simple transcoding tasks (e.g., eighty-two to 82, and vice versa) are often failed. Order and hierarchy errors are observed in number reading, sequential order is often impaired, and the process of carryover is failed. Patients with conduction aphasia can even fail in reading arithmetical signs (Rosselli and Ardila, 1989).

Despite the many ways that patients with conduction aphasia may fail at calculation tasks, they often retain basic computational skills. Benson and Denckla (1969) demonstrated intact computation skills in a patient with conduction aphasia who had a severe verbal paraphasia for numbers. When given multidigit problems, the patient was asked to read the numbers aloud, present his intermediate products aloud, and then write his answer. All responses were incorrect. With the same problem, however, the patient invariably selected the correct response from a written list of possible answers. For example, when he was given a written problem "4 + 5" he read it aloud as 6 and 7, gave a verbal answer of "8" and a written answer of "5." When given a multiple-choice list he immediately (and confidently) chose 9 as the correct answer. This patient performed in a similar manner on considerably more complex multiplication and division problems; despite producing multiple paraphasic and paragraphic substitutions, his ability to select the correct answer from a multiple-choice list was preserved. In this case report of a patient with conduction aphasia, the acalculia was almost entirely based on language-processing disorder, not anarithmetia.

The neuroanatomical site of damage most commonly noted in cases of conduction aphasia lies close to the area suspected in anarithmetia (Benson and Weir, 1972; Takayama et al., 1994). The acalculia seen in the conduction aphasia case reported by Benson and Denckla, however, was apparently based on a language disorder, suggesting variability in the neuroanatomical locus of acalculia in conduction aphasia.

Acalculia in Extrasylvian Aphasias

Almost no reports correlate specific calculation defects with the varieties of extrasylvian aphasia, but calculation problems almost always accompany these aphasic syndromes. In pure extrasylvian motor aphasia, the difficulty in response initiation and/or maintaining the numerical sequence interferes with the calculating process to such a degree that any but the most elementary calculations are failed. The patient's ability to understand the problem and his basic computational knowledge, however, do not appear to be involved. In extrasylvian sensory aphasia the problem is far more complex. Damage to the parietal-temporal area, particularly the posterior angular gyrus (a common locus for extrasylvian sensory aphasia), is associated with anarithmetia plus a variety of aphasic number-gnosis complications. Serious acalculia is almost invariably present in extrasylvian sensory aphasia. Although rarely described in cases of mixed extrasylvian aphasia, the acalculia of this disorder combines the calculation problems of both the motor and sensory varieties of extrasylvian aphasia to produce a global acalculia.

Anderson, Damasio, and Damasio (1990) reported the case of a well-educated, right-handed woman who, following a circumscribed surgical lesion of the premotor cortex, developed a severe alexia and agraphia. Despite this, she easily read and wrote numbers and could perform written calculations without difficulty. Thus, dissociation of the ability to read and write language and to read and write numbers appears possible but is rare.

Alexic Acalculia

Calculation disorders in individuals with alexia vary with the type of reading disorder.

Acalculia in Parietal-Temporal Alexia

Parietal-temporal alexia includes an inability to comprehend written numbers and other written symbolic systems (e.g., computation signs). Acalculia results from this disability. Observation, however, shows that patients with parietal-temporal alexia have greater impairment in the reading of letters than in the reading of numbers and, although their written arithmetical operations may be globally impaired, their mental performance may be considerably better. A distinction between alexia and agraphia for numbers and anarithmetia is conceptually clear but is often difficult to establish. The topography of brain damage in parietal-temporal alexia and anarithmetia is similar (Levin and Spiers, 1985), focused in the left angular gyrus. In most instances parietal-temporal alexia is associated with alexia for both numbers and arithmetical signs plus an acquired disturbance in computation (anarithmetia). The combination produces a mixed and severe acalculia.

Acalculia in Occipital Alexia

The calculation problems seen in patients with occipital alexia are based on disturbances of number reading. They will comprehend individual numbers but they often have difficulty reading numbers composed of several digits. They tend to show decomposition errors (e.g., 27 is read aloud as "2–7") and hierarchy errors (50 is read as "5"). When reading numbers, patients with occipital alexia may read the first several digits of a sequence successfully but omit the remainder (5637 is read as "563"). This omission style suggests right-sided neglect. Written arithmetical operations are painstakingly slow for these patients and are often unsuccessful because of number-reading problems, visual exploration disorders, and/or impaired number alignment.

Unlike language reading, which traverses from left to right (at least in Western languages), arithmetical tasks typically move from right to left. The right visual field is often hemianopic in patients with occipital alexia and difficulties in directing gaze to the right or in attending to the right side of a line can occur. These mechanical difficulties not only produce right neglect but complicate the patient's already compromised performance in written arithmetical operations.

Agraphic Acalculia

Calculation disturbances can result from inability to write and the type of calculation difficulty can be correlated with a particular type of agraphia. In patient's with Broca aphasia, number agraphia will be nonfluent with both perseveration and order reversal. The agraphia for numbers shares the features observed in the patient's writing of letters, words, and sentences. Thus, numbers are written larger than necessary and are crudely formed. Inability to transcode from verbal to numerical, and vice versa, will be observed; both substitutions and omissions are evident. These patients have difficulty writing sequences of numbers (e.g., 1, 2, 3, . . .), a difficulty that is compounded if they are asked to present numbers in reverse order (e.g., 10, 9, 8, . . .).

In Wernicke aphasia, the patient produces a fluent agraphia for numbers that further complicates their number comprehension deficit and combines to produce errors when writing numbers to dictation. Lexical errors (numerical verbal paraphasias) are observed. Numbers that are well known to the patient (the current year, the patient's age) may be written adequately but even in such overlearned activities, lexical substitutions may occur.

In conduction aphasia paragraphic defects are evident in number writing. These patients frequently fail to convert the numbers they have heard into correct graphic form (paragraphia) although what they write is always a number. Order errors, hierarchy errors, inversions, and verbal paraphasias are observed in patients with conduction aphasia.

Frontal Acalculia

Calculation deficits resulting from frontal brain damage have been mentioned in the literature (Grewel, 1960; Luria, 1966) but, in the simple arithmetic operations used in most calculation tests, these mathematical difficulties are not readily evident. Patients with damage in the prefrontal regions display difficulties in mental operations (particularly serial and successive operations) and the solving of multistep mathematical problems (Rosselli and Ardila, 1989).

Difficulties in calculation tasks in patients with prefrontal damage correspond to three different types: (1) attention difficulties, (2) perseverations, (3) impairment of complex mathematical concepts. Some patients with severe frontal-lobe damage become semimute and apathetic; they will not provide an answer to a computation problem, but this may be entirely a motor response failure.

Attentional deficits produce difficulty in maintenance of the conditions of a task. When given the problem of the eighteen books placed on two shelves (Luria, 1973), the patient with frontal damage may make observations that the shelves are too small or may present an impulsive guess ("18 and 36" or "9 and 9"), apparently without monitoring his or her response. Perseveration may lead to incorrect responses; for example, when asked to subtract 7 from 100 and then continue to subtract 7 from the products, the patient may respond "93, 83, 73." Perseveration may also interfere with the reading and writing of numbers and in transcoding tasks. Numerical and verbal codes may be mixed (they begin to write numbers, then continue with number words).

Patients with frontal-lobe damage have difficulty handling multiple-step problems (e.g., "If you have a five-dollar bill and purchase three cans of Coca-Cola at 65 cents each, how much change will you receive?"), tending to lose one

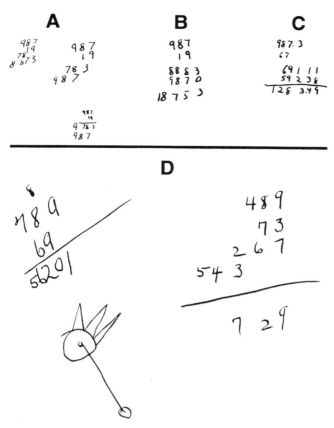

Figure 13.1. *(A,B,C):* Three attempts to multiply 987 × 19 by a young patient who suffered a gunshot wound in the right parietal area. All three show disordered spatial arrangement of numbers. *(D):* Calculation and drawing tests of a 62-year-old patient who suffered a large right-hemisphere cerebrovascular accident. The numbers on the left show disturbed placement of numbers and the "daisy" drawing demonstrates left hemi-neglect. Three years later (numbers on right) there was no improvement in number placement. (From Cohn, 1961).

or more portions. They may correctly analyze and solve each single step but offer a wrong answer based on omission or misplacement of part of the problem. The professional mathematician with a right frontal tumor mentioned earlier in the present chapter provides an example; although he easily performed routine arithmetical tasks, his ability to perform the multiple steps needed to solve advanced calculus problems, his professional activity, was lost (Ardila, personal observation).

Spatial Acalculia

Spatial acalculia has been recognized as a specific type of acalculia (Hécaen, Angelergues, Houiller, 1961), most often occurring after right-hemisphere damage, particularly when the parietal lobe is damaged. Spatial acalculia is frequently associated with left hemi-neglect, topographagnosia, facial recognition disorder, constructional disturbance, and related visuospatial disorders (Grafman et al., 1982; Hécaen, 1962; Rosselli and Ardila, 1989). Patients with a spatial acalculia perform much better in orally presented than in written arithmetical tasks. They have no difficulties in number language, counting, simple mental mathematical operations, or successive operations. When they read numbers, however, left neglect may lead to fragmentation (e.g., 23 is read as 523); their reading of complex numbers in which the spatial position is critical may be impaired (e.g., 1003 read as 103), and numbers may be reversed (e.g., 32 read as 23) (Ardila and Rosselli, 1990a).

The spatial problem becomes evident in the writing of numbers. Exclusive use of the right side of the page, reiteration of numbers (e.g., 227 written as "22277"), production of extra strokes (particularly in writing the number 3), inability to maintain a straight written line, spatial disorganization, and writing over a previously used segment may be noted in patients with spatial acalculia. Reiteration of letters and strokes is observed in transcoding from number to written code and left neglect omissions are common. In the performance of written arithmetical operations, these patients understand how to carry (or to borrow) but mislocate the carried quantity. Their ability to align numbers in columns is often impaired (see Figure 13.1). A difficulty in remembering the multiplication tables, although unexpected, is common in these patients. Whether this problem represents a disorder in the use of automatic language (Luria, 1976b) or indicates a difficulty in spatial visualization of the multiplication tables remains unsettled.

Two additional calculation problems can be observed following right-hemisphere damage. First, these patients may mix computational procedures; for instance, when subtracting, these patients may add. Second, despite the impossible incorrectness of the resulting answers, the patient is neither surprised nor embarrassed. A similar unconcern about mistakes has been reported in children with developmental dyscalculia (Strang and Rourke, 1985).

Summary

Quite different types of calculation disorder can be observed with focal brain pathology. Some of the impairments can be correlated with the patient's language deficits (oral or written) and others are apparently related to visuospatial defect or prefrontal deficit. In some cases, there seems to be a primary deficit in the cognitive task of computation (anarithmetia).

Although calculation has a strong relationship to language, many other factors affect calculation competency. The phrenological concept of a calculation center in the brain cannot be supported; neither can the equally ancient idea of a holistic basis for all higher mental activities. The study of acalculia clearly indicates that many different brain areas participate in calculation and just as clearly shows that damage in one of these areas tends to produce a disorder that is clinically distinct from that produced by damage to another of the areas. By studying the various defects of calculation, one can gain a relatively simple insight into the complex neural patterns needed to carry out cognitive functions.

14

Anomia

· ·

Disordered word finding (anomia) easily ranks as the most common language impairment. Everyone complains from time to time that they are unable to find the appropriate name and this normal problem can be greatly magnified by brain injury. Word-finding deficits are noted and complained about by patients with structural damage to any cerebral area in either hemisphere. Virtually every aphasic patient suffers some degree of naming disturbance; however, the characteristics of the word-finding problem can vary considerably in the different aphasia syndromes. These differences represent a potentially valuable guide in the diagnosis and therapy of aphasia and can be a useful tool for linguistic investigation.

It is important to bear in mind that *anomia* is a term with a double meaning in aphasiology. In one usage, the term is synonymous with naming disorder; in this broad sense all aphasic patients are anomic. Schuell, Jenkins, and Carroll (1962) found anomia to be the most prevalent general factor in aphasic disorders, and naming difficulties are the most permanent residual deficit in chronic aphasics. When used in the broad sense of a word-finding disorder (e.g., decreased performance on a confrontation naming task), *anomia* is not of localizing value (Benson and Geschwind, 1976, 1985). In attempts to be more specific, some aphasiologists limit use of the term to those patients whose word-finding difficulty leads to circumlocutions and/or verbal paraphasias as observed in some patients with fluent aphasia. In this more tightly defined sense, *anomia* becomes synonymous with anomic aphasia (Benson and Geschwind, 1971; Goodglass and Kaplan, 1972; Kertesz, 1985), nominal aphasia (Head, 1926), or amnesic aphasia (Hécaen, 1972; Luria, 1976a,b). It is important to keep in mind that naming difficulties, often called anomia, are present in all aphasics but that the term *anomia* is also used to refer to a particular aphasia syndrome (anomic aphasia).

The complexity of word-finding disorders was illustrated by Kohn and Goodglass (1985), who analyzed and attempted to categorize naming disorders that occurred in five groups of patients with different types of aphasia (Broca, Wernicke, conduction, posterior anomia, and frontal anomia). When these patients were shown pictures to name, they all had problems but the style of naming errors differed between the groups. Verbal semantic paraphasias and multiword circumlocutions were most frequent in patients with posterior anomia; patients with conduction, Broca, or Wernicke aphasia tended to produce more phonemic paraphasias. Failure to respond was most common with Broca aphasia, whole-part errors with frontal anomia, and poor phonemic cueing with Wernicke aphasia. Unrelated responses were occasionally observed in patients with Wernicke aphasia, and perseverations occurred in patients with frontal anomia. Each aphasic group had naming difficulties involving characteristic errors, but the errors were not exclusive to the group.

Naming difficulties can result from a deficit at different stages of the naming process: perception (decoding), storage, selection, retrieval, or actual production of the word (encoding) (Barton, Maruszewski, and Urrea, 1969; Benson, 1979c). Furthermore, acquired naming difficulties can be restricted to a specific semantic category (Benson, 1988a) and even to a particular modality of presentation (Brown, 1972). Naming errors can result from the patient's inability to perceive or to identify the target object and as such can be considered a perceptual or agnosic defect. Chapter 15 includes a clinical view of the neural basis for word finding based on varieties of anomia. Word finding is a complicated process and a simple cataloging of right or wrong answers to a confrontation naming task does not provide an adequate picture of anomia. In this chapter several distinct varieties of word-finding defect will be described.

Classifications of Anomia

Anomia has been classified in various ways (e.g., Benson, 1979c, 1988a; Brown, 1972; Gainotti, 1987; Gainotti, Silveri et al., 1986; Geschwind, 1967b; Kremin, 1988; Weinstein and Keller, 1973). All the schemes are based on clinical distinctions between subtypes of naming disorder. Table 14.1 outlines a differential classification of naming errors compiled from earlier schemes, augmented by more recent information. Wherever possible, the types of naming disorders have been associated with aphasia syndromes.

Table 14.1. Classification of Anomia

TYPE OF ANOMIA	ASSOCIATED APHASIA OR AGNOSIA SYNDROME
Word Production Anomia	
Prefrontal anomia	Extrasylvian motor aphasia-Type I
	Extrasylvian motor aphasia-Type II
Articulatory initiation anomia	Broca aphasia
	Extrasylvian motor aphasia-Type I
	Extrasylvian motor aphasia-Type II
Articulatory reduction anomia	Broca aphasia
Paraphasic anomia	Conduction aphasia
Phonemic disintegration anomia	Wernicke aphasia
Word Selection Anomia	Extrasylvian sensory aphasia-Type I
Semantic Anomia	Extrasylvian sensory aphasia-Type II
Disconnection Anomia	
Category-specific anomia	
Color anomia	Color agnosia
Finger (body part) anomia	Autotopagnosia
Other types	
Modality-specific anomia	
Visual anomia	Visual agnosia
Tactile anomia	Astereognosis
Auditory anomia	Auditory nonverbal agnosia
Gustatory anomia	Gustatory agnosia
Olfactory anomia	Olfactory agnosia
Callosal anomia	

Word Production Anomia

Difficulty in producing (encoding) words is a characteristic of aphasia based on anterior language area damage, specifically Broca's area, the left supplementary motor area, and/or the cortex anterior to or above Broca's area. Difficulties in name production observed in these extrasylvian motor aphasias involve several different aspects of word formulation: the selection of the word, the initiation of the motor speech activity, the production of the required articulatory movements, and, finally, the correct sequencing of phonemes in the word. One or several of these defects are observed in the verbal output of most patients with dominant-hemisphere frontal brain damage.

Prefrontal Anomia

Characteristic word-finding problems are seen in patients with lesions that involve dominant-hemisphere prefrontal areas. A decreased number of words will be produced in category-naming tasks (see Chapter 6) but several other word-finding problems may also be noted. Patients with left prefrontal cortical damage that produces either extrasylvian motor aphasia-Type I or extrasylvian motor aphasia-Type II may show any of three types of naming errors:

1. Fragmentation (whole-part errors) (Kohn and Goodglass, 1985). A fragmented response (e.g., calling a green butterfly "grass") can result from a unilateral attention defect, a visual exploration disorder based on damage to the frontal eye field (Brodmann area 8) and/or from impulsivity (i.e., the response is given without exploration of the whole picture or object) (Yarbus, 1965).

2. Perseveration. The patient tends to repeat a name which he has previously produced (e.g., after correctly naming the ear, a patient calls the mouth an "ear"). Perseveration represents a sign of severe brain damage and may be a particularly important sign of prefrontal damage (Stuss and Benson, 1986).

3. Extravagant verbal paraphasias. These appear to result from a free association of ideas (e.g., a patient names the index finger as "the collector" because it is used for pointing at someone who owes you money).

Articulatory Initiation Anomia

In both types of extrasylvian motor aphasia (that seen with dominant supplementary motor area, and that following frontal cortical involvement), the patient may manifest great difficulty initiating any movements, including utterances. The resulting word-finding disorder has been termed articulatory initiation anomia (Benson, 1979a). The patient produces names only after apparent effort and may use incorrect phonemes. The supplementary motor area appears crucial to the initiation of intentional motor activity, including motor speech (Botez and Barbeau, 1971; Goldberg, 1985). Clinically, patients with damage in the left supplementary motor area show the greatest problems initiating the motor articulatory movements required to produce the words. Considerable clinical evidence indicates that disconnection of the supplementary motor area from Broca's area also interferes with initiation of articulation (Alexander and Benson, 1991; Benson, 1988a; Freedman, Alexander, and Naeser, 1984; Rubens, 1976). In clinical practice, combinations of prefrontal anomia and articulatory initiation anomia are frequent.

Articulatory Reduction Anomia

In Broca aphasia, semantically meaningful names are better preserved than less meaningful names and grammatical words but confrontation naming is routinely defective. A diverse variety of additional naming disturbances can be demonstrated in Broca aphasia patients, some of which can be characterized as evidence of reduced articulatory competency. Kohn and Goodglass (1985) found that patients with Broca aphasia produced phonemic paraphasias, unrecognizable words (nonwords), and even semantic paraphasias when given picture-naming tasks. In addition to prefrontal and articulatory initiation problems, they documented a verbal-output deficit reflected in slow, effortful speech, simplification of syllabic clusters, and phonemic assimilations (i.e., a patient reiterates a previously produced phoneme in a following syllable or anticipates a phoneme intended for a future syllable). Reduction of the repertoire of phonemes and syllables can be so severe in Broca aphasia that expressive language is severely restricted, even to a single syllable.

Negated responses (refusal to name) are frequent in patients with Broca aphasia but can often be overcome with phonemic and/or contextual cues. Phonetic deviations are evident; they may be so severe that the phonemic category is wrongly perceived or sufficiently mild to produce an apparent phonemic paraphasia (Buckingham, 1979a), and unrecognizable words can result from multiple distortions of the target word.

Paraphasic Anomia

In conduction aphasia, the patient's spontaneous language may be relatively preserved whereas naming difficulties become evident. Literal paraphasias (substitution of phonemes) are apparent in spontaneous speech and become even more prominent when the patient attempts to name. The produced name often has the correct number of syllables, but if it contains one or more literal paraphasias the response is clearly incorrect. The patients often attempt self-correction of the deviations, leading to progressive approximations toward the target word (*conduit d'approche*). In contrast, automatized language is produced without apparent effort. A name that cannot be produced during a naming task may be produced easily during casual conversation or when included in an automatized sequence. Cueing is of little help. The patient often states that he knows the target name, but does not know how to say it. In most instances, this can be substantiated by the patient's comprehension of the name (e.g., if the name is offered by the examiner, the patient will correctly point to an object that he could not name).

Phonemic Disintegration Anomia

Naming disorders are common but not consistent in Wernicke aphasia. Semantic substitutions (e.g., head for dog), jargon (e.g., gopf for dog), and augmentations (e.g., dog-wog for dog) may be intermixed with the patient's refusal to answer. In some patients with Wernicke aphasia, a disorder termed phonemic disintegration can be observed. When the problem is sufficiently severe a phonemic jargon

(jargon aphasia) is produced. More often the Wernicke aphasia patient's verbal output is fluent—abundant and well articulated with good prosody and no apparent effort. Grammatical connectors are not only used, but frequently overused; phonetic distortions are not evident, and the number of nouns is reduced in the utterances. The word-finding defect appears most prominently as excessive phonemic paraphasias during attempts to produce names (neologisms). Unrelated responses are occasionally observed in these patients, but cueing is of little help (Kohn and Goodglass, 1985). The patient has difficulty reproducing the phonemic sequence of the target word and may not recognize the word when it is presented by the examiner. The correct decoding and phonological sequence of the lexical units appear impaired (Luria, 1966).

Word Selection Anomia

Word selection anomia, in its purest form, occurs with fully normal language function except for word-finding pauses, circumlocutions, and sheer failure to name. Repetition and comprehension are relatively normal and true language deficit is only observed in tests of naming. Pointing to objects when the name is given is quick and correct, and the patient often describes the use of an object that he cannot name, indicating that the problem is not based on visual agnosia. Almost invariably, structural pathology in cases with word selection anomia involves the posterior inferior portion of the temporal lobe (Brodmann area 37) and/ or the surrounding posterior temporal and anterior occipital tissues (Benson, 1988a; Luders, Lesser, and Hahn, 1991). Word selection anomia can be considered a form of memory retrieval disorder; the patient easily repeats and understands the word when it is presented by the examiner, indicating both intact word processing and word memory storage functions, but cannot retrieve the name (on command or on confrontation). Cueing, either phonetic or contextual, rarely aids the patient's ability to retrieve the name.

Semantic Anomia

The main characteristic that distinguishes semantic anomia and word selection anomia is that the patient with semantic anomia not only fails to name objects but also fails to identify (point to) the object when the name is presented to him. This is a two-way deficit in which it can be said that the word has lost its symbolic meaning. Just as in word selection anomia, the patient's language repetition is normal; he easily repeats the target name but cannot extract the meaning of the word. Semantic anomia is observed in extrasylvian sensory aphasia when the parietal-occipital area, particularly the angular gyrus (Brodmann area 39), is involved. Semantic (verbal) paraphasias and circumlocutions are frequent. Semantic anomia has been described as the aphasia associated with dementia of the Alzheimer type (Cummings et al., 1985). Patients with semantic anomia have difficulty categorizing (e.g., separating items such as clothing, furniture, tools, etc. into conceptual groupings) and cannot produce a representation of an object when presented with the name (e.g., "Draw the image that comes to mind when you hear the word 'dog' ") (Ardila, Lopez, and Montanes, 1983).

A linguistic distinction between word selection anomia and semantic anomia has been proposed by Gainotti and colleagues (Gainotti, 1987; Gainotti, Carlomagno, et al., 1986; Gainotti, Silveri, et al., 1987) who distinguished two varieties of aphasic anomia: (1) Some anomics have no lexical comprehension disturbance. The deficit lies outside the semantic-lexical system, probably at the level in which the lexical item corresponding to the retrieved semantic representation is formed into the appropriate phonological form (word selection anomia). (2) Other anomics have a lexical-comprehension disorder. This indicates a deficit within the semantic-lexical system, either a problem accessing the semantic representation or a loss of information at the level of the lexical representation (semantic anomia). In Gainotti's first variety, the disorder corresponds to a verbal memory retrieval deficit; in the second, the disruption involves the semantic field of the words.

Disconnection Anomia

Three distinct variations of word-finding defect can best be described as examples of specific neural pathway disconnections.

Category-Specific Anomia

In category-specific anomia, the word-finding difficulty involves a specific linguistic or semantic word category. Broca aphasics have greater difficulty naming actions and using verbs than in naming objects. Wernicke aphasics present the opposite pattern: they find it easier to use verbs and to name actions than to produce object names (Luria, 1976a,b; Miceli et al., 1984). These rather gross categorization differences help distinguish anterior aphasias (pre-Rolandic) from posterior aphasias.

Additional, more-specific category-naming problems are seen in some brain-damaged patients. In general, *category-specific anomia* refers to a state in which the patient has more difficulty naming items belonging to one specific category than items belonging to other categories. The best-known example is color anomia. Patients with color-naming disorder based on mesial occipital lesions (frequently associated with occipital alexia), although unable to name colors on confrontation or to select the appropriate color when the name is presented, have little or no difficulty naming objects or body parts. Many of these subjects can use color names correctly in conversation (e.g., "Tomatoes are red") and can demonstrate intact color perception by accurately categorizing colors. The two-way (visual-verbal/verbal-visual) state has been called color agnosia (Benson, 1979a; Schnider et al., 1994) and color anomia (Damasio, 1985).

Other sensory-dependent categories may also be preferentially involved in category-specific anomia. In cases of autotopagnosia, most often based on left parietal damage, an anomia with maximum difficulty naming body parts is observed; the subject can name colors and external objects (e.g., room objects) much better than body parts (Frederiks, 1985). Goodglass and colleagues (1966) gave aphasic patients a naming test divided into five distinct categories: objects, letters, numbers, actions, and colors. They found that selective impairment (or selective sparing) of naming in specific categories was more the rule than the exception. Berndt (1988a) reported a study that corroborated the longstanding clinical observation that naming can be more difficult for some specific word categories. Warrington (1981) has noted that some patients had selective difficulty in understanding abstract but not concrete words, whereas other patients showed the opposite pattern. Some of these patients had difficulty naming animals and foods but no trouble naming inanimate objects (Warrington and Shallice, 1984). One patient could name in the categories of animals, flowers, and food but not in inanimate objects (Warrington and McCarthy, 1983). Hart, Berndt, and Caramazza (1985) described a patient with a naming deficit that involved fruits and vegetables, and Temple (1986) described a 12-year-old child with an anomia that particularly affected the category of animals. In all instances, the subject's naming in other categories was relatively, but not absolutely, superior.

Clearly in the case of color naming and less clearly for the other category-specific anomias, the problem represents a neuroanatomical disconnection in which the properly received and processed perception cannot be transmitted to a brain area essential for the cross-modal association needed for name production.

Modality-Specific Anomia
Modality-specific anomia (Brown, 1972) refers to an inability to name objects presented in one sensory modality but not when the same object is presented via a different sensory modality. Although resembling category-specific anomia, modality-specific anomia involves a single sensory modality, not a cognitive category (Goodglass, Barton, and Kaplan, 1968).

Most objects can be known (recognized) in different ways; relatively few are known solely through a single sensory modality. Thus, although an individual building is identified primarily through visual knowledge and can only be named on visual presentation, many common items (e.g., coins, keys, pens, or combs) are not only recognized visually, but also through tactile and/or auditory sensations. Many coins are designed so that they can be recognized by touch (size, shape, serrated edges). The mental representation of a coin appears more complex than the mental representation of a building because coins are experienced through at least two different sensory modalities. Similarly, experience with food is multimodal. Ice cream is easily recognized through sight, taste, temperature, and texture. A cigarette can be identified (named) when presented through visual, tactile, or olfactory senses and a telephone has visual, auditory, and tactile representations. A subject's knowledge of most objects represents combinations of multiple (two or more) sensory modalities (Corballis, 1991; Konorski, 1969) and one's ability to name objects usually reflects this multiple sensory background. Although a stimulus may be offered in only one sensory modality, other associations may be used in the word-finding process. Unfortunately, in aphasia assessment, naming disorders are often tested only by visual presentation. Rarely are tactile, auditory, olfactory, or gustatory modalities evaluated.

An example of a case of modality-specific anomia would be a patient who can name an object presented visually but not when it is placed in his hands—a tactile anomia. Most such occurrences are called agnosia by clinicians. Visual agnosia is characterized by an inability to name visually presented objects that are readily named when presented for tactile or auditory perception (Farah, 1990; Grüsser and Landis, 1991, Rubens and Benson, 1971). The patient with visual agnosia may not recognize a coin on visual presentation but recognizes and names it when placed in his hands or when hearing the jingling sound made by multiple coins. *Astereognosis* and *auditory agnosia* (Schnider et al., 1994) refer to a patient's inability to recognize tactile or auditory presentations of objects, with a spared ability to recognize (and name) them when visually presented. These modality-specific disorders (visual agnosia, auditory agnosia, and astereognosis) represent unimodal perceptual disorders (Benson, 1994) and give rise to modality-specific anomias. In each instance, preservation of primary sensation must be demonstrated if the naming disorder is to be considered a modality-specific anomia (agnosia) rather than sensory receptive loss (i.e., blindness, deafness, cortical sensory loss).

Gustatory anomia and olfactory anomia are rarely investigated (Konorski, 1969) but both can be demonstrated. For example, Lopera and Ardila (1992) reported a patient with a bilateral mesial temporal-occipital lesion who stated that he could not recognize (or name) what he was eating but could discern tasty from non-tasty food and who maintained his premorbid food preferences. His naming of foods on visual presentation, although impaired, was much better; he could name an apple on sight but not by taste and he noted that when seeing a food he could not imagine what its taste would be.

Olfactory anomia most often represents a peripheral sensory problem but can follow brain damage. The patient cannot name an odor (e.g., coffee, a flower) but does name the substance when it is presented visually. Whether this state can occur in the absence of anosmia remains somewhat uncertain, however, as it is almost impossible to distinguish the peripheral from the central functions.

Modality-specific visual anomia is readily identified as a disconnection syndrome. With proper techniques, examples of modality-specific anomia based on disconnection in other systems can also be proved. In most instances, however, the causative lesion encompasses too large a territory for clear demonstrations.

Callosal Anomia

Following surgical separation of the corpus callosum, the disconnection of the two hemispheres produces a callosal anomia, an inability to name objects palpated by the nonpreferred (almost always left) hand (Gazzaniga and Sperry, 1967; Geschwind and Kaplan, 1962). With this same hand, however, the patient can (by palpation) after-select the item from an array of objects, demonstrating that the object was both recognized and remembered but could not be named. In this situation the right hemisphere has correctly analyzed the tactile information but isolation (separation) from the linguistically dominant hemisphere does not allow matching of the right hemisphere's perception of the object with its spoken name (Bogen, 1969). This clinical state has also been reported following anterior cerebral artery infarction and in cases with acute hydrocephalus producing compression of the corpus callosum (Bogen, 1986; Geschwind, 1965). Tactile naming is not the only disturbed function in cases of total callosal section. Gazzaniga and Sperry (1967) presented pictures of nameable objects to the left visual field (by tachistoscope) of subjects who had undergone callosal section to control epileptic seizures. When visual material was presented to the left visual field only, these patients could not name the pictured object but their left hand could pick up the correct object from an array, demonstrating an anomia based on visual disconnection (Gazzaniga and Sperry, 1967).

Summary

This chapter has looked at word finding on the basis of the discrete variations in naming disturbance that can follow damage to specific brain sites. The broad variety, both of types of word-finding defect and of anatomical sites that play a role in word finding, indicates that the process of providing a name for a perceived item is a complex task which requires activity in many brain regions. The neural system(s) operational in naming appear to have considerable redundancy; isolated lesions may affect one type of naming skill but leave others uninvolved or only mildly disturbed. Anomia is present, to some degree, in all aphasic patients but it cannot be characterized merely as a pass/fail score on a test of naming competency. Qualitative differences in word-finding defects are of significance for both neuroanatomical and linguistic investigations of language.

15

Neural Basis of Language Functions

· ·

At least since the time of Gall, a focal neuroanatomical basis for language has been conjectured. Gall's view of a specific cortical locus for language was substantiated, in spirit if not in precise anatomy, by the clinical studies of Broca, Wernicke, and their followers. However, his full premise that a cortical mosaic consisting of discrete organs (centers), each performing a specific cognitive function, was not substantiated. The brain-as-a-whole interpretation (that all higher mental functions such as language are performed as a single operating unit—the mind) remained standard before and after the nineteenth-century language localization efforts, the holistic explanation has proved equally unsuccessful. Current views, borrowing on information theory and the mechanistic designs of electronic computers but featuring both neuroanatomical and neurophysiological demonstrations, hold that language is a product of cognitive networks with processes distributed over a complex neuroanatomical architecture (Edelman, 1989; Goldman-Rakic, 1990; Mesulam, 1990). The distributed-network concept has considerable potential; to establish a neural basis for language, however, the neural networks underlying language function must be defined. This chapter will attempt to outline parameters of language-dedicated cortical networks based on clinical observations and apply this information to individual language functions.

Hemispheric specialization, a factor that is basic to the distributed processing of cognitive networks, has proved crucial to the study of language function. Hemispheric lateralization of language was discussed in Chapter 3 and only a reminder is needed here. For at least 150 years it has been known that the left hemisphere is crucial for language function. It has become increasingly well recognized, however, that the right hemisphere also participates in language functions, albeit in a different manner. Both the nature and the degree of the right hemisphere's participation remain controversial, and an accurate determination is difficult because both cerebral hemispheres participate in most cognitive networks.

Surgical (or pathological) section of the corpus callosum can effectively interrupt cross-callosal networks and provides evidence that separation of the hemispheres does not produce aphasia. Thus, fibers coursing through the corpus callosum are not essential for basic language functions. Alterations in the overall production of language do occur following section of the corpus callosum, however, and carefully designed experiments have demonstrated that, to a limited degree, the isolated right hemisphere can perform some language functions (Zaidel, 1985). The study of individuals with agenesis of the corpus callosum indicates that pathways other than the corpus callosum can perform interhemispheric transfer of the signals used for language formulation (Gott and Saul, 1978). Both cerebral hemispheres participate in normal language function but in a skewed manner, with a strong left-hemisphere predominance.

Neural Basis of Higher Cortical Function

The brain area most crucial for human language, the cortex, remains largely unexplored. Seventy percent of all neurons in the central nervous system are said to be located in the cortex (Nauta and Feirtag, 1986), and over 75% of these are in what is termed "association cortex." Although the gross topography and cytoarchitectonics of the cortex have been mapped (Brodmann, 1908, 1912; von Bonin and Bailey, 1947; Vogt and Vogt, 1919), the functional interconnections of association cortex areas have only begun to be traced; this work has been hampered by the unavailability of human specimens for in vivo neuroanatomical and functional investigations. Similarly, scientific descriptions of cortical functions remain incomplete. Moderately comprehensive descriptions of elementary sensory and motor functions are available in the basic neuroanatomy literature, but the pertinent components of such high-level cognitive functions as language, verbal memory, and executive control are still being developed. Any attempt to define the cognitive networks that process language, therefore, demands speculation.

Neuroanatomical Divisions of Cortex

The major neural systems for monitoring external sensation—visual, auditory, somesthetic—traverse varied subcortical courses before they reach the cortex. The three neural systems synapse and undergo processing in separate areas of the thalamus; each then proceeds to an area of cortex that is not only separate from the others but dedicated to the processing of a single sensory modality (see Figure 15.1). In a reversed but similar manner, motor responses are conducted out of the cortex from a single totally dedicated cortical area. These four areas of *primary cortex* (visual, auditory, somesthetic, and motor) categorize and transfer stimuli to the next processing step in the neural circuit for that modality.

Pathways from a primary cortical area connect only with neurons in nearby areas, also dedicated solely to a single sensory or motor modality. These secondary processing areas, termed *unimodal association cortex*, occupy a vast amount of the neocortex, from which they carry out essential, albeit modality-restricted, functions. Figure 15.2 presents a graphic outline of the unimodal association cortex. The final product of the many synaptic loops that connect the neural aggregates of the unimodal association cortex is a unimodal percept, a perception of an externally presented stimulus that remains within the single sensory domain.

From the unimodal association cortex, multiple projections interconnect a variety of cortical areas. Most fibers carrying unimodal percepts course to the nearby (posterior) or distant (anterior) *heteromodal association cortex*. The posterior region is also known as cross-modal, polymodal, multimodal, or intermodal association cortex to designate its prime function, the intermixing of unimodal percepts. Posterior heteromodal association cortex occupies a junction where pathways conducting percepts from the three external unimodal sensory areas can be

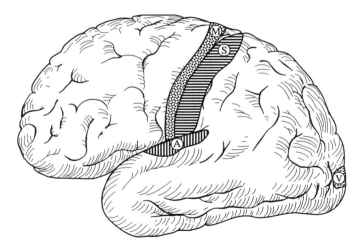

Figure 15.1. Artist's rendition of primary cortex. *(V):* primary visual cortex (Brodmann area 17); *(A):* primary auditory cortex (Brodmann area 41, 42); *(S):* primary somesthetic cortex (Brodmann area 3, 1, 2); *(M):* primary motor cortex (Brodmann area 4).

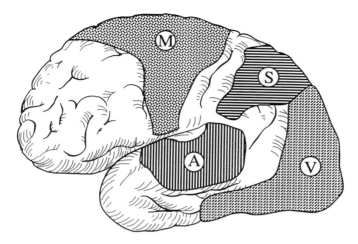

Figure 15.2. Artist's rendition of unimodal association cortex: *(V)* visual association cortex (Brodmann area 18, 19); *(A)* auditory association cortex (Brodmann area 21, 22); *(S)* somesthetic association cortex (Brodmann area 5, 7); *(M)* motor association cortex (Brodmann area 6, 8).

joined. The product of this joining can be described as a crossmodal association; new, more complex associations (concepts) are formed, based on information from multiple modalities. Posterior heteromodal association cortex is not a passive junction, however. It not only receives and synthesizes diverse unimodal percepts but it is connected with vast storehouses of previously processed unimodal and heteromodal percepts and with brain circuits capable of maintaining and manipulating this material. Posterior heteromodal association cortex is an essential contributor to the concept-forming, thought-processing functions of the cortex.

Posterior heteromodal association cortex is intimately connected with anterior heteromodal association cortex. Both clinical experience and animal experimentation demonstrate that this neural site is essential for the maintenance of information in a serial manner for short periods of time, a process currently termed working memory (Baddeley, 1992; Goldman-Rakic, 1990). Within this interplay of newly derived unimodal and heteromodal data associated with older, stored memories of multiple modalities abetted by the ability to maintain bits of information over short time spans, complex, often novel, multiple-modality concepts can be formed. It is in this neocortical arena that thoughts and ideas are formulated and processed. Figure 15.3 presents the present authors' view of the cortical areas dedicated to heteromodal associations.

Language is a product of heteromodal percept processing. Mental impressions based on both auditory and visual input are formed and intermixed with

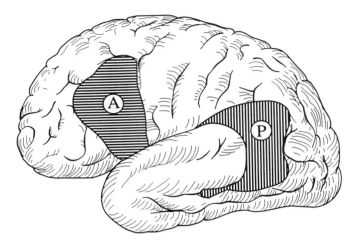

Figure 15.3. Artist's rendition of heteromodal association cortex: *(P):* posterior heteromodal association cortex (Brodmann area 37, 39); *(A)* anterior heteromodal association cortex (Brodmann area 44, 45 and 46).

many other associations to form the semantic aspects of language in the posterior heteromodal association cortex. Language processing, particularly its crucial sequential and relational aspects (syntax), demands and is the product of the time-based control mechanisms of the anterior heteromodal association cortex.

Unimodal and heteromodal percepts are assimilated in complex neural networks which carry out the encoding and decoding activities that are the core of language processing. An additional cortical area, termed *supramodal association cortex*, is of considerable consequence for all higher-level mental activity. Supramodal association cortex, richly connected with limbic, hypothalamic, thalamic, and basal ganglia networks, introduces homeostatic influences that monitor, inhibit, facilitate, and manage the multiple heteromodal percepts constantly being formed. Supramodal association cortex provides a complex and sophisticated mechanism that forcefully influences executive control functions (Fuster, 1980; Newell and Simon, 1972; Stuss and Benson, 1986). Figure 15.4 illustrates the portion of lateral frontal lobe that functions as supramodal association cortex.

All association cortices are, to a greater or lesser degree, dependent upon both subcortical activation and subcortical control. Primary sensory cortex receives almost all of its stimuli directly from external sensory receptors via pathways that emerge from the thalamus. Many other major subcortical areas (e.g., reticular substance, limbic pathways, basal ganglia) are most strongly connected to the supramodal association cortex and selected portions of anterior heteromodal association cortex. The combination of subcortical and prefrontal structures, in-

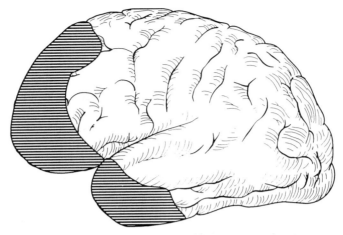

Figure 15.4. Artist's rendition of supramodal (horizontal hatching) association cortex (Brodmann area 9, 10, 11, 47).

cluding the supplementary motor cortex, represent the so-called frontal systems. In contrast to the strong subcortical influences on the primary cortex and the supramodal association cortex, both the unimodal and the heteromodal association cortices receive the vast majority of their sensory-motor and homeostatic information via cortical-cortical pathways. The neural networks formed from the unimodal and heteromodal association cortices receive little but modulatory influences directly from subcortical structures.

Functional Attributes of Association Cortex

Utilizing the matrix of anatomical structures presented above, and accepting the function of the primary sensory cortex as that of reception and transfer of externally produced stimuli, the functions of the three divisions of association cortex can be further postulated.

Each separate region of unimodal association cortex receives fibers from a single primary sensory area and remains dedicated to that modality. In the unimodal association cortex the sensory stimulus (already altered and categorized through a maze of local synapses) is discriminated from and contrasted with other simultaneously received stimuli. The products formed from the multiple discriminations are further compared to previously experienced perceptions of a similar type to form a unimodal percept. As an example, the attributes of size, roundness, color, movement, etc. eventually form a unimodal (visual) percept of a ball in flight. At this stage the unimodal percept is not yet fully identified (i.e., named), a process that demands association across multiple modalities.

In the next processing step, the unimodal percept is transferred to the heteromodal association network. Here, multiple interconnections (associations) can be simultaneously activated. These include linkages to other simultaneously formed percepts in the same modality (e.g., the visual background of the ball in flight) and with previously experienced and stored unimodal percepts (memories) in different modalities. The newly formed multimodal percept is also compared with stored heteromodal associations (memories of previously experienced multimodal percepts), manipulated to allow its use in novel observations (cognition) and maintained in serial order for immediate recall (often called short-term memory). Formation of a heteromodal association (e.g., identification of the ball and its trajectory) demands the interplay of vast multitudes of individual neurons and their interconnections, a working consortium currently identified by terms such as complex cognitive networks, neural matrices, and distributed neural processing networks (Goldman-Rakic, 1990; Mesulam, 1990). It is only through the vast array of potential associations available from these networks that language can be formulated. Although simple cross-modal association can be proposed as a basic semantic activity, vastly more complex networks are actually operant in simple meaning formulation; the performance of the sequential, relational activities of syntax demands the activation of even more networks.

The millions of potential cognitive networks, many hundreds of which are probably active at any given moment, demand considerable control, above and beyond maintenance of serial order. Clinical observations (Levin et al., 1991; Luria, 1973; Stuss and Benson, 1986) indicate that the supramodal association cortex, located in the rostral and orbital prefrontal cortex (see Figure 15.4), monitors and controls polymodal associations. This control is achieved by selection and sequencing of the innumerable simultaneously active neural networks to be activated into consciousness, probably through selective inhibition. Supramodal association cortex, thus, acts to gate heteromodal associations, the process called executive control (Fuster, 1980; Stuss and Benson, 1986). Multiple clinical observations (demonstrating impaired competency) suggest that the supramodal association cortex anticipates, conjectures, ruminates, plans for the future, and fantasizes (Levin and Grossman, 1978; Luria, 1966; Stuss and Benson, 1986). In addition, study of individuals who have suffered frontal-lobe brain damage indicates that the supramodal association cortex is needed for self-awareness and self-analysis, characteristics which are essential for full levels of consciousness.

Language—the decoding, formulation and encoding of linguistic material—is a function of heteromodal association cortex, influenced by both unimodal percept input and supramodal executive control. Focal damage involving heteromodal association cortex can interfere with different aspects of the complex networks needed for language, while allowing many other language functions to operate in a normal fashion. The syndromes of aphasia are based on longstanding observations that a relatively consistent language impairment indicates structural brain damage in a relatively consistent language area. Based on these observations, distinct language-processing activities associated with discrete lesions in unimodal and heteromodal association networks and their connections can be proposed. At best, the functional disorders outlined must remain inexact, as the aphasia syndromes are based on damage to rather large neuroanatomical conglomerates; only relatively crude basic language correlations are possible on this basis. Nonetheless, these correlations strongly demonstrate distinct neural bases for various language functions.

Localization of Individual Language Functions

Conversational Language

One of the most striking correlations between aphasia and neuroanatomy is illustrated by the striking differences in the verbal output of fluent and nonfluent aphasics. An anatomical basis for these aphasic output differences has been recognized for well over a century (Wernicke, 1874, 1908). Early brain-imaging studies (Benson, 1967; Poeck, Kerschensteiner, and Hartje, 1972; Wagenaar, Snow, and Prins, 1975) confirmed the clinically derived anterior/posterior dichotomy for the differences in conversational speech. Nonfluent aphasic output indicates pathology involving the dominant hemisphere's anterior heteromodal cortical structures, whereas fluent aphasic output, particularly when associated with paraphasia, suggests a lesion involving the posterior language area (see Figure 15.5). Many language-based subdivisions can be made within the fluent and nonfluent verbal outputs but the basic dichotomy remains. Although some exceptions to this rule are recognized (e.g., left-handedness, acute brain pathology, or childhood aphasia may produce an unclassifiable verbal output), the anterior/posterior differentiation of conversational verbal output decisively demonstrates that anatomically specific variations exist for language functions.

Repetition of Spoken Language

Another well-studied dichotomy of language function concerns success or failure in the ability to repeat spoken language. As noted in Chapter 8, patients with aphasia following pathology involving cortical tissues in the dominant-hemisphere

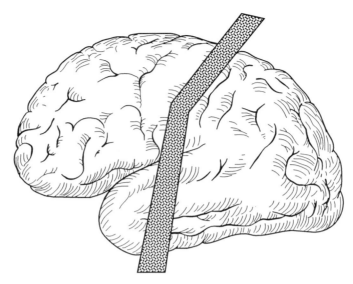

Figure 15.5. Artist's rendition of separation of fluent (anterior brain) from nonfluent (posterior brain) areas.

sylvian fissure area will have repetition disturbance whether their output is fluent or nonfluent. Figure 15.6 presents a crude neuroanatomical guide to the location of brain areas critical for repetition.

In contrast, patients with pathology involving the extrasylvian area of the dominant hemisphere (see Chapter 9) have clearly delineated language syndromes in which the ability to repeat spoken language is relatively well preserved.

Combining information from the two dichotomies (fluency/nonfluency and repetition/nonrepetition) provides powerful data for localization of language functions within the language-dominant hemisphere.

Comprehension of Spoken Language

Unlike conversational speech or repetition of spoken language, the comprehension of a spoken language demands a number of interacting functions and cannot be presented as a simple dichotomy. Four different dysfunctions of auditory-verbal processing can be outlined, based on recognized clinical aphasia syndromes, and a neuroanatomical basis can be demonstrated for each dysfunction. By combining the anatomical correlates of the dysfunctions, a neural network for the comprehension of spoken language can be postulated. The prime deficit of each of the separate auditory-comprehension dysfunctions can be considered to represent impairment in a separate function of auditory comprehension.

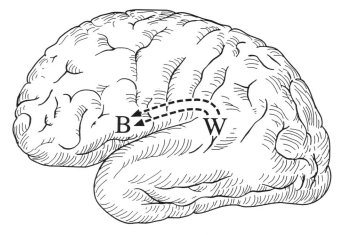

Figure 15.6. Artist's rendition of primary perisylvian language network: *(W)* Wernicke's area; *(B)* Broca's area; dotted lines indicate arcuate fasciculus.

One distinguishable dysfunction concerns disturbance of the reception of auditory language stimuli at the appropriate cortical site. Damage to the primary auditory cortex of the language-dominant hemisphere, or to fibers bringing stimuli to this area, will produce pure word-deafness (see Chapter 8); if auditory language symbols cannot be received in the cortex, heard language cannot be processed. The subject can be considered deaf, but only to verbal sounds.

A second dysfunction, closely related to pure word-deafness but both functionally and clinically distinct, is a disturbance of the unimodal processing of auditory language signals. Wernicke's aphasia is the clinical syndrome that occurs when the auditory signal is received by the subject but cannot be sufficiently analyzed (discriminated and compared) to form a unimodal percept. Although the subject's hearing is normal, reliable percepts based on language sounds cannot be produced. Comprehension of spoken language is significantly disordered.

A third distinct comprehension dysfunction occurs through faulty formation of cross-modal associations. When a unimodal percept can be formed from auditory language sounds but cannot be further processed because of the subject's inability to form cross-modal associations, an extrasylvian sensory aphasia occurs. The purest examples of extrasylvian sensory aphasia have pathology that involves dominant-hemisphere parietal association cortex.

The fourth distinct dysfunction concerns the comprehension of multiple bits of spoken language (e.g., phrase or sentence length), a process that demands the maintenance and short-term storage of temporally graded auditory signals plus the ability to reproduce these sequences, accurately, for cognitive manipulations.

This complex function may be impaired by pathology involving many different areas of association cortex but the most notable (at least the most pure) examples of disordered comprehension of serial speech despite good ability to process individual language elements is most often noted to follow frontal-lobe damage. In particular, pathology affecting prefrontal heteromodal association cortex of the language-dominant hemisphere can disturb the relationship (syntax) of elements of language, thus producing an auditory verbal comprehension disorder.

Figure 15.7 outlines the basic neuroanatomical localizations of the four types of disordered auditory language comprehension derived from clinical observations. Most of the areas involved in the first three dysfunctions in auditory language decoding are located in close proximity to each other; damage involving one area often affects several. Mixtures of the three posterior auditory language comprehension disturbances are common but pure examples of each type can be seen. The fourth auditory comprehension disorder is separate and often overlooked, as it is often obscured by obvious motor speech disruptions.

Word-Finding Ability

The ability to name, to produce the correct word for an object, appears simple and so elementary that even young children learn to perform the task easily. Neuroanatomical correlation studies, however, suggest that simple confrontation naming demands the integrated function of a number of separate regions compris-

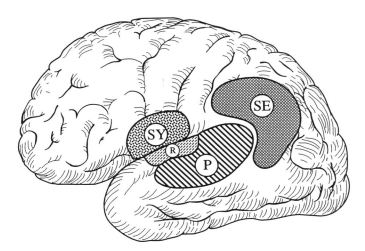

Figure 15.7. Artist's rendition of the four areas involved in comprehension of spoken language: (R) receptive area (Heschl's gyrus); (P) perceptive area (auditory association cortex); (SE) semantic interpretation area (angular gyrus); (SY) syntactical interpretation area (Broca's area).

ing a complex neuroanatomical network. Four clinically distinct aspects of naming have been outlined (see Chapter 14), each with a more-or-less dedicated anatomical localization. As the clinical aspects of these clinical disorders were described earlier, the types of anomia will be presented only by name and anatomical location in the present chapter.

Three types of *disconnection anomia*—category-specific, modality-specific, and callosal—are readily identified. In each, the basic disturbance is a disconnection in which essential information processed in an area of unilateral or heteromodal association cortex is separated from the language processing cortex of the dominant hemisphere. Although they produce clinically significant naming disorders, the disconnection anomias are often the products of brain damage outside the classic language area.

Pathological involvement of the posterior heteromodal association cortex of the dominant hemisphere produces a distinct disturbance called *semantic anomia;* although unimodal percepts are fully formed in all relevant modalities and nonverbal cross-modality associations are processed, the percepts cannot be integrated into the verbal aspects of language (i.e., the subject cannot associate intact unimodal and heteromodal percepts with semantically appropriate language symbols). Words that can be processed and even repeated have no meaning for the subject. Semantic anomia most often follows damage to the dominant-hemisphere angular gyrus.

A somewhat more specific naming disturbance, called *word selection anomia,* occurs with involvement of the posterior lateral temporal lobe of the dominant hemisphere. Patients with word selection anomia readily recognize objects, as proved by their ability to give descriptions of the object's function, but fail to produce the specific name. The word selection problem involves generation of the name only, not recognition or identification (other than by name).

Finally, two clinically distinct varieties of anomia can be related to verbal production disturbances, or *word production anomia.* These disorders occur with pathology located more anteriorly in the language-dominant hemisphere. In paraphasic anomia the pathology disconnects the more posterior language area from the motor cortex dedicated to language production. In articulatory initiation anomia the pathology involves the motor speech cortex or its prefrontal connections. Figure 15.8 presents, in simplified form, the primary neuroanatomical areas associated with word production disturbance.

Reading

Chapter 11 presented clinical varieties of acquired reading disturbance (alexia) along with the neuroanatomical loci of damage typically associated with the alexia syndromes. To define the neural networks involved in reading, three varieties of

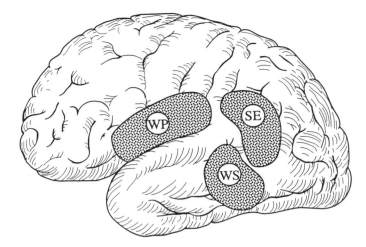

Figure 15.8. Artist's rendition of cortical areas crucial to word finding. *(WP)* word production area; *(WS)* word selection area; *(SE)* semantic processing area.

alexia will be considered. The first, *occipital alexia*, follows disconnection of an intact (unimodal) visual language percept from the posterior heteromodal language cortex of the dominant hemisphere and thus resembles the modality-specific and category-specific anomias. A second variation, *parietal-temporal alexia*, follows damage to that portion of the heteromodal association cortex needed to carry out cross-modal associations. In this situation a correctly processed unimodal visual language percept cannot be associated with other stored information (e.g, auditory, somesthetic) to provide full meaning to the visualized word. The causative lesion typically involves the angular gyrus of the dominant hemisphere, and the disorder resembles semantic anomia.

The third variety, *frontal alexia*, features disturbed ability to maintain the linguistic sequences and to recognize the relationships of cortical networks that are essential for the comprehension of sentence-length written material. Simple language forms (semantically specific words) may be interpreted properly but crucial relational structures (e.g., "in" versus "on") and longer passages or grammatically complex relationships cannot be maintained for processing. The characteristic lesion is located in the frontal heteromodal association cortex of the language-dominant hemisphere. Figure 15.9 outlines the neuroanatomical areas involved in the three major varieties of alexia.

Writing

As was demonstrated in Chapter 12, writing is a relatively poorly defined, multifactorial, and functionally complex language form. To localize the neural func-

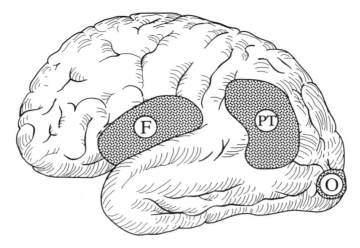

Figure 15.9. Artist's rendition of three cortical areas involved in reading. *(F)* frontal area (site of damage causing frontal alexia); *(PT)* parietal-temporal area (site of damage causing parietal-temporal alexia); *(O)* occipital area (site of damage causing occipital alexia).

tions active in graphic language production, the two types of breakdown—aphasic agraphia and mechanical (nonaphasic) agraphia—deserve separate attention. Aphasic agraphia is a complex disorder that may contain any one or several of the types of verbal processing disturbance seen in aphasia. In general, the locations of the lesions which produce aphasic agraphia correspond to the sites associated with the lesions that produce similar disturbances in oral language. In many cases of aphasic agraphia the problem is further complicated by overlying mechanical writing disturbances, often based on damage to subcortical motor circuits. Mechanical agraphia can cause production of a wide variety of clumsy, poorly formed written marks that often defy interpretation. Although aphasic agraphia can in general be outlined in the manner of the aphasias, mechanical agraphia complicates the clinical findings sufficiently that simple neural networks dedicated to writing are not readily postulated.

Calculation

Acalculia has come under fairly intense study and its relationship to language is becoming better understood. Both aphasic and spatial varieties of acalculia follow damage in relatively focal brain areas (see Chapter 13). *Aphasic acalculia* occurs when damage involves the language-dominant hemisphere to produce disturbances in the processing (decoding or encoding) of spoken or written number language. *Spatial acalculia* is most often associated with posterior nondominant-hemisphere pathology causing disorderd visuospatial relationships. A third type of calculation disorder—*anarithmetia* (the acquired loss of the ability to perform computations)—can be demonstrated (Hécaen, 1962). Early studies (Critchley, 1953; Grewel, 1960) suggested that anarithmetia occurred in disorders which caused "diffuse brain pathology." Alzheimer disease or related dementing disorders were cited as prime examples. The few cases of anarithmetia based on focal brain damage described in the literature (Benson and Weir, 1972; Spiers, 1987) had pathology involving the dominant-hemisphere posterior heteromodal association cortex (parietal-temporal junction area). A neuroanatomical network that includes the neural strata for language (aphasic acalculia), visuospatial discrimination (spatial acalculia), and cognition (anarithmetia) indicates that a complex, bihemispheric neural matrix is active in calculation.

Ideomotor Praxis

The ability to carry out, on command, a specified motor activity demands language function, at least for interpretation of the command. Acquired disturbance of the ability to perform the motor act, when not based on primary comprehension disorder or primary motor dysfunction, is called *ideomotor apraxia*. The mandatory language factor demands a neural base that can involve various language-dedicated brain areas.

First, the oral command must be processed into a unimodal percept which in turn must undergo cross-modal interpretation. Disordered formation of the unimodal percept or disrupted transfer for processing by appropriate heteromodal association cortex areas obviates comprehension of the command. In contemporary neurological practice this is classed as an aphasia and not a praxis disturbance. When it can be proved that a subject can comprehend a command but cannot carry it out despite fully normal motor functions, a disconnection (language comprehension cortex separated from motor association cortex of the dominant hemisphere) can be surmised. This variety of ideomotor apraxia has been called *parietal apraxia*, as most individuals with this problem have damage involving the supramarginal gyrus or brain tissue just beneath this portion of the dominant parietal cortex.

Another well-described variety of ideomotor apraxia, a clumsiness or incompetency of the nonpathological left hand in a patient with right hemiplegia, has been termed *sympathetic apraxia* (Geschwind, 1967a; Liepmann, 1900, 1905). In this situation the command is comprehended but the damage causing the right hemiplegia involves the synapses necessary to pass this language-based information to the motor area of the right hemisphere. The message is not conveyed.

A third variety of ideomotor apraxia, *callosal apraxia*, also refers to an inability of the subject's left limbs to follow a command that is understood and easily carried out by the right limbs. In this situation, destruction of left-to-right-hemisphere connections through the corpus callosum produces the disconnection. Varieties of ideomotor apraxia are discussed further in Chapter 17. Figure 17.2 illustrates the three neuroanatomical regions where interruption to the neural network needed to carry out a verbally presented command can occur and produce ideomotor apraxia. In each of these varieties (or syndromes) of apraxia, the intact motor cortex region has been separated from the brain area in which an auditory command was accurately comprehended.

Summary

This chapter has outlined a neuroanatomical hierarchy of higher cortical functions and presented some of the cortical and subcortical structures that subserve various aspects of language function. The correlations are relatively crude but clearly demonstrate that language function, while demanding much of the cortex for overall operation, depends on the specific interrelationships of different anatomical areas that have specific language-oriented functions. Dedicated neural networks execute individual language functions. Interrelationships between these networks are responsible for language.

III

RELATED DISORDERS

. . . .

16

Speech Disorders

. . . .

Speech and language can be separated both by definition and by assessment, at least technically. In the terminology defined in Chapter 1, speech disorders are not included as aspects of aphasia. For the clinician, however, language disorders and speech disorders are superficially similar and so often coexist that a working knowledge of both is needed. In addition, some speech disorders mimic the verbal output of aphasics to a sufficient degree that an ability to separate the two becomes essential. In this chapter, a number of the more common speech disorders will be described, with particular emphasis on those likely to co-occur with aphasia. Table 16.1 outlines the disorders that will be discussed.

Mutism

Strictly speaking, mutism does not co-occur with aphasia. Aphasics must produce some verbal sounds; without them, it is impossible to determine that an individ-

Table 16.1. Speech Disorders

Mutism
Motor Speech Disorders
Scanning Speech
Reiterative Speech Disorders

ual has a disorder of language. Certain types of mutism, however, do occur in the early stages of brain damage that causes aphasia; other types of mutism should be considered for differential diagnosis. Table 16.2 presents an outline of the types of mutism to be discussed. Mutism indicates a total lack of voice; hypophonia refers to an abnormally low voice volume. Although hypophonia is not mutism by this definition, the two conditions are so intimately connected, essentially as points on a single spectrum, that hypophonia deserves discussion with mutism.

Laryngitis

The most common cause of decreased voice volume is laryngeal pathology. This is usually inflammatory (laryngitis) but laryngeal hypophonia may have other causes such as damage to the superior pharyngeal nerve, nodules or polyps of the larynx or vocal chords, or carcinoma involving the larynx. None of these disorders are functionally related to aphasia, but any one of them can occur in a patient with aphasia. For instance, one patient whose pure word-deafness was carefully investigated and reported (Albert and Bear, 1974) subsequently became hypophonic and eventually mute. Investigation demonstrated a carcinoma of the larynx that eventually led to death. For many months the patient's language abnormality obscured the slowly progressive change in voice volume.

Elective Mutism

Elective mutism is a rare occurrence most often reported in young, school-age children (Wilkins, 1985). The individual is said to speak "normally" to his peers, to his siblings, or even to his parents but refuses to speak to others such as teachers, other relatives, physicians, etc. Most reports of this condition stress the transient nature of the disorder and the need to counsel the parents, teachers, and other significant figures to help the patient overcome a disabling sense of inadequacy (Atoynatan, 1986; Salfield, 1950). However, following "recovery" from elective mutism many subjects are found to have abnormal verbal output (Reed,

Table 16.2. Types of Mutism

Laryngitis
Elective Mutism
Psychogenic Mutism
Aphemia
Hypophonia

1963). In some cases, the abnormal output that follows a period of mutism represents a "new" language for the immigrant child (Schvartzman et al., 1990). In other cases the abnormal output identifies a motor speech disorder. Crucial to the diagnosis of elective mutism is demonstration of normal or at least reasonable speech output at some time during the period of mutism. Too often the family members are so familiar with the individual's nonverbal communication efforts that they misinterpret and misreport it as normal speech. Obviously, teachers, counselors, etc. are less adept at interpreting the subject's nonverbal communications, leading to misinterpretation as elective nonresponses. Some young children are so shy and sensitive that they offer only limited amounts of speech for examiners. In this situation, even modestly careful attempts by the examiner will bring out sufficient speech to demonstrate that the child is not mute (Schvarztman et al., 1990).

Psychogenic Mutism

Psychogenic mutism is often considered synonymous with elective mutism, but it is more accurately defined as a distinct entity. Psychogenic mutism can occur at any age and may or may not be related to a brain abnormality. Mutism has been reported as a primary finding of conversion reaction, most often in patients with significant underlying psychiatric disorder (Altshuler, Cummings, and Mills, 1986). It is important to realize, however, that acute language impairment (aphasia) in young children often produces an initial period of mutism (Alajouanine and Lhermitte, 1965; Hécaen and Albert, 1978; Satz and Bullard-Bates, 1981). Psychogenic mutism, like psychogenic amnesia, represents an inefficient response to stress and most often signifies the presence of a serious underlying mental disorder.

Aphemia

One speech disorder featuring mutism and/or hypophonia and often classed with the aphasias is aphemia (Broca aphasia-Type I) (see Chapter 8). The individual with aphemia has an initial but transitory mutism, being unable to verbalize, to name, to repeat or to read aloud. Comprehension of spoken language, however, is intact and the patient can produce written language with full linguistic competency. Total mutism is almost invariably transient in cases of aphemia, lasting from a few days to a week or more. It is usually followed by a low-volume (hypophonic), inadequately articulated (mushy) verbal output that is difficult for the listener to understand. With continuing recovery the individual will produce sufficient verbal output to demonstrate that language functions are intact. As recovery continues it is usually noted that the individual's motor speech has changed;

the altered rhythm and abnormal inflection have been termed dysprosody (Monrad-Krohn, 1947) and often suggest a foreign-language background, the "foreign-accent syndrome" (Alexander, Benson, and Stuss, 1989a). Aphemia should be classed as a speech, not a language, disorder but, inasmuch as the prosodic quality of verbal output provides considerable communication value, aphemia stands between pure speech and pure language disorders.

It has been proposed that lasting mutism requires bihemispheric involvement (Cappa et al., 1987; Groswasser et al., 1988; Pineda and Ardila, 1992; Sussman et al., 1983), whereas transient mutism can be observed following unilateral left lower motor cortex damage (Alexander, Benson, and Stuss, 1989; Schiff et al., 1983). With unilateral lesions, a compensatory action of the contralateral unaffected brain appears to allow recovery of basic speech production. Levine and Mohr (1979) reported four cases with bilateral lesions associated with a severe verbal production defect. On recovery, three of the patients exhibited dysarthric speech; only one suffered a lasting mutism. In the case with permanent mutism, a relatively complete destruction of the pre-Rolandic region was present bilaterally. It can be suggested that unilateral frontal opercular damage can be associated with transient mutism but that bilateral frontal opercular damage is necessary for a lasting mutism.

Hypophonia

Hypophonia (abnormally low voice volume) is a disturbance that is seen commonly in neurological practice; many neurologic disorders can produce hypophonia without affecting language competency. Damage to the reticular substance of the mesencephalon can produce an akinetic mute state (Botez and Barbeau, 1971; Segarra, 1970) but more often produces degrees of hypophonia (Alexander and Schmidt, 1980; Masdeu et al., 1978). Hypophonia can occur after lesions that involve the thalamus and basal ganglia (Alexander and Benson, 1991; Damasio et al., 1982; Riklan and Levita, 1970). Many of the causes of subcortical dementia (e.g., Parkinson's disease, progressive supranuclear palsy) also produce decreased voice volume. Hypophonia can also be seen following bilateral motor system damage that produces pseudobulbar palsy. Hypophonia is a characteristic feature of Broca aphasia-Type I and of extrasylvian motor aphasia-Type I and Type II but tends to be transient in these language syndromes. Low voice volume may also coexist with any of the other aphasic syndromes, based on multiple lesions, particularly if the brain damage is bilateral. In summary, hypophonia is found in many types of brain disease and often coexists with language disorder.

Finally, it is well to note that extrasylvian motor aphasia-Type I is routinely associated with reduced verbal output involving both the quantity of words produced and the ability to initiate speech. The resulting lack of verbal production can superficially resemble mutism but some hypophonic output can usually be demonstrated.

Tissue destruction or neurochemical (neurotransmitter) disorder affecting the upper brain stem and/or the frontal septal area bilaterally can interfere with the initiation of both behavior and verbal output. When severe, this status is called *akinetic mutism* (Plum and Posner, 1982; Segarra, 1970), but far more often a hypokinetic (bradykinetic) status with severely limited verbalization that is notably hypophonic is produced. A hypokinetic-hypophonic state suggests brain-stem and/or medial-frontal dysfunction.

Motor Speech Disorders

A complex and often confusing group of motor speech disorders, based on impaired motor control of the speech musculature, is often referred to under the term *dysarthria*. Dysarthria has traditionally been used to describe only those motor speech problems based on neurologic dysfunction (thus excluding laryngitis, laryngeal nodules, etc.). Dysarthria itself occurs exclusive of language disturbance but in actual practice dysarthria and aphasia frequently co-exist (Critchley, 1952). Some aphasiologists (Tonkonogy and Goodglass, 1981; Trost and Canter, 1974) have suggested that some types of dysarthria have a cortical source and may be directly involved in aphasia. The relationship between cortical damage and articulatory defect is particularly noted in cases of pure aphemia (Lecours and Lhermitte, 1976), and many individuals with anterior aphasia will have some degree of dysarthria (Alexander, Benson, and Stuss, 1989). Although most types of dysarthria are not associated with aphasia, the frequency of co-occurring motor speech disorder and aphasia is considerable and the clinical findings of the two disorders are sufficiently similar that the clinician must recognize varieties of dysarthria. Table 16.3 presents a traditional classification of variations of motor speech disorder based on the underlying neurologic disorder or locus of neuroanatomical involvement. The following descriptions are derived from the seminal work of Darley, Aronson, and Brown (1969, 1975) and the later revision of this work by Metter (1985).

Flaccid Motor Speech Disorder

Weakness of the vocal chords and/or supporting structures will produce a notable alteration of motor speech output; two variations are recognized. One is *flaccid dysphonia*, a motor speech disorder featuring breathy, harsh output, reduced vol-

Table 16.3. Etiologies of Motor Speech Disorders

DISORDER	TYPICAL ETIOLOGY
Flaccid	
Dysphonia	Superior laryngeal nerve palsy
Dysarthria	Bulbar poliomyelitis, bulbar palsy, myasthenia gravis
Spastic	Pseudobulbar palsy
Ataxic	Cerebellar disease/damage
Hypokinetic	Parkinson's disease
Hyperkinetic	
Choreiform	Huntington's disease, Sydenham's chorea
Dystonic	Dystonia musculorum deformans, tardive dyskinesia
Mixed	Multiple sclerosis, Wilson's disease, amyotrophic lateral sclerosis

ume and a tendency to speak in short phrases. Damage to the superior laryngeal nerve produces a classic flaccid dysphonia. The second variation is a *flaccid dysarthria,* producing a breathy, hypernasal verbal output, again with reduced loudness and short phrases. This is the output noted in bulbar palsy, myasthenia gravis, and bulbar poliomyelitis. Flaccid motor speech disorders are not associated with aphasia.

Spastic Dysarthria

Spastic dysarthria is a motor speech problem characterized by a harsh, low-pitched, slow, monotonous verbal output that appears strained or strangled in output. This is the verbal output that characterizes pseudobulbar palsy (bilateral spasticity) and may be present to a lesser degree following significant unilateral upper motor neuron disturbance. Spastic dysarthria is frequently associated with motor aphasia, particularly Broca aphasia.

Ataxic Dysarthria

Ataxic dysarthria is manifested by striking alterations of normal rhythm with slowness, irregular breakdowns, and improper stress producing an uneven, jumpy, unpredictable output. Ataxic dysarthria is most classically seen in cases of acute cerebellar damage.

Hypokinetic Dysarthria

Hypokinetic dysarthria is characterized by a monotonous output based on decreased variation of both pitch and volume (monotone). Speech output tends to be somewhat faster than in the previously described dysarthrias but is characterized by a striking lack of normal inflection. This is the verbal output that is seen in advanced Parkinson's disease.

Hyperkinetic Dysarthria

Two varieties of motor speech disorder can be classified as hyperkinetic. The first, *choreiform dysarthria*, features prolonged phoneme and sentence segments, intermixed with silences and showing variable, often improper stress (phoneme inflection). This speech output is characteristically seen in choreiform disorders such as Huntington's disease. The second type, *dystonic dysarthria*, produces a slower speaking rate with prolongation of the individual phonemes and segments and with abnormal, unexpected appearances of stress or of silence. Dystonic dysarthria is the motor speech problem seen in dystonia musculorum deformans and, to some degree, characterizes the verbal output of the tardive dyskinesia syndrome. In both types of hyperkinetic dysarthria the breakdowns in verbal output are inconsistent in occurrence.

Mixed Motor Speech Disorder

In clinical practice a mixed dysarthria syndrome showing the characteristics of several types of motor speech disorder is common. Several classic neurologic disorders (e.g., multiple sclerosis, Wilson's disease, advanced amyotrophic lateral sclerosis) produce several identifiable variations of dysarthria concurrently.

Table 16.4 presents some of the differential features of the motor speech disorders and illustrates how difficult it is to adequately define and characterize the various types of motor speech disorder in written descriptions. In contrast, most clinicians have little difficulty in recognizing the variations of motor speech that characterize the common neurologic disorders. Thus, the verbal output of Parkinson's disease is easily distinguished from that of pseudobulbar spastic dysarthria or the flaccid dysphonia of superior laryngeal nerve palsy.

An underlying language disorder will complicate identification of the variety of dysarthria, and vice versa. It is easy to mistake the abnormal verbal output produced by a speech disorder for an intrinsic language disorder, particularly when short utterances with abnormal stress or inflection, decreased pitch, and low volume are present. An individual's pure motor speech disorder is easily

Table 16.4. Characteristics of Motor Speech Disorders

TYPE	RESPIRATION	PHONATION	RESONANCE	ARTICULATION	PROSODY
Flaccid Dysphonia	Reduced loudness, inspiratory stridor, short phrases	Breathy, harsh; diplophonia	—	—	—
Dysarthria	Reduced loudness, inspiratory stridor, short phrases	Breathy	Nasal emission, hypernasality	Imprecise consonants	—
Spastic	Short phrases	Harsh, strain-strangled, low pitch	Hypernasality	Imprecise consonants, distorted vowels	Slow, reduced stress, monotony
Ataxic	—	Harsh, monotonous pitch, monotonous volume	—	Imprecise consonants, distorted vowels, irregular breakdowns	Dysrhythmia, slowness
Hypokinetic	Short phrases, short rushes	Monotonous pitch, monotonous volume, decreased volume, breathiness	—	Imprecise consonants	Mild slowing, reduced stress, monotone
Hyperkinetic Choreiform	Sudden inspiratory or expiratory sighs	Harsh, loudness variations, strain-strangled, monotonous pitch, monotonous volume	Hypernasality	Imprecise consonants, distorted vowels, irregular breakdowns, prolonged phonemes	Prolonged segments, silences, short phrases, variable rate
Dystonic	—	Harsh, strain-strangled, voice stoppage, excess volume	—	Imprecise consonants, distorted vowels, irregular breakdowns, prolonged phonemes	Slow rate, short phrases, prolonged segments, silences

misdiagnosed and treated as a language disorder, particularly Broca aphasia, and the opposite is also true. The therapy for the two disorders—aphasia and dysarthria—is distinctly different and their differentiation is important.

Scanning Speech

For many years neurologists have recognized scanning speech as one leg of "Charcot's triad" (ataxia, nystagmus, and scanning speech), a set of findings considered pathognomonic for multiple sclerosis. Based on this observation, scanning speech has long been interpreted as due to malfunction of the cerebellum. Scanning speech does occur in some patients with multiple sclerosis, but usually only after the disease is far advanced; even in this situation there is little direct evidence to specify a cerebellar localization for scanning speech.

Scanning speech is characterized by a slow, deliberate, segmented, and monotonous verbal output presented as individual words or major segments of words. The output retains both grammatical and semantic competence and articulation remains relatively normal. It is the prosodic quality, particularly rhythm and inflection, that are disrupted. The slow, fragmented rhythm of scanning speech superficially resembles a nonfluent output and is often interpreted, incorrectly, as an anterior aphasia.

Kremer, Russell, and Smyth (1947) reported a group of patients who had suffered significant brain trauma with prolonged coma, third-nerve palsy, a combination of cerebellar ataxia and spasticity affecting the same limb, and, following recovery, a scanning speech. Based on this unusual cluster of neurologic findings, the authors suggested that the major pathology was located at the level of the decussation of the brachium conjunctivum in the mesencephalon. Motor fibers in the cerebral peduncle, the third nerve as it exited the brain stem and the crossed efferent cerebellar pathway could all be involved by a relatively small lesion. The prolonged coma reported in their patients would also imply a midbrain lesion. The mesencephalic localization of pathology was circumstantially substantiated by demonstration of an enlarged aqueduct of Sylvius in three of their patients. Boller and colleagues (1972) confirmed the occurrence of aqueductal enlargement in a series of post-trauma patients. Characteristic scanning speech is most often seen in individuals recovered from a prolonged period of unconsciousness based on brain trauma. Against this background it has been suggested that scanning speech follows midbrain trauma (Benson, 1979; Kremer, Russell, and Smyth, 1947) but the localization remains without absolute verification. Scanning speech is not a sign of cerebellar damage, however; none of the patients in the study by Kremer, Russell, and Smyth had other evidence indicating direct cerebellar pathology. Although scanning speech is easily misinterpreted as a nonfluent aphasia, careful evaluation reveals that there is no true language impairment in these cases. Scanning speech will respond, to some degree, to speech therapy efforts.

Reiterative Speech Disorders

Stutter

The tendency to stutter (repeatedly iterate an uttered sound) is common, particularly among developing males. Although stutter is a distinctive, easily recognized speech disorder, when it is superimposed on a language disorder a confusing clinical picture is produced. It is now well recognized that a stutter can appear following brain damage in an individual who never previously stuttered (Helm, Butler, and Benson, 1978; Rosenbek et al., 1978; Rosenfield, 1984) and the co-occurrence of acquired stutter and aphasia has been reported (Farmer, 1975). Two types of stutter—developmental and acquired—are subtly different and deserve separate consideration (Canter, 1971).

By far the most common of the two is developmental stutter, characterized by silent or audible involuntary repetitions and/or prolongations of an uttered sound. Bloodstein (1981) characterized stuttering as a speech behavior combining a sound that is improperly patterned in time with the speaker's reactions to the problem. Developmental stuttering is present in 1% to 2% of the populations of all nationalities, is considerably more common among males than females, and shows a strong multiple-generation familial component. Characteristically, the dysfluency of developmental stutter involves the first syllable of a word. Initiation of the word is either followed by a machine-gun-like repetition (stutter) or the presentation of the syllable followed by a prolonged silence (stammer); both situations are accompanied by physical and emotional discomfort (stress). The degree of stutter tends to decrease with the subject's advancing age, often seeming to disappear following puberty; an ongoing tendency to stutter, however, can occur at times of fatigue or stress and, to some degree, the problem tends to return as the subject reaches advanced age. If an individual with an acquired aphasia is found to stutter, an immediate question for the clinician concerns whether the individual stuttered in childhood.

One rather simplistic but still popular theory concerning developmental stutter holds that bihemispheric language function (rivalry) is present. This theory was supported by a report of four neurosurgical cases in which developmental stutter disappeared following a surgical procedure on one hemisphere (in two of the cases, the left; in the other two, the right) (Jones, 1966). A repeated study of brain surgery on stutterers (Andrews, Quinn, and Sorby, 1972) did not, however, fully corroborate these observations. Most current theories of stuttering propose a basic neurophysiologic disturbance, not a simple hemispheric competition (Deal and Cannito, 1991; Rosenfield, 1984), but both theories may be correct.

Of concern to the clinician evaluating aphasia is the patient with a newly acquired stutter following brain damage (Caplan, 1972). When acquired stutter appears acutely following insult to the brain, the patient's verbal output tends to show repetitions, prolongations, and blocks that are not restricted to the initial syllable. The stutter can involve grammatical as well as substantive words, and although the speaker may be somewhat annoyed by the stutter the problem does not produce the significant anxiety that characterizes developmental stuttering. In the patient with an acquired stutter there is little or no grimacing, fist-clenching, body tenseness, or other evidence of anxiety. Studies of acquired stutter (Helm, Butler, and Benson, 1978; Rosenbeck et al., 1978) suggest that acquired stutter most often occurs following bilateral brain abnormality but has been reported following either unilateral damage to the right hemisphere (Ardila and Lopez, 1986) or the left (Helm, Butler, and Benson, 1978). Acquired stutter may be transient or permanent, probably dependent upon the degree of brain abnormality. No focal neuroanatomical site or sites have been associated with acquired stutter.

Palilalia

Palilalia is a comparatively unusual speech disorder characterized by the involuntary reiterative repetition of words or phrases during verbal output. It resembles stutter but involves words and phrases rather than syllables. The reiterative elements most often appear at the end of a spoken phrase but may occur at the beginning or midportion of an utterance. There is a tendency for the repeated utterance to increase in speed but decrease in volume until it finally fades. Early descriptions of palilalia were in patients who had suffered von Economo's encephalitis. Later studies demonstrated the disorder in patients with calcification of the basal ganglia (Fahr's disease), and it was considered that palilalia indicated bilateral basal ganglia involvement (Brain, 1961). Identical verbal-output problems (palilalia) can be seen in patients with untreated schizophrenia, in patients with paramedial thalamic damage (Yasuda et al., 1990), in severe aphasia (particularly in patients with mixed cerebral dominance), in the later stages of degenerative brain diseases such as Alzheimer's disease (Cummings et al., 1985; Hier, Hagenlocker, and Shindler, 1985), following electrical stimulation to a variety of left-hemisphere sites (Lecours, Vanier, and Lhermitte, 1983), or following right-hemisphere damage (Horner and Massey, 1983). Paroxysmal palilalia has been observed in association with epilepsy (Ardila and Lopez, 1988). Palilalia, like most of the speech disorders described in this chapter, is best demonstrated by clinical measures. If palilalia is concurrent with aphasia, the two disorders deserve individual treatment.

Echolalia

Echolalia, the tendency for a patient to repeat words or phrases just addressed to him, is the best known and one of the easiest to recognize of the reiterative speech disorders. Although echolalia represents a characteristic, almost pathognomomic, finding in the extrasylvian aphasias, the disturbance is also a feature of many degenerative brain diseases (Cummings and Benson, 1989; Neumann and Cohn, 1953). Both Chapters 6 and 9 contain additional descriptions of echolalia.

Logoclonia

Logoclonia, the tendency for a patient to repeat the final syllable of a word when speaking, most often indicates bilateral brain dysfunction. Logoclonia is reported in many patients in late-stage dementia with severe mental deterioration (Bayles, Tomoeda, and Boone, 1985; Cummings and Benson, 1989).

The reiterative speech disorders (except for echolalia) are of primary interest as indicators of significant bilateral brain disorder that usually involves subcortical structures. The reiterative speech disorders, as well as most of the other speech disorders outlined in this chapter, can be considered the product of disturbance within a series of finely tuned motor speech circuits. The characteristics of the speech output disorder tend to vary, dependent upon the subcortical area or areas damaged.

Summary

Speech disorders, although technically distinct from language disorders, resemble and may coexist with the language impairments of aphasia. Both diagnosis and treatment for speech disorders and for aphasia demand different approaches and the clinician must be aware of speech dysfunction when evaluating language problems. Mutism, varieties of motor speech disorder, scanning speech, and several types of reiterative speech disorders can occur in brain-damaged patients who are potential aphasics.

17

Associated Neurologic and Behavioral Problems

· ·

Most approaches to aphasia focus on disordered language and rarely take into account complicating behaviors. In actuality, aphasia almost never occurs as an isolated finding. Language functions are performed by consortiums of cells located in many sites scattered across the dominant (usually left) hemisphere that are further influenced by connections with nondominant-hemisphere neuronal networks. Brain damage of sufficient scope to produce a disorder of language is almost bound to interfere with circuitry needed for other behavioral functions that operate in or through the same cerebral areas. Almost every patient with aphasia will have additional neurologic or behavioral problems that complicate the aphasia picture.

The neurologic and behavioral complications of aphasia are incompletely understood and behavioral complications that often go unrecognized interfere with both the diagnosis and the treatment of aphasia. Recognition of the behavioral complications is essential for understanding and treating language disorder. Fortunately, in the past decade the fields of behavioral neurology and neuropsychiatry have grown rapidly. Professionals with expertise in both the neurologic and the behavioral complications that accompany aphasia can be found at many medical centers. A multidisciplinary approach utilizing the expertise of neurologists, language therapists, and specialists in neurorehabilitation provides the most effective treatment for the aphasic patient.

Only a few of the neurologic and behavioral problems associated with aphasia will be discussed in this chapter. Each description will be limited and the reader is advised to consult the current literature, including *Organic Psychiatry, 2d Edition* (Lishman, 1987), *Clinical Neuropsychiatry* (Cummings, 1985b), *Handbook of Clinical Neurology, Vols. 45 and 46* (Frederiks, 1985), *The American Psychiatric Press Textbook of Neuropsychiatry, 2d Edition* (Yudofsky and Hales, 1992), *Behavioral Neurology: 100 Maxims* (Devinsky, 1992), and *Clinical Neuropsychology* (Heilman and Valenstein, 1993). Disorders of speech, an extremely important complication in many cases of aphasia, were discussed in Chapter 16.

Disorders of Awareness

Most patients with aphasia suffer some degree of disordered awareness at the onset of the disease. Many have an ongoing awareness problem that significantly interferes with rehabilitation. Only three of the more common of these problems will be discussed here.

Confusional State

Although it is easy to state that almost every aphasic patient initially suffers some degree of confusion, what this means is not clear. Identical clinical phenomena are called confusional state by neurologists, delirium by psychiatrists, and metabolic or toxic encephalopathy by internists and surgeons, and the state called confusion is difficult for each group to define. The most cogent definition—*inability to maintain a coherent line of thought*—is simple but far too broad. One pertinent aspect is the degree of alertness (wakefulness) in the confused state. Many aphasic patients show some degree of lethargy, drowsiness, obtundation, or even stupor, particularly in the early stages after a brain insult.

The problem of disordered alertness improves spontaneously in most aphasics but a residual degree of attention abnormality is often present. Although the patients may appear alert and easily pass standard tests of attention (e.g., digit span), their attention wanders and their ability to maintain interest is decreased. The somewhat dated term *clouding of consciousness*, indicating a dulling of the intellectual processes, muddled reasoning, and disorganized behavior, can be used to characterize this state. The significantly confused patient appears bewildered or perplexed; lesser degrees may not be conspicuous but still prove detrimental to rehabilitation efforts.

Many patients in confusional state have perceptual disturbances; they can misinterpret environmental stimuli (illusions), can suffer vivid hallucinations that lead to agitation, and can show striking emotional and personality alterations (e.g., anxiety, fear, depression, paranoia). Even more common than these florid disturbances, the patient's normal sleep pattern is often disturbed—agitated wakefulness at night and long periods of sleep during the day. Psychomotor activity varies; some patients become pathologically hypoactive, others become hyperactive. The symptoms of acute confusion tend to fluctuate and the course is usually self-limited. It must be recognized, however, particularly in elderly patients, that the onset of acute confusion is a sign of danger. The mortality rates for geriatric individuals admitted to hospital in a confusional state run high (from 25% to 40%) (Lipowski, 1990).

Inattention

Closely related to confusional state, but tending to be much more prolonged, is the condition called inattention. In most aphasic patients inattention is unilateral, manifested by a tendency to neglect one side (usually the right side in the aphasic patient) and show unconcern about all or part of the body on one side. In more severe states, unawareness of all but intense stimuli occurring in one side of space may be seen and the patients may even show outright denial of any difficulty with that side (anosognosia) (Benson and Geschwind, 1975; Critchley, 1953; Heilman and colleagues (Heilman, 1985a,b,c); Mesulam, 1985). Table 17.1 presents four gradations of unilateral inattention that may occur following brain injury.

Most of the current literature implies that unilateral neglect is far more common following right-brain damage than left-brain damage (Heilman, Valenstein, and Watson, 1985; Mesulam, 1990), largely predicated on the fact that almost all tests for neglect are based on visual stimulation. In many investigations the visual stimuli are complex, demanding high-level visuospatial discrimination, a function that the right hemisphere performs better (Benson, 1994; Grüsser and Landis, 1991). Patients with right-brain damage and significant left inattention easily comprehend relatively complicated language structures. In contrast, linguistically complex language tasks are not performed well by many left-brain-damaged individuals who easily perform the visuospatial tasks used to demonstrate unilateral neglect. Unilateral visual inattention in individuals with damage to the language-dominant hemisphere may appear subtle, at least in contrast to the language de-

Table 17.1. Gradations of Unilateral Inattention

Neglect
Unconcern
Unawareness
Anosognosia

fect, but can be disabling (Cutting, 1978; Heilman and Valenstein, 1972). The aphasic patient tends to ignore persons on their right side, prefers to perform unimanual tasks with the left hand and may use only the left-hand portion of a sheet of paper for writing. Much stronger right-sided stimuli (visual, auditory, somesthetic) are needed to attract and maintain their attention. Most experienced aphasiologists have learned to seat themselves on the patient's left side to attain maximum attention for all stimuli, including language clues.

Inintention

Closely related to unilateral inattention is a motor disturbance termed inintention (Heilman, Valenstein, and Watson, 1985a), a disorder in which a neurologically intact limb is not used (motor neglect). Some aphasic patients who, although they have no right-limb paralysis, use only their left arm for gesture, eating, picking up items, pointing, and other tasks usually performed by the dominant limb. If specifically told to use their right limb they perform successfully, but when left without direction they return to performing with their left limb. If consciously attending to motor acts, some aphasic patients with right inintention can use both limbs but, when not specifically attending to the motor response, will not use the right limbs. Inintention represents a significant problem for rehabilitation.

Many theories have been formulated in the past several decades to explain the neuroanatomical basis for attention and intention (Heilman, Valenstein, and Watson, 1985a; Mesulam, 1985). Multiple sites within the central nervous system (frontal cortex, parietal cortex, thalamus, cingulate gyrus, and mesecephalic reticular areas) are involved in the maintenance of attention (see Figure 17.1). These different anatomical areas are interconnected by a complex network of pathways that course through both hemispheres (Mesulam, 1990). Either the nuclear centers or the pathways that connect them can be damaged by the lesions that produce aphasia. Inattention and inintention commonly co-occur with aphasia.

Motor Disorders

The most obvious neurologic disorder complicating aphasia is the presence of motor disorder. While often obvious, motor dysfunction may be subtle and demand special testing techniques for demonstration.

Hemiparesis

About 80% of nonfluent aphasic patients have some degree of hemiparesis, and a smaller but still significant number of fluent aphasics also show unilateral motor

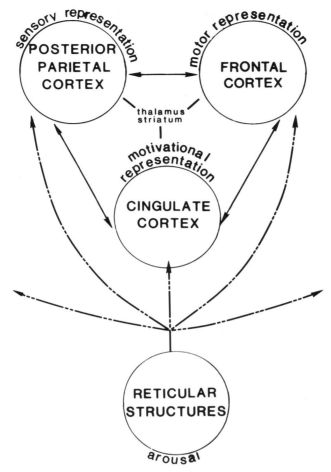

Figure 17.1. Diagrammatic representation of prime neural areas active in attentional behavior. (From Mesulam, 1985).

disturbance (Benson, 1979a; Howes and Geschwind, 1964). Considerable variation in the degree of paralysis can be seen, ranging from total hemiplegia (total inability to move the limbs on one side—usually right) to a mild slowing of rapid repetitive movements of the fingers. Most aphasic patients show some degree, albeit often mild, of unilateral motor disturbance. Until the examiner has gained appropriate experience in testing for these disturbances, they can easily be misinterpreted; the patient's poor performance is likely to be considered a lack of cooperation, poor motivation, or even malingering.

Rehabilitation measures are often effective for the paralysis, and the resulting improvement may prove to be a significant factor in the course of aphasia therapy. Thus, the aphasic patient who can be taught to operate a wheelchair is a better language therapy candidate than the totally bedridden aphasic. Initial successes at ambulation are often associated with improvements in language. All patients with hemiparesis deserve active physical therapy, and it is often beneficial to combine motor rehabilitation with language therapy.

Pseudobulbar Palsy

An extremely troublesome motor control problem that is present in some aphasics has been termed pseudobulbar palsy, spastic bulbar palsy, or supranuclear bulbar palsy. The terminology arises from the similarity of the clinical symptoms to the motor disturbances that occur when the bulbar musculature is paralyzed (hypophonia, difficulty in swallowing, lack of oral agility). In addition, and often the most dramatic and most troublesome manifestation, is an inability to inhibit emotional responses, leading to a striking excess of emotional expression called *pseudobulbar affect*.

The motor symptomatology in patients with pseudobulbar palsy can vary considerably. Some patients will show significant bilateral motor disability, involving not only the bulbar musculature but also the limbs, producing paralysis and bradykinesia. Some even suffer double incontinence. Others manifest few limb motor problems but have major bulbar malfunction including difficulty in swallowing, a tendency to drool or choke, a hoarse, hypophonic voice, a masklike expressionless face, and decreased eye-blinking. Pseudobulbar affect—the tendency to laugh uncontrollably in happy situations or to cry and sob following an unhappy stimulus—can be seen with either type of motor dysfunction and even when there is little or no obvious motor disorder. Some patients with pseudobulbar affect will vacillate from one type of excessive emotional outburst (laughing) to the other (crying) in a period of seconds. Although the emotional response tends to be in the appropriate direction, the excessive degree of the response is obviously abnormal.

The pseudobulbar state is a product of bilateral brain insult involving either motor or frontal control pathways (Lieberman and Benson, 1977; Tilney and Morrison, 1912). Damage to the cortex (particularly premotor or prefrontal), subcortical (primarily frontal) white matter, the internal capsule, or the midbrain cerebral peduncles bilaterally can produce the pseudobulbar symptoms. Pseudobulbar palsy must be acknowledged as a serious complication for the aphasic patient. Not only does their bulbar weakness interfere with oral-facial acts such as phonation but their emotional overflow interferes with communication efforts to such a degree as to be almost totally disabling. Language therapy in these cases must be combined with behavioral conditioning, but the result is probably most dependent upon some degree of spontaneous recovery to allow retraining.

Extraocular Motor Palsies

True paralysis of the extraocular musculature (EOM) is not common as a complication of aphasia. The aphasic patient who does show an EOM disorder (e.g., squint) is often found to have a developmental eye muscle imbalance that was overcome during adult life but recurred following unilateral brain damage. On the other hand, disturbance of conjugate (bilateral) eye movements may occur, particularly in patients with anterior aphasia. Following the acute insult, a full *conjugate deviation* may be present; the patient's eyes move only toward the side of the lesion (e.g., to the left with left-hemisphere lesions) and cannot move, or move only weakly, toward the other side. Full conjugate gaze disturbance is almost invariably short-lived, usually lasting a few days to several weeks. During early recovery from conjugate deviation, the patient easily moves his eyes in either direction when following a moving target, but when given commands to "look to the right" and "look to the left," the patient readily carries out the command looking to the left but will fail or have great difficulty looking to the right (a failure of language directed movement, an *apraxia of gaze*). An lesser degree of eye movement difficulty, a problem called *gaze paresis*, is relatively common in patients with anterior aphasia following recovery from the acute eye deviation problem. Gaze paresis is analogous to limb paresis, a weakness but not a total paralysis of movement; right hemiparesis is often accompanied by right gaze paresis. In addition, even if successful in performing lateral gaze, patients with gaze paresis will have difficulty maintaining their gaze toward the paretic side. Even though recovery from conjugate deviation is relatively rapid, a residual gaze paresis may be demonstrated for months or even longer (Holmes, 1918).

Unilateral gaze paresis most commonly follows pathology involving the frontal eye field (Brodmann area 8) (Benson, 1977; Crosby, Humphrey, and Lauer, 1962; Fuster, 1989; Kennard, 1939). The reverse situation—a state in which the ability to follow moving visual stimuli is lost while there is no difficulty moving the gaze on command—can occur in patients with lesions that involve posterior parietal cortex (Brodmann areas 18 and 19) (Crosby et al., 1962). Pathology in the left posterior parietal area may not be associated with aphasia but can affect the ability to read (Holmes, 1918) as the patient has difficulty moving his gaze from left to right along a printed line. Gaze paresis secondary to a dominant-hemisphere Brodmann-area-8 lesion can also interfere with reading (Benson, 1973).

Apraxia

Although long recognized as a neurological disorder (Liepmann, 1900), apraxia remains a mysterious, controversial, and hard-to-define motor abnormality. For much of the twentieth century the term *apraxia* was applied to any disorder, short of gross paralysis, that interferes with complex motor activities. Thus, oral apraxia, verbal apraxia, gait apraxia, oculomotor apraxia, ideational apraxia, constructional apraxia, and dressing apraxia were all explained as breakdowns of patterned motor functions (engrams). In many of these disorders, however, the motor act cannot be performed normally under any circumstance. A pervasive clumsiness indicates underlying disorder of the motor system (a subtle paralysis). One contemporary definition of apraxia excludes any primary motor (or sensory) disorder; only failure to carry out a maneuver competently on oral or written command is accepted as apraxia (Geschwind and Damasio, 1985). A patient's inability to carry out a motor act when verbally commanded although the act is easily performed spontaneously is of obvious significance in the evaluation of aphasia. Apraxia is a common complication in aphasia (De Renzi, Pieczuro, and Vignolo, 1966; Tognola and Vignolo, 1980). Although many varieties of apraxia have been suggested in the literature, only one—ideomotor apraxia—is firmly related to language.

Ideomotor Apraxia

Ideomotor apraxia has been defined as an acquired inability to carry out on command a motor activity that is easily performed spontaneously (Benson and Geschwind, 1985). As many as 40% of aphasic patients, when properly tested, show this problem (Benson, 1979a). Inherent in the definition of ideomotor apraxia is competence, not only in comprehension of language but also in the motor acts necessary to carry them out. Obvious causes of failure such as Wernicke's aphasia, cerebellar ataxia, or hemiplegia are easily excluded. More subtle difficulties are not so readily noted.

Evidence of ideomotor apraxia can be sought by testing the patient's motor responses in three spheres: buccofacial activities (e.g., whistling, coughing, sucking, blowing, winking, smiling), limb activities (e.g., making a fist, waving goodbye, saluting, shaking hands), and whole-body activities (e.g., standing up, sitting down, turning around, kicking a ball). If the aphasic patient comprehends spoken language but fails to perform these acts on command, ideomotor apraxia can be suspected.

Additional tests for possible ideomotor apraxia include requests to imitate the examiner in the use a real object (e.g., a comb, toothbrush, or hammer). When a patient is asked to pretend the use of an object but substitutes his finger or his hand for the object (body part for object), a subtle form of ideomotor apraxia is present.

Ideomotor apraxia is common in the anterior aphasias (Broca aphasia, extrasylvian motor aphasia, conduction aphasia) but is easily misinterpreted as a comprehension disturbance, particularly when tests of language comprehension are limited to responses to a few commands.

Many investigators have attempted to provide mechanistic explanations of apraxia (Geschwind, 1967a; Hécaen and Albert, 1978; Heilman and Gonzalez-Rothi, 1993; Liepmann and Maas, 1907) but most attempts have become complicated by the need to explain the variations of motor response failure. The basic disturbance is illustrated in Figure 17.2, a simple drawing that outlines three neuroanatomical areas in which tissue damage (cortex or white-matter pathways) can produce ideomotor apraxia. One of the areas includes tissues in or deep to the supramarginal gyrus of the dominant parietal lobe involving the superior longitudinal fasciculus, particularly the arcuate fasciculus. A second commonly in-

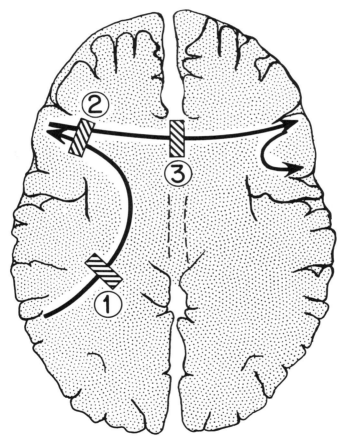

Figure 17.2. Diagrammatic representation of the neural pathways active in carrying out an oral command (e.g., "make a fist with your left hand"). The three areas in which damage can produce ideomotor apraxia are indicated: *(1)* arcuate fasciculus; *(2)* dominant-hemisphere motor association cortex; *(3)* corpus callosum. (From Benson and Geschwind, 1985).

volved area is the dominant-hemisphere motor association cortex, or the white-matter tissues underlying this region. A third brain area includes the anterior corpus callosum and/or the pathways that traverse this interhemispheric connector. Damage to either the arcuate fasciculus or Broca's area of the dominant hemisphere is routinely associated with significant aphasia. Ideomotor apraxia is commonly demonstrated in both Broca and conduction aphasia cases and can interfere with both assessment and rehabilitation.

Sensory Disorders

Although far less obvious than motor impairments, disorders of sensory reception and analysis can produce significant disability for aphasic patients (Beauvois et al., 1978). The underlying problem is easily overlooked unless careful testing of sensory modalities is carried out. Such testing is difficult and the problem is increased by the patient's language disorder.

Hemisensory Loss

Unilateral sensory loss (decreased realization of pain, temperature, and position; poor ability to locate a stimulus on the body; poor texture recognition; and abnormal two-point discrimination) is common, at least as common as motor disorder in the aphasic patient. Hemisensory loss often complicates the clinical findings and may even produce a unilateral inattention state, a state called amorphosynthesis by Denny-Brown and colleagues (Denny-Brown and Banker, 1954; Denny-Brown, Meyer, and Horenstein, 1952).

Demonstration of sensory loss is not easy in the aphasic patient who is unable to give precise verbal responses to sensory tests. Crude estimations of patient response including right/left comparisons and careful observation for subtle indications following stimulation (e.g., grimacing, limb withdrawal, pupil dilation) may provide suggestions of a unilateral sensory impairment. Sensory changes are most common following damage to the parietal lobe or the pathways connecting the parietal sensory cortex with the thalamus. Sensory changes may occur, however, over a broader neuroanatomical spectrum; many patients with anterior aphasia show some degree of unilateral sensory disorder (Benson, 1973). The extent of body area involved (full hemibody or only a portion of the contralateral side) depends on the site and extent of brain damage. Decreased sense of joint movement limited to one or several fingers of the right hand may be the only sensory loss in some patients with conduction aphasia (Geschwind, 1965).

Although not as evident as paralysis, hemisensory loss is at least as disabling and must be considered in rehabilitation plans for the aphasic patient. Blaming poor cooperation (motivation) by the patient for failure of language therapy without realization of the extent of a sensory impairment remains a common problem in neurorehabilitation. Some degree of compensation for sensory impairment can be learned by the patient if the therapist is aware of the problem and provides appropriate training.

Visual-Field Defect

Decrease in the extent of the visual fields (homonymous hemianopia, quadrantopia) is common in aphasic patients, particularly if the underlying pathology involves the posterior hemisphere. Visual-field defects have been correlated with the presence of behavioral problems, and it has been suggested that the presence of a visual-field defect gives rise to a more guarded prognosis for recovery of language disability (De Renzi, Faglioni, and Scotti, 1970; Smith, 1972). In general this is true, probably because the presence of a visual-field defect in addition to an aphasia indicates that a larger area of brain has been damaged.

In some circumstances the visual field defect and/or unilateral visual neglect are of considerable consequence in language processing. In particular, individuals with alexia and a right visual-field defect almost always show both unilateral inattention and occulomotor inintention, producing a mechanical difficulty in the scanning of a printed line that hampers reading retraining. Visual-field defects are relatively easy to demonstrate but most often are not open to improvement through therapy. Only compensatory functions can be taught.

Agnosia

Agnosia, like *apraxia*, is a term that has been sufficiently overused to have lost meaning. In its broadest definition, *agnosia* indicates lack of recognition, and a broad variety of behavioral disturbances can be placed under this rubric. A better definition, "a percept stripped of its meaning" (Milner and Teuber, 1968), implies that even though an intact percept is present (in a single modality) it cannot be recognized but when the same object is presented in another sensory modality, it is readily recognized. Thus, a patient with agnosia may fail to name an object on visual confrontation but readily names the object when it is placed in his hand for palpation. Three types of agnosia will be discussed—visual, auditory, and tactile.

Visual Agnosia

In pure form, visual agnosia is relatively rare, but less isolated visual recognition problems are probably present in many patients with posterior hemisphere damage. By definition, the patient with visual agnosia must have sufficient visual competency to visualize the object (form a percept) and sufficient language to use the object name. The classic visual agnosia occurs when the patient fails to name on visual confrontation but easily succeeds when the object is presented through another sensory modality (Milner and Teuber, 1968; Rubens and Benson, 1971). A separate syndrome related to visual agnosia—optic aphasia—has been suggested (Freund, 1888; Lhermitte and Beauvois, 1973; Schnider et al., 1994) but the distinction between optic aphasia and visual agnosia remains technical and controversial.

Two distinct varieties (or syndromes) of visual agnosia have long been accepted (Lissauer, 1889): (1) *apperceptive visual agnosia,* in which the visual image is sufficiently distorted that it cannot be recognized by the subject (Critchley, 1953; Farah, 1990, Grüsser and Landis, 1991); (2) *associative visual agnosia,* in which the visualized object is perceived normally (as demonstrated by the subject's preserved ability to copy or draw the object) but cannot be identified through visual stimulus alone (Farah, 1990; Grüsser and Landis, 1991; Rubens and Benson, 1971; Teuber, 1968). Most recorded cases of visual agnosia show a hemianopic visual-field defect (usually right-sided); many have prosopagnosia (the inability to recognize familiar faces) (Benson, Segarra, and Albert, 1974; Lhermitte, Chain, and Escourelle, 1972) and constructional disturbance; posterior alexia, color-naming disturbance, amnesia, and anomia have also been reported in patients with visual agnosia. It seems probable that in many cases of posterior aphasia (and/or other brain disorders with significant cognitive disturbance) visual agnosia may be present but masked by many other thought-processing disorders (Benson, 1994).

Auditory Agnosia
Auditory agnosia has been used to describe two clinically distinct disorders (Albert et al., 1972; Goldstein, 1974; Vignolo, 1969). *Verbal auditory agnosia,* also known as pure word-deafness (see Chapter 8), is a state in which language sounds can be heard but not comprehended (Goldstein, Brown, and Hollander, 1975). The opposite, *nonverbal auditory agnosia,* defines a rarely described disorder in which an individual can hear environmental sounds (of a typewriter, a telephone's ring, a dog's bark) but cannot recognize them (Schnider et al., 1994). Individuals with nonverbal auditory agnosia can understand spoken language; those with verbal auditory agnosia can identify nonverbal auditory stimuli. The auditory recognition deficits appear hemisphere-specific (left-verbal; right-nonverbal) (Vignolo, 1969). The pathology in cases of unilateral auditory agnosia involves the primary auditory cortex (Heschl's gyrus) or connections between the thalamus and this area. A few cases of global auditory agnosia based on bitemporal damage have been described. Individuals with global auditory agnosia comprehend written language but cannot readily recognize either spoken language or nonverbal environmental sounds (Kaufer and Benson, 1994). Most individuals with global auditory

agnosia have numerous other disturbances based on brain damage and are often considered psychotic or demented because of the many problems.

Tactile Agnosia

Tactile agnosia is even more difficult to define. Often called *astereognosis*, tactile agnosia most often stems from a primary sensory-processing disorder. Traditionally, the individual with astereognosis fails to recognize an object being palpated but readily names the object when it is visualized. Determining whether the patient's failure represents true agnosia or merely a cortical sensory loss has always proved difficult. Recognition of the presence of a significant sensory disturbance is of importance for aphasia rehabilitation.

Disorders of Cognitive Function

A number of problems in overall cognitive function, either caused by the language disorder or by independent disorders superimposed on the aphasia, deserve careful consideration.

Amnesia

Amnesia, disturbed ability to learn, is a serious complication for the aphasic patient. Amnesia has four consistent clinical characteristics: (1) normal immediate recall (digit span, etc.); (2) significant (not always total) defect in the ability to learn new material; (3) relatively good ability to retrieve old, overlearned material except for a notable gap (called retrograde amnesia) in the recall of material learned long before the onset of the amnesia; (4) relatively intact intelligence and personality functions (Benson and McDaniel, 1991).

Although representing an apparently distinct mental disorder, amnesia becomes far less distinct when a language disorder is superimposed. The distinction between amnesia (inability to learn a name) and anomia (inability to remember a name) appears nebulous, at least superficially; in fact, many patients with anomia complain of a memory disturbance. It is relatively easy, however, to distinguish an individual with a pure anomia from an individual with an uncomplicated amnesia. The individual with anomia does learn new material; and the individual with amnesia easily performs confrontation naming tasks. Although the two conditions are not based on the same underlying problem, distinction becomes difficult when both conditions are present. The boundaries between problems based on learning disorder (amnesia) and those due to language disorder (aphasia) may be almost impossible to define.

The presence of amnesia is of considerable importance in aphasia rehabilitation; the aphasic patient with a significant amnesia will not benefit from language therapy. Rehabilitation measures for such a patient must stress motor retraining and behavioral modification. If, as often happens, the ability to learn improves over time, standard language therapy can then be initiated.

Amnesia can be caused by a number of disorders (Brierly, 1966). The most common is brain trauma where the outlook for eventual recovery of memory function is quite good. Even in cases in which brain trauma has caused both aphasia and amnesia, the possibility of eventual memory improvement is good. Other causes of amnesia, such as stroke, brain tumor, Korsakoff's disease, herpes encephalitis, epileptic surgery, or hypoxia, have less favorable prognoses. Nonetheless, when any of these is associated with aphasia the possibility of sufficient improvement in memory function to merit eventual aphasia therapy warrants ongoing evaluations.

Dementia

Dementia, an acquired impairment of intellectual capacity, is said to be present when there is significant disturbance of at least three of the following functions: (1) speech and/or language, (2) memory, (3) visuospatial skills, (4) cognition (manipulation of the fund of knowledge), (5) personality/emotion (Cummings, Benson, and LoVerme, 1980).

Hundreds of different disorders are known to cause dementia (Cummings and Benson, 1992). The categorization of dementia into cortical or subcortical (Albert, Feldman, and Willis, 1974; Cummings and Benson, 1984) utilizes the difference between speech disorders and language disorders as a distinguishing criterion. Thus, dementias considered to be cortical (e.g., Alzheimer's disease, Pick's disease) have early onset of language disorder but well-preserved motor speech. In contrast, those considered subcortical (e.g., vascular dementia, Huntington's disease or other movement disorders) show early and progressive speech problems but retain language competency. A number of dementing conditions (e.g., head trauma, brain tumor, major strokes) produce a mixed cortical/subcortical picture and show both speech and language impairment.

The language disorders that occur in cortical dementia have been characterized and thoroughly studied (Bayles and Kazniak, 1987; Cummings et al., 1985; Holland et al., 1985; Kertesz, Polk, and Carr, 1990). One of the earliest defects heralding the onset of Alzheimer's disease is a problem with naming. In the earliest stages this is demonstrable only with category naming tasks (e.g., generating a list of names of animals, cities, words beginning with a specific letter of the alphabet). Very early in the course, patients with Alzheimer's disease will perform poorly on word generation tests but show no emptiness in conversational speech and perform normally in confrontation naming tests. As the disease progresses, an emptiness is noted in conversation but the patient still performs adequately in confrontation naming. Eventually, confrontation naming becomes abnormal; by this time the patient also has some comprehension disturbance and tends to use paraphasic substitutions. Eventually a full-blown extrasylvian sensory aphasia syndrome develops, with fluent verbal output and excellent repetition but significant comprehension disturbance, and great difficulty with naming, reading, and writing (Cummings et al., 1985). Along with the progression of the language disorder, other features of Alzheimer's disease are demonstrable, including amnesia, visuospatial dysfunction, personality change, and problems in the manipulation of knowledge.

The combination of dementia and aphasia is probably most troublesome in vascular cases. Following several large strokes, a patient is likely to be both aphasic and demented. The symptom picture varies, based on the areas of brain infarcted. Herpes encephalitis, a less common cause of combined aphasia, amnesia, and dementia, is based on significant temporal-lobe damage. Those patients who survive an initial herpes infection will show a broad dementia. This is followed by a period in which both aphasia and memory disturbance are prominent. With ongoing recovery some patients with herpes encephalitis have little residual aphasia, although a significant memory (learning) disturbance continues (Cermak, 1982; Rose and Symonds, 1960).

As would be anticipated, the presence of dementia makes aphasia rehabilitation extremely difficult. If the cause of the dementia is static (e.g., stroke, brain trauma), however, and some degree of spontaneous recovery can be anticipated, language therapy may prove useful.

Gerstmann Syndrome

Since first fully defined, the Gerstmann syndrome (Gerstmann, 1931) has remained a topic of controversy. The syndrome is defined as the combination of four clinical findings—right-left disorientation, finger agnosia, agraphia, and acalculia (Kinsbourne and Warrington, 1962a). Schilder (1931) and Stengel (1944) noted that all patients who showed the four components of the Gerstmann syndrome also had some degree of constructional disturbance. Early investigators agreed that the syndrome occurred following dominant-hemisphere parietal-lobe disturbance.

The very existence of the Gerstmann syndrome was strongly disputed by Benton (1961, 1977, 1991), Critchley (1966), Heimburger, Demyer, and Reitan (1961), and others who noted that the full syndrome is rare and that the presence of one or several of the components does not indicate dominant-hemisphere parietal-lobe pathology. The pertinence of the syndrome, particularly attempts to explain the four defects by a single psychological mechanism, fell into question. Poeck and Orgass (1966, 1969) demonstrated that the Gerstmann syndrome was almost invariably associated with aphasia and suggested that it was merely a subtle form of language impairment. This was not helpful, however, as an explanation of the syndrome, because most aphasic patients show none or only one or two components of the Gerstmann syndrome.

Ongoing clinical experience has supported the original contentions of Gerstmann, Stengel, and others that when all four clinical findings co-occur, dominant-hemisphere parietal-lobe dysfunction can be strongly suspected. When the Gerstmann syndrome, parietal-temporal alexia and anomic aphasia are all present, dominant angular gyrus damage is probable (Benson, Cummings, and Tsai, 1982). Each of the individual components of the Gerstmann syndrome can occur with pathology located elsewhere in the brain, but co-occurrence of all four components (particularly when associated with parietal-temporal alexia and anomic aphasia) provides strong localization information.

Epilepsy

Convulsive seizures represent a significant complication for the aphasic patient. The frequency with which seizures co-occur with aphasia has proved difficult to ascertain but the common association of aphasia and cerebrovascular accident (CVA) provides some data. It has been estimated that as many as 25% of patients with a cerebrovascular accident will eventually develop seizures; CVA is recognized as the most common cause of an initial seizure in individuals over the age of 70 (Adams and Victor, 1989). Seizures occur more often following hemorrhage than other types of CVA, but infarcts, emboli, tumors, cerebral trauma, neurosurgical procedures, or almost any other invasion of brain tissue can cause epileptic seizures (Engel, 1989).

Most of the seizures in individuals with aphasia can be controlled adequately by use of antiepileptic drugs (AEDs). It must be remembered, however, that almost all AEDs produce some degree of cognitive impairment (Dodrill and Troupin, 1977; Trimble and Reynolds, 1984). The risk of having a seizure must be weighed against the effects of the AEDs when deciding whether an epileptic patient should be treated or not. Most aphasic patients are not given AEDs unless they have had a seizure, but most who do have a seizure will be treated.

Summary

A wide variety of neurologic and behavioral disorders can co-occur with aphasia. In fact, it is the exceptional aphasic patient who does not suffer one or more of the associated disorders discussed in this chapter. These disorders confound the diagnosis of both language and behavior disorders, complicate attempts at aphasia rehabilitation, and seriously hamper the accuracy of pure linguistic investigations of aphasia.

18

Communication Disturbances in Aging and Dementia

· ·

As a cognitive ability, language is relatively insensitive to age effects (Bayles and Kaszniak, 1987). In fact, an individual's language capabilities commonly increase during the lifespan, with continued improvement observed into the 60s. Some deterioration in language capability can be seen during normal aging, however, becoming evident around age 75 (Albert, 1988) to 80 (Benton, Eslinger, and Damasio, 1981). In addition, linguistic decline is evident in some types of dementia. Language disorder is a distinguishing feature of Alzheimer's disease (Cummings and Benson, 1992) and it can be the initial, and for some time the only, cognitive impairment in progressive aphasia (Kirshner et al., 1984; Mesulam, 1982). In contrast, speech disorders are features of a number of subcortical disorders that produce dementia (e.g., Parkinson's disease, Huntington's disease). To characterize the communication disturbances of dementia, the language alterations that occur with normal aging must first be reviewed.

Speech and Language Alterations in Normal Aging

With advancing age, most individuals develop medical problems that broadly affect physical and neurobehavioral function. "Normal" aging becomes almost impossible to define and many of the characteristic features of aging must be acknowledged as indirect effects of disease. It is recognized that some general alterations do occur in normal aging, particularly a pervasive slowing, that can alter both motor and mental functions of the elderly (Cummings and Benson, 1992). Depending on the specific aspect of language considered, aging can be associated with more or less evident language changes (Ardila and Rosselli, 1989; Beasley and Davis, 1981). For instance, it is well known that in the Wechsler Adult Intelligence Scale (WAIS) there is a greater decrement with advancing age in the scores on Performance subtests than on Verbal subtests (Storandt, 1977). Verbal subtest scores, particularly the Vocabulary subtest, tend to remain stable and may even improve with age. Mild word-finding difficulties, reflected as latency during naming, are often the earliest sign of language involvement but are not routinely noted until people reach their 70s. Simplification of grammar and difficulties in phonologic discrimination also occur with advancing age but are usually even more delayed. The language changes in aging are subtle and diverse, involving lexicon, phonology, grammar, language comprehension, and language production. Changes are usually observed only after the seventh decade of life and for most individuals remain mild except in the presence of dementia or other brain pathology.

Lexicon

Vocabulary tends to increase during most of a person's life, with increasing lexicon still evident into the 60s (Bayles and Kaszniak, 1987). Age-dependent decrements in verbal learning can be observed, however, particularly in tasks such as paired associate learning (Ruch, 1934) but this mild verbal learning difficulty suggests a short-term memory deficit. A decline in verbal-memory function can be observed, apparently beginning in or after the 50s (see Table 18.1). Eysenck

Table 18.1. Mean Number of Trials Required to Recall Ten Words in 346 Normal Aging Subjects

YEARS OF SCHOOLING	AGE				
	56–60	61–65	66–70	71–75	>75
0–5 years	8.39	9.05	9.75	9.90	10.14
6–12 years	6.75	7.89	8.45	8.92	9.00
>12 years	6.65	7.24	7.52	7.57	7.86
Average	7.26	8.06	8.57	8.80	9.00

Adapted from Ardila and Roselli, 1989.

(1974) has suggested that the age decrement in verbal memory might indicate that the subject has developed problems with the deeper semantic forms of encoding. Whether the problem with verbal learning is memory dependent or language dependent is probably not a rational distinction. Age-related deficits are more pronounced for connected prose material than for word lists (Craik, 1984; Gilbert and Leveer, 1971). At least some of the memory decline noted with advancing age appears to be associated with increased problems with depression (Speedie et al., 1990).

Total vocabulary is well maintained during old age, at least into the 70s (Fox, 1947; Owens, 1953). Wallach and Kogan (1961) reported a decline in scores on vocabulary tests associated with aging but the decline was relatively late, becoming evident only after the 70s. Although older subjects are slower to make lexical decisions, the lexicon appears intact (Cerella and Fozard, 1984). Increased latencies in verbal tasks probably reflect the general psychomotor slowing of increasing age, not language loss. Bayles, Tomoeda, and Boone (1985), using the Peabody Picture Vocabulary Test-Revised (Dunn, 1965b), found no significant change in subject performance between the third and the eighth decade of life. Obler and Albert (1981) contend that during normal aging, active as opposed to passive vocabulary may deteriorate; thus, the lexicon that the subject can understand is better preserved than the lexicon available for expression.

Although the lexical representation of the words (lexical repertoire) may be intact, semantic representation (meaning of the words) may be disrupted. Botwinick and Storandt (1974) observed differences in the extent of semantic knowledge between young (mean age 18.42) and old (mean age 70.58) "normal" subjects. The younger subjects were frequently able to give superior synonym responses in the WAIS vocabulary subtest; subjects in the seventh and eighth decade were more likely to produce multiword responses (explanations, descriptions, and illustrations). Thus, although the aging subject's repertoire of words is maintained, the semantic field of the lexical items may be narrowed.

Confrontation naming competency has been observed to decrease with age (Au, Albert, and Obler, 1989; Goodglass, 1980; LaBarge, Edwards, and Knesevich, 1986). When subjects are unable to correctly name an item, they often use semantically related associations (semantic paraphasias) or circumlocutions. Table 18.2 shows the scores on naming performance in a shortened version of the Boston Naming Test administered to 346 normal older subjects in different age ranges and with different educational levels (Ardila and Rosselli, 1989). Naming difficulties were strongly dependent on the subject's educational level. Between the youngest (56–60 years) and the oldest (>75 years) age ranges, a decrease of more than 10% is observed in the naming ability of the low-educational-level group in contrast to only about a 2.5% drop in the university-level group. On the

Table 18.2. Naming in the Elderly

Boston Naming Test—shortened version (15 figures). For each figure, 3 points were given when the illustration was correctly named; 2 points when semantic cueing was required for correct naming; 1 point when phonologic cueing was required for correct naming. (Maximum score = 45)

YEARS OF SCHOOLING	AGE				
	56–60	*61–65*	*66–70*	*71–75*	*>75*
0–5	42.05	41.78	41.40	39.84	37.70
6–12	43.25	43.54	42.38	41.64	39.57
>12	44.04	44.48	43.88	43.35	43.29

Adapted from Ardila, Rosselli and Puente, 1994.

Boston Diagnostic Aphasia Examination (BDAE), a negative correlation of −.24 between subject age and Confrontation Naming subtest score, and a negative correlation of −.18 between age and Animal Naming subtest score has been demonstrated (Rosselli et al., 1990).

Phonology

Phonology is well preserved during aging and even in some forms of dementia (Bayles and Kaszniak, 1987; Cummings and Benson, 1992). Emery (1985) did not find differences in the phonological-level subtest scores of the BDAE in a sample of elderly subjects. Phonemic changes in words are not usually observed in the language of the elderly, except for very low frequency words (with the latter, phonemic paraphasias can appear across ages, particularly in low-educational-level subjects who attempt to use low-frequency words). Peripheral nonlanguage problems (e.g., edentulousness, poorly fitting dental prosthesis) or central nervous system disorders (e.g., incipient Parkinson's disease; pseudobulbar palsy) affecting oral agility can produce mild problems in the production of rapid articulatory movements, a disorder sometimes known as "elderly speech." Mild phonetic (but not phonemic) changes can be present.

Phonological discrimination apparently remains normal with advancing age but some decrement in the perception of speech sounds has been reported with increased age (Botwinick, 1978). Aging is often associated with some degree of hypoacusis, particularly affecting higher auditory frequencies; many of the defects in verbal output of the elderly can be attributed to hearing impairment (Botwinick, 1978), not to altered phonemic discrimination. Reduced speech perception may also reflect the increased time required to process information by the higher auditory centers in the elderly (Corso, 1971).

Grammar

The term *grammar* usually encompasses both morphology (word composition rules) and syntax (word order rules); in general, neither morphology nor syntax are particularly sensitive to aging (Botwinick, 1978). Nonetheless, sentences produced by older subjects tend to be simplified. Emery (1985) points out that even though vocabulary reduction is not particularly evident during normal aging, tests that probe internal morphology of words are highly sensitive to aging. The subject's ability to make use of word composition rules may decrease during normal aging.

Emery (1985) also found that aging is associated with difficulties in using and understanding complex syntax. In a test for syntactic complexity, the performance of subjects in the eighth decade was about 80% of that of subjects in the fourth decade. This demonstrable decrement supports the observation that older subjects use simplified grammatical constructions.

Language Comprehension

Emery (1985) compared the performance of normal elderly subjects (mean age 78.5) with young subjects (mean age 36.4) on the Token Test, a sensitive measure of sequential language comprehension, and found a decrement of around 12% in the elderly group. The oldest subjects (those from 78.5 to 88.2 years) showed an additional decrease of about 18%. In the same study, a group of patients with a diagnosis of "Alzheimer-type" dementia scored only about 20% as well as the normal elderly groups. An age effect can be demonstrated in the Auditory Comprehension subtests of the BDAE (see Table 18.3), more evident in subtests such as Complex Material, and less in simple subtests like Commands (Rosselli et al., 1990a).

Language comprehension deficits reflect many superimposed factors: decreased speed in processing information, auditory deficits, decrements in handling complex grammar, and mild difficulty with word meaning. General aging factors (e.g., slowed information processing), sensory deficits (e.g., mild hypoacusis), and actual language deficits (e.g., decreased comprehension of complex grammar, mild word-finding difficulties) are all involved in the language comprehension deficits of the elderly. Language comprehension in the elderly may improve if these factors can be controlled. Thus, when whoever is speaking to the subject speaks at a slower rate, with decreased syntactic complexity, and avoids unusual

Table 18.3. Influence of Age on Auditory Comprehension

Scores on auditory comprehension subtests of the Boston Diagnostic Aphasia Examination in different age ranges. (Mean and standard deviation in parentheses.)

	AGE		
	16–30	*31–50*	*51–65*
Word discrimination	70.9	70.7	68.2
	(3.4)	(4.1)	(8.3)
Commands	15.0	15.0	15.0
	(0.0)	(0.0)	(0.0)
Body part identification	19.4	19.7	18.8
	(1.6)	(0.6)	(3.0)
Complex material	10.5	10.5	9.9
	(1.8)	(2.0)	(1.9)

Adapted from Rosselli et al., 1990a.

and sophisticated words, and when sensory (auditory) loss is controlled for, the older subject demonstrates good language comprehension.

Language Production

Generative naming (verbal fluency) tests in which the subject is asked to produce as many words as possible belonging to a specific category in a specific period of time (usually one minute) show a decrease with age (Obler and Albert, 1981). Table 18.4 presents the word production of normal elderly subjects in two modes: semantic (animals and fruits), and phonological (words beginning with *s* and *a*). In the highest age range, production in the semantic categories was about 70%, and in the phonological categories about 60% of the word production was observed in the youngest subjects. It has been proposed that a normal young adult can name some 18 ± 6 animals in one minute (Goodglass and Kaplan, 1972), and some 15 ± 5 words beginning with a particular letter (Benton and Hamsher, 1976). However, the effect of educational level is so great that "normal" performances are found only in better-educated subjects (Ardila and Rosselli, 1989). Diminished performance in generating names by the elderly can be attributed not only to impairments in verbal search but also to decreased speed in performing the task. General psychomotor slowing represents one of the most basic factors of aging (Van Gorp and Mahler, 1990) and affects many different performances including language.

Bayles and Boone (1982), using a battery of language tests (story-retelling, naming, sentence disambiguation, verbal expression, and sentence correction), discriminated dementia from normal aging; a discriminant analysis disclosed sentence correction and verbal expression tasks to be best at distinguishing patients with senile dementia from normal aged subjects; semantic functions were found to be more sensitive to the effects of aging than phonologic and syntactic activities.

Although repetition is usually preserved (Cummings and Benson, 1989), elderly adults show performance decrements in measures of phonological competence (Benjamin, 1981), auditory comprehension (Goodglass, 1980; Rosselli et al., 1990a), and in speed of encoding and decoding language (Salthouse and Somberg, 1982). The deficits, however, are mild.

Speech and Language in Dementia

Abnormalities in speech and/or language characterize almost all dementia syndromes but both the type and the degree of the communication defect varies considerably among the different syndromes (Cummings and Benson, 1983, 1989). Cortical dementia, particularly dementia of Alzheimer type, is characterized by language disorders, whereas the typical subcortical dementias feature speech disorders (Cummings and Benson, 1983; Cummings et al., 1985). Because of growing public interest and the subsequent availability of research funds, most research effort in the past few years has been devoted to the analysis of the language disorders of dementia of the Alzheimer type (Bayles and Kaszniak, 1987;

Table 18.4. Influence of Age on Verbal Fluency

Results with verbal fluency tests: Scores on semantic (animals and fruits) and phonological (S and A) testing. (Phonological scores in parentheses.)

YEARS OF SCHOOLING	AGE				
	56–60	*61–65*	*66–70*	*71–75*	*>75*
0–5 years	25.65 (18.83)	24.43 (16.81)	22.42 (14.58)	22.55 (14.55)	18.91 (14.05)
6–12 years	32.00 (24.59)	31.87 (24.21)	26.78 (19.85)	25.41 (18.68)	21.91 (14.43)
>12 years	32.30 (26.72)	32.20 (25.85)	31.63 (25.09)	27.55 (24.86)	23.44 (18.17)

Adapted from Ardila and Rosselli, 1989.

Cummings et al., 1985; Diesenfeldt, 1989; Emery, 1985; Kontiola et al., 1990; Murdoch et al., 1987; Shuttleworth and Huber, 1988).

Dementia of the Alzheimer Type

From a rare neuropathological curiosity, Alzheimer's disease has been catapulted into prominence as the fourth or fifth most common cause of death in the United States and one of the most expensive of all current medical health problems (Cummings and Benson, 1992; Katzman and Karasu, 1975; Max, 1993; Plum, 1979).

Often defined merely as a progressive memory disturbance in the elderly, dementia of the Alzheimer type (DAT) has become the label for any dementia syndrome of the elderly that occurs without obvious cause (e.g., stroke, tumor). Current conceptions indicate that at least two varieties of DAT exist, each with clinical features that are clearly distinct from the mental impairments of normal aging and from many other disorders that cause dementia (Saunders et al., 1993). One variety (familial Alzheimer's disease—FAD) features a relatively early onset (before age 60), a progressive course, and in many cases a family history of the disorder. The second variety, senile dementia of the Alzheimer's type (SDAT), also called sporadic Alzheimer's disease, has a later age of onset, a somewhat more indolent course, and less evidence of a familial basis. Most clinicians, however, classify the two varieties as a single disorder—DAT. Unfortunately, most investigations, including many excellent language studies, fail to distinguish between the two varieties of DAT, grouping all progressive dementias of the elderly with the FAD cases as a single entity—Alzheimer's disease. This has produced confusing, indistinct, and often incorrect results.

Both varieties of DAT are characterized by a progressive failure in mental functions that includes defects in language, memory, cognition, visuospatial skills and insight/judgment. Both varieties of DAT lack the motor disorders (speech defects, psychomotor retardation, instability) that are frequently seen with other causes of dementia. The combination of positive and negative verbal-output signs (i.e., abnormal language but normal speech mechanics) provides a fairly distinct and readily diagnosed clinical picture for DAT (Cummings and Benson, 1992; McKhann et al., 1984).

The language disorder in DAT varies with the progression of the disease, ranging from mild word-finding difficulties (demonstrated only by careful testing) to severe global aphasia. Seltzer and Sherwin (1983), based on study of a small population of patients with organic brain disorders, concluded that language disturbances are more prominent in DAT with a presenile presentation; Folstein and Breitner (1981), also in a limited study, proposed that language deficits are found more frequently in dominantly inherited DAT than in the sporadic inheritance variety of DAT. Neither of these assumptions has been consistently confirmed.

In their inventory of clinical features separating cortical from subcortical dementia, Cummings and Benson (1986) proposed that language deficits represented one of the major characteristics of the cortical disorder. In patients with cortical disorders, spontaneous verbal output was described as empty, lacking specific content, and accompanied by naming and comprehension impairments; repetition was well preserved, but paraphasic errors (most often semantic but also phonological) would appear when the disorder became advanced. Aphasia is a constant and systematic manifestation in virtually all patients with DAT (Cummings et al., 1985; Kertesz, 1985).

The evolution of the language dissolution in DAT is consistent. Word-finding difficulty is always present first, often one of the earliest definable defects. The first demonstrable problem is deficient category naming but eventually the word-finding problem produces a notable emptiness (lack of specific substantive words) in the verbal output. In the early stages of DAT, when word-finding defects are obvious in conversation, confrontation naming may remain intact. Finally, with progression of the disease the patient with DAT will show problems with confrontation naming, and as the disorder advances, perceptual defects (difficulty in language comprehension) and paraphasic substitutions occur (Bandera et al., 1991; Diesenfeldt, 1989). At this stage, repetition and motor speech (articulation, syntax) remain intact so the patient with DAT shows an extrasylvian (transcortical) sensory aphasia syndrome on aphasia testing (Cummings et al., 1985). With further progression, the patient's output becomes sparse (except for echolalia) and in the terminal stages the DAT patient will become mute. Differences in naming difficulties range from lexical retrieval problems to agnosia (impaired perceptual analysis) (Goldstein et al., 1992; Shuttleworth and Huber, 1988; Sommers and Pierce, 1990). Both lexical retrieval and perceptual problems can usually be demonstrated as the disorder progresses but word-finding problems appear first and are more evident than the perceptual disorders (Bayles and Kaszniak, 1987).

Although it can be stated that DAT produces an aphasic disorder, this does not mean that DAT is characterized by a typical aphasic syndrome. Instead, at various stages DAT resembles different aphasia syndromes. The progressive variability of the disordered language features has led to disagreement as to the name used to describe the language disturbance of DAT. Critchley (1964) proposed the term *dyslogia*, implying the existence of a generalized cognitive deficit underlying the language problem. Halpern, Darley, and Brown (1973) also considered the language disorder of dementia to represent a generalized intellectual deterioration. Emery (1985) considered that the aphasia syndromes most closely related to the language disorder of DAT were semantic aphasia and transcortical sensory aphasia; she proposed, however, the term *regressive aphasia*, based on the difficulty of fitting the DAT language disturbance into any single established aphasic category.

Whitworth and Larson (1988) administered the Boston Diagnostic Aphasia Examination (BDAE) and the Boston Naming Test (BNT) to a sample of patients with DAT and to a group of other patients who had a dementia not based on DAT. Good correlations were found between Mini-Mental State Examination (Folstein et al., 1975) scores and naming subtests (animal naming, BNT) and the word discrimination subtests that they used. In fact, the scores on the language tests correctly reflected the stage of the dementia of all subjects. Whitworth and Larson suggested that aphasia is an early, pervasive symptom of DAT and that language testing provides differential diagnostic information separating DAT patients not only from the normal elderly but from patients with other causes of dementia.

Most patients with "probable Alzheimer's disease" (McKhann et al., 1984) present a fluent output with occasional paraphasias, some impairment in auditory comprehension, preservation of the ability to repeat, and naming difficulties with both circumlocutions and semantic paraphasias (Appell, Kertesz, and Fisman, 1982; Bayles and Tomoeda, 1983; Kontiola et al., 1990). As spontaneous output remains normal in grammatical competence, phrase length, and melodic line, the semantic system is obviously more impaired than either phonology or syntax (Bayles, 1982).

As DAT progresses, reading and writing deteriorate and are eventually lost; reading aloud remains better preserved than reading comprehension during progression of the disorder. In fact, at one stage in the progression of DAT the patients will read aloud fluently but totally fail to comprehend what they have just said out loud, as though they were reciting a foreign language. Neither phonological paraphasias nor echolalia are evident in their oral reading.

The performance of DAT patients on overlearned verbal tasks (such as the recitation of the alphabet) and completion tasks is generally poor. As the disease continues to progress, repetition eventually deteriorates, the verbal output becomes simplified in grammatical form, and altered mechanical aspects of speech become evident, decreasing the intelligibility of their output. Echolalia, palilalia, logoclonia, and semimutism can be observed in the late stages of DAT and total mutism eventually sets in. Table 18.5 summarizes the language and speech characteristics found in the evolution of DAT.

Other Types of Dementia

Both speech and language disturbances represent important diagnostic criteria in other types of dementia but the different dementia syndromes tend to be associated with different speech and language disturbance profiles (Cummings and Benson, 1983; Gainotti et al., 1989; Kontiola et al., 1990; Murdoch, 1988; Troster et al., 1989).

Table 18.5. Language and Speech
Characteristics of Dementia of
the Alzheimer Type

Initial Stage

Word-finding difficulties

Mild comprehension deficits

Semantic paraphasias and circumlocutions

Good repetition

Phonology preserved

Grammar preserved

Normal articulation

Reading aloud better than reading comprehension

Writing mildly impaired

Middle Stage

Language comprehension deficits

Empty speech

Phonological paraphasias

Repetition span decreased

Grammatical simplification

Reading and writing impaired

Decreased speech volume and intelligibility

Final Stage

Severe anomia

Echolalia

Palilalia

Logoclonia

Semi-mutism to mutism

Reading and writing impossible

Dysarthria

Pick's Disease

Pick's disease features language disturbances as one of the more important clinical signs (Holland et al., 1985). The initial language defect in Pick's disease is a disorder of semantic competence. The patient not only shows difficulty in word-finding but an equally severe problem in word comprehension. For these patients, many substantive words appear to have lost their symbolic meaning. Except for difficulty in interpretation of semantic meaning, language comprehension is preserved. In the early stage of Pick's disease, aphasic signs are infrequent, but iterations in spoken language become common. Some patients tend to retell, endlessly, details of selected aspects of their life; later, iteration of words, echolalia, and logoclonia develop (Tissot, Constantinidis, and Richard, 1985). Paraphasias are rare, but paraphrasing is frequent. The writing of these patients shows the same tendency for iteration observed in spoken language, with seemingly endless repetitions of the same idea in sentences and phrases.

Multi-infarct Dementia

Multi-infarct dementia (MID) is a heterogenous syndrome of mental impairments with symptomatology dependent upon the cerebral area involved by infarction. A wide range of language deficits can be observed in MID (Kontiola et al, 1990). As vascular infarction can involve both cortical and subcortical tissues, language disorders in MID can range from pure speech disorders (dysarthria) to varieties of aphasia syndromes. Cummings and Benson (1989) found a near-normal performance on the language subtests in a group of patients with vascular lacunar disease; these subjects presented short, grammatically simple phrases and some degree of dysarthria was usually present. Table 18.6 compares the speech and language characteristics of DAT, MID and Parkinson's disease subjects.

Subcortical Dementias

Subcortical dementias, when in the pure state, feature a severe speech disorder, without language deficit; the patient will present clinically significant dysarthria but no aphasia (Albert, Feldman, and Willis, 1974; Cummings and Benson, 1983, 1984). Parkinson's disease (PD) and Huntington's disease (HD) are typical degenerative disease states with major pathology focused in subcortical cerebral structures and are almost invariably associated with a progressive dementia. In comparison to DAT, intellectual impairment in the subcortical dementias appears less severe, at least partially because language competency is retained in the subcortical disorders.

In *Parkinson's disease* (PD), dysarthria, disordered writing mechanics, abnormal speech melody, and decreased phrase length and grammatical complexity are seen (Cummings et al., 1988, Cummings and Benson, 1989). PD patients have difficulty repeating complex words and verbal sequences. They show a significant impairment in verbal memory; when presented with a series of words they show limited verbal learning curves with intrusions and increased sensitivity to interference (Ostrosky-Solis et al., 1988). All speech measures tend to be impaired, whereas except for some syntactical simplifications, disorders in language are not

Table 18.6. Comparative Speech and Language Disturbances in Dementia of the Alzheimer Type (DAT), Multi-infarct Dementia (MID), and Parkinson's Disease (PD).

Scale Scores Range from 0 (normal) to 6 (most abnormal)

LANGUAGE TEST	DAT	MID	PD
Spontaneous Speech			
Information content	2.80	0.72	1.18
Melodic line	0.40	2.67	2.56
Phrase length	0.40	1.05	2.31
Grammatical complexity	0.20	—	1.06
Auditory Comprehension			
Word discrimination	0.80	—	0.06
Yes/no questions	0.90	—	0.18
Sequential commands	0.70	—	0.37
Complex commands	1.30	—	1.00
Repetition			
Numbers	0.00	—	0.12
Phrases	1.10	—	0.50
Naming (confrontation)	2.10	0.77	0.43
Paraphasia			
Literal	0.40	—	0.12
Verbal	0.80	—	0.18
Neologistic	0.10	—	0.00
Reading Aloud			
Words	0.00	—	0.00
Sentences	0.60	0.00	0.25
Reading Comprehension			
Word	0.70	—	0.00
Commands	1.30	—	0.56
Sentences	1.20	—	0.37
Writing			
Mechanics	0.60	1.83	3.62
Dictation	1.50	—	2.43
Narrative	3.70	—	3.25

(*continued*)

Table 18.6. Comparative Speech and Language Disturbances in Dementia of the Alzheimer Type (DAT), Multi-infarct Dementia (MID), and Parkinson's Disease (PD). (*Continued*)

Scale Scores Range from 0 (normal) to 6 (most abnormal)

Automatic Speech			
Alphabet recitation	1.00	—	0.87
Counting (1–20)	0.00	—	0.25
Sentence completion	0.40	—	0.00
Nursery rhymes	2.00	2.44	0.86
Speech Characteristics			
Loudness	0.50	1.77	3.81
Pitch	0.20	1.83	2.18
Articulation	0.50	1.88	2.75
Rate	0.30	1.72	2.81
Intelligibility	0.30	—	2.62
Reiteration			
Stuttering	—	0.00	0.70
Mini-Mental State Examination (mean)	17.90	18.77	20.25
Word List Generation			
Animal names per minute (mean)	5.50	—	10.62
Age (mean)	73.20	67.38	71.81

Adapted from Cummings et al., 1985; Cummings et al., 1988; Cummings and Benson, 1989.

evident. Speech monitoring skills are impaired in PD patients (McNamara et al., 1992), but whether this represents a language dysfunction remains unsettled.

Huntington's disease (HD) presents a distinctly different form of dysarthria (ataxic, hyperkinetic) but resembles PD in the minimal degree of language disturbance present during most of the course (Rosselli et al., 1987). In HD patients, word generation becomes impaired but confrontation naming ability remains intact (Butters et al., 1978). Obler and Albert (1981) reported mild naming difficulties in late-stage HD patients but, in general, language function is not significantly impaired (Caine and Fisher, 1985).

In several other traditional subcortical dementing disorders (*Wilson's disease, progressive supranuclear palsy, olivopontocerebellar degeneration*), speech disorder is a notable finding.

One speech characteristic, hypophonia, becomes a significant difficulty in all subcortical dementias; decreased voice volume usually occurs early, and unless the disease process is appropriately treated the hypophonia will progress to total mutism.

Posterior Cortical Atrophy

Crystal and colleagues (1982) reported a patient who was eventually given a diagnosis of Alzheimer's disease but who originally presented with a right parietal-lobe syndrome, and De Renzi (1986) reported a single case of a patient with visual agnosia and apraxia without other evidence of dementia. Benson, Davis, and Snyder (1988) described three cases with an atypical dementia that featured initial symptomatology indicating involvement of posterior cortical (occipital and parietal) structures and suggested that the disorder be called posterior cortical atrophy (PCA). Alexia was an early finding in these cases and became an outstanding clinical sign. Although oral language testing revealed anomia and some decrease in language comprehension in the later stages, repetition remained normal—the pattern of extrasylvian (transcortical) sensory aphasia. Visual agnosia, constructional disturbances, environmental agnosia, and the Balint syndrome (sticky fixation, visual ataxia, and simultanagnosia) were dramatic findings that separated this disorder from DAT. Even more distinguishing, the patients with PCA retained both memory and insight until the very late stages.

Progressive Aphasia

Since the initial, tentative report by Mesulam (1982), a progressive language disturbance known as slowly progressive aphasia, progressive aphasia without dementia, primary progressive aphasia, nonfamilial dysphasic dementia, or progressive language disturbance has attracted considerable attention (Basso, Capitani, and Laiacona, 1988; Craenhals et al., 1990; Duffy and Peterson, 1992; Graff-Radford et al., 1990; Green et al., 1990; Heath, Kennedy, and Kapur, 1983; Kempler et al., 1990; Kirshner et al., 1987; Lippa et al., 1991; Mehler, 1988; Mendez and Zander, 1991; Northen, Hopcutt, and Griffiths, 1990; Poeck and Luzzatti, 1988; Sapin, Anderson, and Pulaski, 1989; Tyrrell et al., 1990; Wechsler, 1977; Weintraub, Robin, and Mesulam, 1990). Progressive aphasia has been defined as a language deficit of insidious onset and gradual progression, with a minimum of a two-year history of progressive language disorder (Weintraub, Robin, and Mesulam, 1990), and prolonged course in the absence of evident generalized cognitive impairment. A real or presumed involvement of the left perisylvian brain region is present, but no focal-nervous-system disease such as infarct, tumor, or abscess can be demonstrated.

Poeck and Luzzatti (1988) emphasized that reports of degenerative conditions selectively affecting language, with sparing of other cognitive functions, extend to at least the beginning of the twentieth century. They list nineteen cases reported in the early neurology literature. Only recently, however, as aphasia and dementia studies have become more sophisticated, has the problem of progressive aphasia attracted medical attention. Between 1977 and 1990, twenty-eight papers appeared in the medical literature on this topic, with a total of fifty-four cases reported (Duffy and Peterson, 1992). Progressive aphasia is not rare.

In 1977, Wechsler reported a case of a patient with presenile dementia who presented with a progressive aphasia and developed a more global mental impairment only in the late end-stage. Mesulam (1982) reported six cases of progressive language deterioration without evident associated intellectual deficit. The observation that a monosymptomatic (language) deterioration can be present for some time as the initial manifestation of a progressive dementia has been further confirmed (Duffy and Peterson, 1992; Kirshner et al., 1987; Poeck and Luzzatti, 1988). Isolated, progressive, monosymptomatic language impairment has also been found in other dementia syndromes such as Creutzfeldt-Jakob disease (Mandell, Alexander, and Carpenter, 1989) and Pick's disease (Graff-Radford et al., 1990). Aphasia may represent the initial, and in some cases the only, sign of dementia (Assal, Favre, and Regli, 1984; Benson and Zaias, 1991). Duffy and Peterson (1992) summarized the main characteristics of progressive aphasia:

1. Age of onset ranges from 40 to 75, with a mean of 59.3 years.
2. Involvement of males predominates over females, with a ratio of 2:1.
3. The duration of isolated language symptoms can range from 1 to 15 years with a mean of 5.3 years.
4. Autopsy findings reported for 14 cases disclosed Pick's disease in four, Creutzfeldt-Jakob disease in three, Alzheimer's disease in 3, focal spongiform degeneration in 2, and nonspecific cellular changes in 2. The diversity of pathology does not support the existence of a specific disease underlying isolated language decline.
5. Of the 47 cases with CT scan, 13 were normal, 5 showed diffuse abnormality, 10 had greater left than right abnormality, and 19 had left-hemisphere abnormality only.
6. Most of the reported cases had predominantly fluent, anomic or Wernicke-like aphasia, but 12 cases with nonfluent or Broca's aphasia have been described.

Snowden and colleagues (1992), reporting on their extensive clinical experience with this disorder, divided progressive aphasia into three varieties—fluent, nonfluent, and mixed.

Progressive aphasia has a variable clinical presentation, probably based on the neuroanatomical locus of the initial pathological breakdown. Progressive aphasia consists of a heterogenous group of symptoms and, as mentioned above, the progressive disorder can begin with isolated neurobehavior disorders, such as alexia, visual agnosia, or apraxia (Benson, Davis, and Snyder, 1988; Crystal et al., 1982; De Renzi, 1986). Current experience suggests that progressive mental impairment may be produced by many different etiologies and may have either focal or widespread (both anatomical and symptomatic) onset; progressive aphasia is one possible occurrence.

Summary

With advancing age, subtle but real decrements in language function can be demonstrated. Both speech and language problems can become disabling in cases of progressive mental impairment (dementia). Dementia of the Alzheimer type, both the familial and the sporadic varieties, is always associated with a language impairment. The degree of language disturbance varies, changing with progression of the disorder; occasionally language disorder may be the only clinical sign of DAT. In multi-infarct dementia, impairment varies depending on the site or sites of brain infarction. Frequently, both cortical and subcortical sites are damaged, producing unique combinations of speech and language disturbances. In pure subcortical dementia, speech dysfunction is present early and language is not significantly impaired until the terminal stages; some naming difficulties, shortened phrase length, decreased grammatical complexity, and verbal learning deficits may be observed but are insignificant in comparison to the speech disorder.

19

Psychiatric Aspects of Aphasia

· ·

The acute loss of the ability to communicate through language produces obvious psychological difficulties for both the patient and those close to him or her. Psychiatric complications are important not only in the overall clinical status of aphasic patients but also in determining the success of rehabilitation. Despite the facts that aphasia has been actively studied for well over a century, that it represents a major arena for subspecialists within psychology (e.g., psycholinguists, neuropsychologists), and that most early treatment methods stressed psychological support (sympathy and understanding), relatively little attention has been given to the psychiatric problems confronting the patient with aphasia.

There may be two reasons for this lack of interest in the psychiatric complications of aphasia. First, it is an obviously "organic" disorder, not basically psychogenic. Under the old and now discredited functional/organic division of behavioral disorders, aphasia was clearly a problem for the neurologist, not the psychiatrist. Second, aphasia obviously interferes with a person's ability to communicate. Both factors tended to exclude the aphasic patient from the purview of most mid-twentieth-century psychiatrists; the "talk therapy" that prevailed during that period was difficult to conduct with an aphasic subject.

The psychiatric problems of the aphasic patient can be severe and, when they occur, are almost invariably significant for the long-term management of a patient with aphasia. These problems will be discussed under two major headings—psychosocial aspects and neurobehavioral aspects—with additional points presented concerning the risk of suicide and the legal ramifications of disordered language function.

Psychosocial Aspects

Many potentially significant psychosocial complications can affect the aphasic patient and family members. Although not the primary concern of most members of the rehabilitation team, these problems are often of paramount concern for the patient and family. Recognizing these problems and using environmental and social changes to improve them can be crucial rehabilitation measures.

Altered Life Style

Easily overlooked is the fact that most individuals with acquired aphasia have a sudden, unexpected, and truly calamitous alteration of their lifestyle. Any impairment of language function is of obvious concern but in many aphasic patients the loss of language, particularly in the early stages, is an overwhelming blow. Language is so basic to human function that its abrupt loss ranks, in shock value, with the sudden onset of blindness, quadriplegia, or an incurable, rapidly fatal malignancy. The loss of language and the concomitant disturbances in physical status (e.g., hemiplegia) seriously jeopardize the stabilizing currents of personal existence: work, social life, recreational activities, family relationships, sexual competence, etc. Even such simple pleasures as reading the newspaper, understanding television, or carrying on a conversation may no longer be possible. The aphasia itself is an adversity but the abrupt change in lifestyle that accompanies the disorder is often the source of the most serious personal problems.

Economic Status

Of real concern for the aphasic, and for family members, is the acute alteration of economic status that can accompany the onset of aphasia. Aphasia often occurs at an age when the individual's earning capacity is at its prime. Most aphasics are financially independent and self-sufficient at the time the disorder occurs. This desirable economic status suddenly disappears. Even though medical and/or disability insurance may be available, family savings and other sources of support are liable to be strained. The aphasic has a growing awareness that economic independence is permanently lost; for many this represents a crushing blow, a loss of lifetime efforts. Problems of financial solvency become a matter of deep concern. In addition, family members, particularly the patient's spouse, may find their financial security dissolved or seriously threatened by the sudden alteration, a situation that adversely affects the patient as well.

Social Status

By the stage of life in which aphasia strikes, most individuals have established fixed, relatively secure, and generally satisfactory patterns of both work and social activities. They have established stable relations with their co-workers, neighbors, social and recreational associates, and many others in their community. The onset of aphasia changes this status but the change does not occur immediately. It is over a period of weeks or months that the degree of change becomes clear. As a patient fully recognizes his altered social position, yet another vexation caused by the aphasia must be acknowledged.

Family Status

In a manner resembling the alteration of social position, aphasia also tends to alter the patient's family status. Most aphasics will have developed a stable role in a family setting, either as the leader or as a major contributor to family activities. If the language disturbance is relatively mild, the aphasic may retain or eventually regain premorbid family status. If the language disturbance remains severe and is permanently disabling, however, the patient's spouse or some other family member will be forced to assume much of the leadership and decision-making role. The onset of aphasia can place an individual in a passive, childlike position within his or her own family. Assistance may be needed to enable the patient to carry out everyday activities (e.g., eating, dressing) and most family decisions will have to be made by others. The patient's reaction to this downgrading of status can be violent, with negative, hostile, paranoid, and downright cruel behavior directed toward close family members. The patient's realization of the alteration of position within the family is often delayed, however, and if family members manage the situation intelligently adverse reactions can be minimized. Unfortunately, many (perhaps a majority) of families are not capable of gracefully carrying out changes in family status for the patient. Spouses often feel (and express) anger and hostility because they now suffer decreased income, altered social position, and have many added responsibilities forced on them. Instead of providing emotional support for the individual who has become aphasic, family members often cause additional psychological problems. Altered family status affects most aphasic individuals and must be recognized as a potential psychosocial complication.

Physical Status

For some aphasics, the onset of the language disorder is accompanied by a significant alteration in physical capability. A previously active, fully self-caring individual may be paralyzed, and must learn to stand and to walk again. The disability may be such that the patient can never hope to regain competence in physical activities such as athletics, dancing, hiking, or even just walking. Less obvious functional changes are common and may be just as disabling as a full paralysis. Insecurity in balance, visual-field defect, unilateral inattention, paresthesias, vague (or not-so-vague) pain, epileptic seizures, the need for surgical treatment, and many other medical problems associated with the brain lesion produce an additional concern for many aphasic patients. Physical disability routinely demands a considerably more confined lifestyle than was enjoyed prior to the onset of the aphasia. The onus of impairment, the threat that additional impairment may occur, and the individual's realization that he or she is truly mortal produces a significant psychological burden. Even more than language impairment, the physical disability that accompanies some cases of aphasia threatens the patient's self-esteem.

Recreational Status

Based on the complications occurring with the onset of aphasia, most patients are forced to change established recreational patterns. Such demanding physical activities as hunting, hiking, swimming, tennis, golf, or bowling may be impossible because of physical problems concomitant with the onset of aphasia. Even less-demanding recreational activities such as card games, reading, or attending parties may not be possible because of communication difficulty. Both the physical disabilities and the language limitations that accompany aphasia cause serious problems for continued recreational activities.

Sexual Status

Frequently overlooked but of considerable significance among the psychosocial problems distressing the aphasic individual is the real or imagined loss of sexual capability (Benson, 1992). Aphasia-producing pathology does not, by itself, affect sexual competency. Nonetheless, a major degree of paralysis, inability to communicate one's feelings, and uncertainty about residual sexual competency can significantly hinder healthy sexual relationships. Many aphasics suspect that they will never regain sexual competency, a belief often shared by their spouse. Most often, the self-imposed moratorium on sexual activity following the onset of aphasia is physiologically unfounded, but if both partners believe that sexual relations are no longer possible, a considerable sexual maladjustment may be present. The patient's problem is often complicated by concern on the part of the spouse that partaking in sexual activities may cause additional brain damage to the patient.

Often, the patient and the spouse are unable or unwilling to communicate their sexual problems to the physician, adding yet another psychosocial restriction to the aphasic patient and the spouse.

From the foregoing resume, it is obvious that the aphasic patient and the involved family members must face a considerable alteration of lifestyle. Recognition of the problems by caretakers can, in many instances, lead to a satisfactory resolution and thus represent a significant rehabilitation measure. The patient's progress in formal language therapy will be greatly improved if the many psychosocial problems are recognized and relieved as well as possible.

Neurobehavioral Aspects

The brain of the aphasic patient has suffered structural damage to important centers of function. Significant behavioral changes, including mood alteration, are common following brain damage (Folstein, Maiberger, and McHugh, 1977). A temporally determined division of the behavioral consequences of aphasia-producing brain damage is presented below. The first section will describe the more general neurobehavioral complications that are particularly notable in the early, post-onset stages. The second will present neuropsychiatric complications that appear to be anatomically based, differing in characteristics depending on the location of the aphasia-producing lesion (Benson and Ardila, 1993).

Early Post-Onset Behavioral Complications

Most stroke patients suffer lethargy and/or confusion in the early stage after onset. The combination of decreased mental functioning and disturbed ability to decode language produces a period of incomplete understanding of their problem. The residual clouding of full consciousness can be somewhat prolonged in aphasics, a period in which they fail to realize the alterations that have occurred. This impairment eventually clears, sometimes in days but often after many weeks. Even after aphasic patients become fully alert, many remain unaware of the full extent of the problem. Neither the consequence of the language defect nor the full extent of physical disability is fully appreciated. Some aphasics appear to deny disability (anosognosia) and many fail to see the problem in appropriate perspective. This early unawareness-unconcern stage provides temporary psychological protection for the patient that makes the initial period following aphasia onset somewhat easier for the family and friends. During this period, however, the patient is unable to participate in plans for the future. Appreciation of reality is significantly decreased. In some patients, particularly those with large posterior, dominant-hemisphere lesions, difficulties in language comprehension (and, presumably, comprehension of their own problem) may persist. In others, the comprehension disorder is more short-lived. In either instance, recovery to a fuller realization of the significance of their problem can lead to a reactive depression.

Reactive Depression

Based on the many personal losses incurred, it would appear appropriate for an aphasic patient to have a period of bereavement, a grief reaction. Altered self-image can lead to feelings of self-deprecation, worthlessness, and severe dysphoria. As a rule, serious reactive depression does not develop with the onset of acquired language impairment. For many aphasic patients, these feelings, if they occur at all, build over a prolonged period, actually measured in weeks or even months. It could be expected that most aphasics would experience reactive depression at some stage, but this is not always so. In some cases, the patient's apparent lack of personal concern reflects the mental deterioration produced by brain injury, but absence of a depressive reaction cannot be automatically accepted as evidence of brain damage or the presence of a strong intrinsic ego strength. Many aphasic patients, particularly those with more posterior language area involvement, do not experience a reactive depression. Many others do develop a characteristic depression with intense feelings of personal worthlessness and hopelessness (Benson and Ardila, 1993). Obviously, this depressive reaction becomes an important, almost an overwhelming, complication for patient management.

The post-onset aphasic reactive depression typically begins with feelings of futility, producing a lack of personal motivation and leading to unwillingness to participate in self-care or in rehabilitation activities. The patient tends to sink within himself or herself, sometimes refusing to eat, and turning away from social interaction with the therapist, with other patients, or even with family members. A strong but passive noncooperation with withdrawal and negativism as key features is seen. The negative reaction may become intense, leading to a catastrophic reaction (Goldstein, 1948), a severe emotional breakdown in which the aphasic patient may cry and moan for hours at a time, increasing the intensity of the outbursts if any effort is made to divert attention or to provide emotional support. The patient forcefully avoids attention, refuses to eat or take medications, and actively declines aid from therapists or family. The catastrophic depressive reaction may be sufficiently severe to produce exhaustion and represents a threat to the patient's health.

Catastrophic reactions are rare in aphasia and need not occur at all. Appearance of the features of a reactive depression in an aphasic patient should immediately alert family members and medical staff to institute strong support measures. Demanding activities such as language therapy and new challenges in occupational or physical therapy should be halted and replaced by activities that the patient can perform successfully. Considerable praise should be given for these successes but, more important, the patient should not be allowed to fail, particularly at tasks considered simple and mundane. The real treatment of catastrophic reaction is prophylactic; by recognizing the patient's increased awareness of his deficits and then by avoiding damaging failures during therapy exercises, the care team can obviate serious catastrophic reaction (Benson, 1992).

Early recognition and prompt response to the onset of the problem by medical personnel and family members are critical elements in the treatment of reactive depression in patients with aphasia. Rehabilitation personnel and family members should be alerted to the possibility of a reactive depression and at the first signs of negativism, withdrawal, sleep problems, or poor appetite, countermeasures should be taken. Sizable amounts of sympathy and personal attention ("tender loving care" in the best use of this term) represents the best treatment and is usually rewarded with the patient's rapid recovery. In truth, reactive depression is a healthy psychological phenomenon and should be allowed to run its course, within limits. It is a painful period, however, for both the patient and those who provide nursing care and rehabilitation. Not only is the aphasic patient significantly depressed, but the problem affects all family members and even medical staff. Support and understanding must be available for all concerned.

The reactive depression seen during aphasia recovery is best controlled by intelligent management. The disorder is self-limited and has a basically favorable prognosis. In most instances the full course is run within ten days. During a period of reactive depression, ongoing language therapy should be continued but should be directed toward positive demonstration of the patient's language competency. Few failures in language function should be allowed. Similar manipulative approaches should be carried out in both physical and occupational therapy. The patient's eating and sleeping patterns may need to be altered and pharmaceutical support offered (e.g., hypnotic medication). Antidepressant medications are rarely necessary or helpful. In fact, these medications are needed primarily to reassure the concerned family, the nursing staff, and physicians that everything possible is being done. Inasmuch as antidepressants are slow to provide response and have powerful, undesirable side effects for many patients in the aphasia age group, they must be used with caution.

Reactive depression is a healthy sign in the aphasic patient. It indicates the recovery of sufficient intellectual competency for the patient to recognize the severity of his problem and the need to alter lifestyle; reactive depression is usually followed by an increased ability to benefit from therapy modalities. The rehabilitation process can then become less involved with overall behavior and more oriented toward specific problems, with an improved potential for success.

Long-Term Neuropsychiatric Complications

Two distinct patterns of psychiatric symptomatology can be seen in aphasic patients and correlated with the neuroanatomical locus of pathology. One disturbance accompanies nonfluent (anterior) aphasia whereas the other occurs in fluent (posterior) aphasia (Benson, 1973).

Frustration/Depression of Anterior Aphasia
The psychiatric reaction associated with anterior (nonfluent) aphasia is time-related. At some time following onset, most individuals with nonfluent aphasia become aware, to a considerable degree, of their new problems. They often know exactly what they want to say but have a verbal output that is restricted and barely intelligible. Their inability to explain their wishes or thoughts is frustrating. Many patients with nonfluent aphasia experience both frustration and depression, problems that interact and aggravate each other. This is the patient in whom a catastrophic reaction may develop, but most often the degree of depression does not reach this dramatic level. The depression in nonfluent aphasia can, however, extend well beyond the reactive depression described above and can represent a serious problem, both in its own right and as a impediment to rehabilitation efforts. The depression is characterized by slowed, almost retarded responses, lack of interest and motivation, and a helpless and hopeless attitude. No effort is expended by the patient. Rumination, although difficult to monitor, appears to dominate the patient's mental efforts. Thoughts of suicide are often voiced by the patient; this threat must be considered seriously by those caring for the patient.

Just as with reactive depression, the depression of anterior aphasia can be combated by recognition of the problem and appropriate alteration of rehabilitation measures. Nursing personnel and family members should be alerted to the patient's problem, including the potential for suicide, and should offer sincere attempts at meaningful interrelationships. Careful monitoring of the patient's emotional status, difficult because of the language impairment, is essential; suicide precautions may be needed. The institution of appropriate antidepressant medication may be of value. The depression of anterior aphasia resembles the depression that follows stroke (Robinson and Chait, 1985; Starkstein and Robinson, 1988, 1993) but physical treatments such as drugs or electroconvulsive therapy must be prescribed with caution in patients with brain damage. The language therapist has a significant potential as psychotherapist, a potential that can be used intelligently in managing the frustration-depression syndrome of anterior aphasia.

Depression is considerably more common in anterior aphasia than in posterior aphasia (Robinson and Benson, 1981). Figure 19.1 illustrates this observation by demonstrating that in a group of brain-damaged stroke patients the distance from the frontal pole of the left hemisphere to the anterior portion of the stroke pathology correlated with the presence of depression (Robinson and Szetela, 1981). The more anterior the lesion the more likely was the patient to have depression.

Several explanations have been suggested for the relationship between left frontal lesions and depression. One, a psychodynamic explanation, centers on the anterior aphasic patient's relatively clear understanding allowing recognition of the significance of the disability coupled with frustration at inability to express their own thoughts and desires (Benson, 1973). This state is further complicated by realization that this undesirable status may be permanent. A more scientific explanation for the depression has also been offered. Robinson et al. (1975) suggested that an asymmetry of neurotransmitter supply, particularly damage to dopamine or norepinephrine channels, could produce the depression. Hemispheric asymmetry of the neurotransmitter distribution has been demonstrated in animals (Robinson et al., 1975; Robinson and Chait, 1985), but whether asymmetry is a source of the problem in humans remains conjectural. Whether the depression is

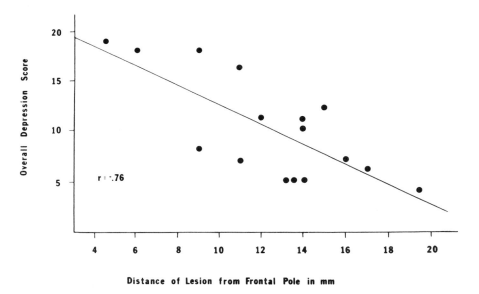

Figure 19.1. Correlation of overall depression score with proximity of lesion site to the frontal pole of the left hemisphere in sixteen left-brain-damaged stroke patients. (From Robinson and Szetela, 1981).

explained neurochemically or psychodynamically, its frequency is high in left anterior stroke patients and represents a factor of consequence in their care.

Unawareness/Unconcern/Paranoia of Posterior Aphasia

Patients with posterior aphasia tend to have a dramatically different behavioral problem. Most not only have notable difficulty in comprehending spoken language but remain unaware of their comprehension problem. This produces a true anosognosia (unawareness, unconcern, and denial). Many patients with posterior aphasia cannot monitor their own verbal output and fail to realize that their verbal output is an incomprehensible jargon. When tape recordings are made of their verbal output and immediately replayed for them, patients with jargon aphasia often deny that it is their output.

Patients with posterior aphasia, unaware of their own problems, tend to blame their communication difficulties on those around them. These patients will complain that the person they are talking to is not speaking clearly (because they themselves cannot understand) or is not attending to what the patient is saying (because they are not being understood). Some posterior aphasia patients suspect that persons in their environment are talking in a special code (which the patient cannot understand), leading to suspicion that these individuals are discussing the patient. This tendency for the patients to place the blame outside of themselves represents a paranoid reaction and is similar (possibly identical) to the well-recognized paranoia seen in patients with acute acquired deafness. In addition, many posterior aphasia patients show impulsive behavior. The combination—unawareness, paranoia, and impulsiveness—can be potentially dangerous. Physical attacks against medical personnel, against family members, against other patients, or against themselves can occur in this group. Almost all aphasic patients who need custodial management because of dangerous behavior suffer from a fluent aphasia (Benson and Geschwind, 1976).

Why patients with posterior aphasia suffer these behavioral abnormalities remains conjectural. Impulsive, paranoid behavior is particularly common when the left temporal lobe is damaged. Thus, almost all patients with pure word-deafness will display significant paranoid responses. The problem is less common when damage is limited to the posterior temporal lobe, producing a Wernicke aphasia, and is much less common with parietal lesions that produce extrasylvian sensory aphasia. Paranoid response is virtually unknown in aphasia based on purely anterior lesions. One possible psychodynamic interpretation, based on patients' unawareness of their own disability leading them to place the blame on others, has been suggested (Benson, 1973). A more neurological interpretation notes that the paranoid disturbance is most striking when more-anterior temporal-lobe tissues are involved, an anatomical locus that is often associated with behavioral dyscontrol (Blumer and Benson, 1982; Elliott, 1992). The language problem in posterior aphasia patients may be further complicated by a tendency toward agitated, impulsive responses. The psychodynamic and neurological interpretations of aphasic paranoid reaction are not necessarily exclusive.

One additional factor further complicating the neurobehavioral disorders occurring with aphasia deserves consideration. Loss of cerebral tissues and their connections alters a number of brain functions, including both basic and higher-level mental control (Benson, 1994). The patient's ability to monitor, manage (inhibit), and control cognitive operations tends to be decreased following brain lesions. *Aphasia should never be considered a disorder affecting language only*. The manifestations of a structurally damaged mental apparatus encompass many non-linguistic behaviors that significantly affect the patient. The aphasic patient is likely to show alterations of personality and/or mental competence similar to those seen in patients with traumatic brain injury.

Suicide

Although the occurrence of suicide is relatively rare in aphasia, the possibility that an aphasic patient will consider, attempt, and/or succeed in suicide deserves serious attention. The depression/frustration/catastrophic reaction seen in patients with anterior aphasia would appear to be the primary suicide concerns, but suicide is rare in this group. Patients with posterior aphasia, on the other hand, particularly those who are paranoid and impulsive, have a tendency toward suicide. In these aphasics, an increasing awareness of their own disability, the probable permanence of a disabling language problem, and the profound alteration of lifestyle based on this disability can lead to premeditated self-destruction. Impulsiveness, also more characteristic of posterior than anterior aphasics, may be a vital factor in producing a rash, life-ending act.

The potential for suicide in patients with aphasia must be recognized and appropriate management modalities considered. This is not easily managed, particularly in patients with posterior aphasia; the language disorders of posterior aphasia make free communication difficult, if not impossible, and preclude or grossly hinder most traditional person-to-person supportive psychotherapy measures. Routine suicide precautions should be put into effect whenever the possibility is suspected. Potential self-destructive devices should be removed, the activities of the patient should be monitored, and if necessary the patient should be transferred to a secure situation such as a locked ward or seclusion room. Intense efforts should be made to establish and maintain interpersonal relationships with the patient; frustrations should be minimized. Even when suicide potential is recognized and appropriate measures are taken, a well-planned life-ending act may still occur. Although suicide is relatively rare in aphasia, about 1 in 2,000 cases (Benson, 1992), the possibility demands recognition. Potent psychotropic drugs such as thorazine, haloperidol, or other neuroleptics may be useful. These drugs, used judiciously in the posterior aphasic patient, are often helpful adjuncts to aphasia therapy and, in the potentially suicidal patient, may be of considerable value. Although neuroleptic dosage should be kept relatively low in the brain-damaged patient, in the treatment of a potential suicide in an aphasic patient the dosage should be sufficient to produce some degree of sedation, at least temporarily.

Legal Aspects

An expert opinion concerning the mental competency of an individual with aphasia may be requested for purely legal (testamentary) purposes. Two aspects of the problem—intelligence in aphasia, and mental competency for legal purposes—deserve consideration.

Intelligence in Aphasia

The relationship between language disorder (aphasia) and mental incompetence (dementia) has produced considerable disagreement (Hoops and LeBrun, 1974). Bastian (1869) dogmatically stated, "We think in words," and many experts use this aphorism to emphasize that the defective use of language symbols automatically produces defects in thinking. Such a view was strongly stressed by the proponents of Gestalt psychology. Goldstein (1948), Brain (1945, 1961), and Bay (1962) accepted that the presence of aphasia indicated abnormal, regressed, or concrete thinking. Most aphasic subjects do perform poorly on standard tests of intellectual competency; this can be demonstrated in the nonverbal as well as the verbal portions of the IQ tests. Many aphasic patients, however, retain nonverbal capabilities to a near-normal degree. There is little doubt that standard IQ tests penalize an aphasic patient, tending to exaggerate any intellectual problems that may be present. Specially designed studies to determine the level of intelligence in aphasia have been reported (Basso, De Renzi, and Faglioni, 1973; Lebrun, 1974; Tissot, Lhermitte, and Ducarne, 1963; Zangwill, 1969). At best, however, these studies provide only nebulous results. Most of these tests treat aphasia as a single, unitary disturbance, failing to note that intellectual dysfunction will vary tremendously, depending on the neuroanatomical locus of damage. Posterior language area pathology is more likely to interfere with intellectual competency than anterior area damage (Benson, 1979b), a clinical observation that has yet to be systematically documented.

Crucial to any discussion of intelligence in aphasia is the definition of intelligence. At best, this remains inadequate. Hamsher (1981) reiterated a broadly held notion: "In civilized cultures, the concept of intelligence has appeared self-evident" (p. 334). Attempts to provide a more precise definition of intelligence are invariably controversial. The term *intelligence* was coined by Cicero, but the concept can be dated to the discourses of Plato, Aristotle, and other early philosophers (Burt, 1955). It can be suggested that intelligence equals stored knowledge, but the ability to manipulate this knowledge is usually included in the definition (Benson, 1994). The definition has been obscured by the use, misuse, and abuse of intelligence testing (Gould, 1981). Some contemporary investigators define intelligence simply as the complex trait that is measured by intelligence tests (Wechsler, 1971). If this approach is used, aphasic patients are severely penalized by the verbal bias of most intelligence tests and their intelligence will be scored as defective. If, however, intelligence is equated with thought processing or with other performance capabilities, some aphasic patients will perform in the normal range and almost all will possess more mental competency than language-based IQ tests can demonstrate. In actual clinical practice the examiner must base any decision concerning the intelligence of an aphasic patient on observations of many different mental capabilities as demonstrated by interpersonal actions (Orgass et al., 1972). Formal test results, although of some usefulness as a base, are not capable of measuring the mental competency of an aphasic patient.

One approach to the administration of neuropsychological testing, the process method (Kaplan, 1990), stresses observation of the strategies used by the subject to solve problems. It appears that the process method could provide useful information for the interpretation of an aphasic patient's intellectual capabilities but, to date, the method is neither fully developed nor widely practiced. Many other less formal observations can be of great usefulness in testing for intelligence in aphasia. Information concerning the patient's retention of social graces; the ability to count and/or make change; the exhibition of appropriate concern about family, business, and personal activities; competency in finding their way in the environment; the ability to socialize; and the presence of self-concern provide valuable indications of residual intelligence in the aphasic patient.

Benson (1979a) stated that "most aphasics comprehend more than they can indicate and think more clearly than their expressive capability demonstrates." Most aphasiologists agree that the demonstration of intellectual competency in the aphasic patient remains difficult and a strong tendency to underestimate the patient's capabilities is still prevalent.

Mental Competency

The clinician may be requested to give an informed opinion concerning an aphasic patient's competency to sign checks or business papers, to dispense money, to manage their own property or other holdings, or to make a will or other testamentary document (Critchley, 1970a). Such a determination demands judgment of both the extent of the patient's language disability and the comprehensibility of the legal document.

Many aphasic patients are fully capable of managing their own affairs; many others are obviously unable to make important decisions and deserve the protection of a conservator or guardian; another group of aphasic patients, intermediate to the first two, can prove troublesome for the clinician who is asked to provide judgment concerning their competency. Even though these patients may have serious language disability, with appropriate aid many of this group are capable of making their own decisions.

When a legal act is to be performed by an aphasic patient (such as the signing of a will or entering into a contract), both thorough evaluation and careful recording of the patient's ability to comprehend spoken and written language and to express their own decisions is necessary. If a clinician is asked to aid an attorney in assuring that the patient understands the legal action, the document in question should be carefully reviewed with the patient on a bit-by-bit basis until both the clinician and the attorney are satisfied that the patient understands the basic meaning of the document. The procedure may require several sessions and, for practical reasons, the document should be kept short, simple, and as free of legal jargon as possible. It is advisable to have the process of explaining the document to the patient videotaped to provide documentation of the explanation and of the patient's response (Benson, 1980, 1992). Although techniques such as this are time consuming, they may allow the aphasic patient to participate in legally complex decision making.

A more difficult problem arises when a clinician is asked to provide testimony concerning an aphasic patient's mental competency in retrospect. Whether the patient was or was not able to understand a legal document consummated after the onset of aphasia is the usual question. Significant testimony can relate only to the observations of the patient's mental and language capabilities recorded at or near the time that the patient signed the document in question. A judgment based on the clinician's review of medical records concerning observations by other physicians or caretakers may be requested. The physician's testimony should attempt to define the patient's ability to understand spoken and written language and to express ideas; it cannot include a firm opinion concerning either the mental competency or the specific desires of the patient at the time in question. The final decision will depend upon whether the document reflected the patient's wishes at the time of signing, a legal, not a medical, determination.

For both legal and personal decisions, aphasic patients should be given the benefit of the extra effort needed to allow them to maintain as much control of their own affairs as possible. A sizable number of aphasic patients are far more intelligent than general appearances would indicate, and many are capable of making their own decisions in significant legal matters.

IV

REHABILITATION

20

Recovery from Aphasia

· ·

Almost from the first observations of language loss due to brain injury, clinicians have been concerned with recovery and rehabilitation. There have been reports of spontaneous or directed language recovery in aphasic patients since at least the sixteenth century (for historical review, see Benton, 1964; Sarno, 1981). It was not until immediately after World War II, however, that hospital units were developed for the rehabilitation of brain-injured patients. A few fundamental observations about aphasia were made in patients injured during World War I, but formal language therapy was not instituted then.

Experience gained from the care of soldiers wounded in World War II gave a major impetus to both the analysis of aphasia recovery and the development of rehabilitation techniques. Medical units devoted to the treatment and rehabilitation of brain damage caused by war injuries were organized, including several units dedicated to the treatment of aphasia. Many of the procedures still used in aphasia rehabilitation were developed from the WWII experience.

Stages of Language Recovery

A perplexing question concerns why some degree of language function returns in most aphasic patients. Two different stages in this recovery of function following brain damage have been suggested (Kertesz, 1988a):

Stage 1: Initial recovery from the acute damage state may reflect recovery from the initial membrane failure that has caused ionic imbalance, edema, hemorrhage, and other cellular disorders. Depending on the type and size of the brain lesion, recovery can commence within a few days of injury and continue for weeks. Some investigators (e.g., Darley, 1975b) suggest a one-month duration for this type of recovery but others believe it can extend further.

Stage 2: Long-term recovery may take place for months or even years. Late recovery suggests the reorganization of language function in the brain. This may involve increased participation of unimpaired areas of the nervous system in language and/or the effects of re-learning.

Figure 20.1 illustrates the two stages of language recovery.

Early (Spontaneous) Recovery Stage

Recovery that occurs naturally, without special treatment, deserves careful consideration. Spontaneous improvement does occur in most aphasia patients and it must be acknowledged that much of the improvement attributed to aphasia therapy, particularly in the early stages, is actually spontaneous recovery. In addition, as Weisenburg and McBride (1935–1964) noted, many aphasic patients carry out a program of self-training; they respond to their language problem by seeking and developing, almost automatically, successful strategies of communication, and most aphasics develop one or more substitute means of communication. Furthermore, aphasics live in a linguistic world and are exposed to a constant program of relearning. Some spontaneous recovery results from naturally evolving neuro-

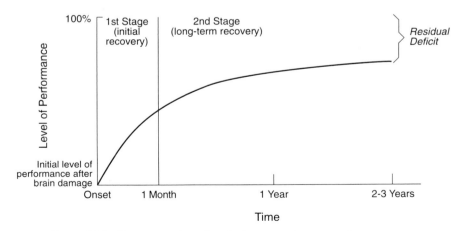

Figure 20.1. Representation of typical course of recovery from aphasia.

physiological processes, but spontaneous recovery is also a consequence of the relearning that occurs naturally from living in a linguistic milieu.

A number of examiners have investigated the course of spontaneous recovery that follows onset of aphasia with generally consistent observations (Culton, 1969; Hanson, Metter, and Riege, 1989; Lomas and Kertesz, 1978; Sarno and Levita, 1971; Smith, 1972; Yarnell, Monroe, and Sobel, 1976). Although all agree that physiological recovery is responsible for the major extent of early language improvement in aphasia, disagreement is found as to how long this spontaneous recovery can be expected. Most investigators suggest that the first one-to-three months is the period of maximum language recovery (Darley, Aranson, and Brown, 1975; Kertesz and McCabe, 1977; Vignolo, 1964). Spontaneous recovery drops precipitously by six to seven months post-onset (Luria, 1963; Sands, Sarno, and Shankweiler, 1969; Vignolo, 1964) and very little spontaneous recovery is demonstrated after one year (Kertesz, Harlock, and Coates, 1979; Kertesz and McCabe, 1977). Thus, spontaneous recovery has a negatively accelerated curve, with maximum increase during the first weeks and months followed by consistent decrease in rate until about one year post-onset, when the curve becomes a virtual plateau. From his review of many reports of untreated aphasia, Darley (1975b) concluded that most spontaneous language recovery occurs in the first month after onset and can be interpreted as neurophysiological changes occurring in the damaged brain. Although spontaneous improvement continues for additional months, the degree was sufficiently limited that in his opinion any significant improvement occurring after this time could be credited to language therapy. Other investigators, however, contend that the patient's self-development of new communication strategies and the benefit of ongoing exposure to language deserve recognition as sources of late "spontaneous" recovery (Penn, 1987).

Late Recovery Stage

Two to three years post-onset, any observed brain damage deficits in the aphasic patient can be considered permanent. A few investigators, however, particularly Geschwind (1985), have suggested that recovery following brain damage can have great individual variation, and in some instances striking improvement may be observed many years after the initial insult. All reports of very late recovery are anecdotal, however, and no long-term investigation supports this view. It is generally agreed that for best results language therapy should be initiated within the first two to three years after aphasia onset.

Analysis of the mechanisms underlying late-stage recovery, when based on rehabilitation, has attracted serious attention (Finger et al., 1988; Stein, 1989). Determination of the mechanisms underlying late recovery has been difficult and several different explanations have been proposed. Much evidence suggests that the right hemisphere plays a role in language processing, an idea originally proposed by Wernicke (1881). Zangwill (1960) analyzed the available evidence and concluded that the two hemispheres were equipotential—that either hemisphere could develop dominance for language, depending on circumstances during early language development. If left hemispherectomy is performed early in life, a nearly normal language development occurs (Basser, 1962). Subtle linguistic deficiencies may be observed in such cases, however; for instance, hemidecorticated subjects demonstrate poor performance in the understanding of complex language syntax (Dennis and Kohn 1975). This observation suggests that one fundamental role of the left hemisphere in language processing concerns phonemic decoding and syntactic organization of language (Zaidel, 1978). The ability of the right hemisphere to acquire language appears to decrease with maturation but does not totally disappear (Cummings et al., 1979).

Right-hemisphere involvement in language has been demonstrated in recovered aphasics in several ways. For instance, some patients who suffer left-brain damage with aphasia but recover language and then sustain a right-brain injury will show a recurrence of the language deficit (Cambier et al., 1983). Similarly, injection of sodium amobarbital into the right carotid artery of recovered aphasics often produces increased language impairment, demonstrating right-hemisphere involvement in language; this finding is rarely present in non-brain-damaged subjects (Kinsbourne, 1971). Evoked-potential studies suggest increasing participation in auditory interpretation by the right hemisphere in left-hemisphere-damaged aphasic patients (Papanicolaou et al., 1988) and studies of cerebral blood flow with Xenon 133 in recovered aphasics disclose increased right-hemisphere participation in language functions (Knopman et al., 1984). Finally, occasional individual case reports have demonstrated late recovery from aphasia in individuals with brain-imaging evidence of total left-hemisphere language area destruction (Cummings et al., 1979). Right-hemisphere participation in the recovery from aphasia can be considered a reasonably well established mechanism (Cappa and Vallar, 1992).

Several investigators, particularly Luria (1963, 1976b), emphasized that functional reorganization of language occurred during aphasia recovery. Functional reorganization refers to the aphasic patient's development of new strategies to compensate for deficits caused by brain damage. Patients with phonemic discrimination deficits learn to rely on proprioception and visual information to compensate for their deficits; patients with difficulties in expository language rely on automatized and emotional language. The patient uses less impaired functions to compensate for the language deficit, a reorganization of the functional system (Luria, 1966; Tsvetkova, 1973); thus, a useful function can be obtained by following a different route. Luria's theory has received support (Goodglass, 1987).

Factors Influencing Recovery

An array of factors that can influence the degree of recovery from aphasia have been proposed. Some appear more crucial than others, but it is probable that they all interact to influence the final language recovery for an aphasic. Basso (1992) distinguishes two groups of prognostic factors related to recovery from aphasia: biographical (age, gender, and handedness), and neurological (etiology, site and extent of lesion, and severity and type of aphasia). Biographical factors appear to play only a minor role in recovery from aphasia whereas neurological factors are crucial. Table 20.1 presents the authors' suggested list of major factors influencing recovery from aphasia.

Lesion Size/Lesion Site

Study of in vivo brain lesions makes it possible to correlate lesion size and lesion location with the degree of recovery. The most elementary factor is lesion size, where a significant negative correlation has been demonstrated between the amount of brain damage and the extent of recovery, with the correlation highest for recovery of fluency in comparison to comprehension (Kertesz, 1988b). Lesion location has also been found to be significant. In Wernicke aphasia, poor recovery

Table 20.1. Factors Influencing Recovery in Aphasia

Lesion size/lesion site	There is a negative correlation between the total amount of brain damaged and the degree of recovery.
Age	In general, the younger the patient, the better the prognosis.
Handedness	Recovery may be better in left-handers.
Gender	Recovery may be better for females than for males.
Etiology	In general, traumatic aphasias have better prognosis than vascular aphasias. Prognosis in tumor cases is variable, but often poor.
Aphasia profile	Anomia represents the most constant residual defect for most aphasic disorders. Comprehension defects have a better prognosis than poor fluency.
Temporal factors	Slow-developing lesions produce a milder aphasia than acute-onset brain damage, but recovery following acute onset is often better.
Time from onset	Greatest recovery occurs in the first weeks or months post-onset, with lesser improvement in the following months. Individual aspects of language may improve to different degrees.
Treatment	Aphasia therapy can prove effective at any period following onset.

has been correlated with middle temporal gyrus, supramarginal gyrus, postcentral gyrus, or insula involvement (Kertesz, 1988a; Kertesz and McCabe, 1977).

Age

The age of the subject has long been considered a crucial factor in language learning. For instance, after a certain age, a second language can no longer be acquired without distinct phonological and syntactic shortcomings. The critical age for language acquisition has been suggested as 12 years by Lenneberg (1967), 5 years by Krashen and Harshman (1972) and even earlier by other investigators (Brain, 1961). In all probability, there is considerable individual variation among subjects. The ability to learn a second language and, by inference, to relearn the first one after aphasia, decreases with age. Sexual maturation and the biological effects of reproductive hormones on the brain are said to produce decreased capacity for language recovery (Kertesz, 1988a). Hemispheric lateralization of language begins early and appears to continue until well after puberty (Bryden, 1963). With increasing lateralization, the speed and efficiency of relearning language after brain damage decreases. The idea that the behavioral effects of brain damage may be less deleterious if sustained early in life, when the nervous system is still immature, has been known as the Kennard principle (Schneider, 1979). However, one study demonstrated that middle aged (50–64) aphasics who had suffered acute onset showed significantly better language recovery than older (65–80) aphasics after a similar acute onset (Taylor, 1992).

Handedness and Gender

Two additional factors for predicting language recovery are frequently mentioned in the literature. Handedness (personal and familial) has been proposed by some as pertinent in aphasia outcome (Geschwind, 1974; Luria, 1966). Some aphasiologists believe that left-handers possess a more bilateral representation of language so that recovery after brain damage would be faster and better. Some proof to support this contention comes from study of World War II brain-injured aphasics (Luria, 1947/1970).

It has also been proposed that gender differences may influence the pattern of recovery in aphasia. Specifically, some investigators posit that females have a more bilateral representation of language (McGlone, 1980); if so, aphasia in women would have a better prognosis. Pizzamiglio and Mammucari (1985) found no initial differences in aphasia severity based on gender in a group of ninety adult aphasics, but three months after onset of aphasia a significantly better improvement was observed in females. The assumption that the prognosis for recovery from aphasia is better for left-handers or for women has not been consistently confirmed (Basso et al., 1990; Kertesz, 1988a). Although gender and handedness may be significant variables in large samples, these factors appear to be of limited significance in individual cases.

Etiology

There can be no question that the etiology underlying the onset of the aphasia is of immense importance in the recovery process. Put simply, progressive disorders progress; gliomas and degenerative processes (e.g., Alzheimer's disease, progressive aphasia) show progressive deterioration. Acute-onset, static disorders (e.g., infarcts, hemorrhages, encephalitis, trauma, resected benign brain tumors) have a better potential for recovery than progressive disorders. Bilateral brain pathology impedes recovery, and, depending on localization, the presence of right-hemisphere lesions tends to limit recovery following left-hemisphere damage that has produced aphasia. As a whole, trauma and hematoma cases appear to recover best. The effects of trauma are often widespread, but if there is no long-term residual amnesia the potential for recovery from post-traumatic aphasia is relatively good. Whether the brain injury is open or closed, head trauma patients appear to do better than those who suffer occlusive vascular accidents or tumors; this is at least partially explained by age difference—trauma usually affects younger individuals (Kertesz, 1988a). Table 20.2 summarizes the influences that various etiologies of aphasic disorders have on the recovery outcome.

Differences in the long-term prognosis between patients suffering vascular accidents and those with invasive brain tumors appear obvious but exceptions are important. The outcome with tumor depends more on the course of the disease than on other recovery factors. Most intracerebral tumors have a poor prognosis and the long-term outcome for a tumor-generated aphasia is limited. Some intracerebral tumors, however, such as oligodendrogliomas or low-grade astrocytomas are slow growing and may respond to surgical debulking, radiation, or chemotherapy and have the potential for relatively long-term aphasia recovery. Extracerebral tumors may have an excellent general prognosis, dependent on type and location; aphasia, if it occurs at all in such cases, often shows a gratifying response to language therapy. Finally, even patients with malignant intracerebral tumor often have a life expectancy of several years or more; language therapy can be just as beneficial for them as it is for patients with aphasia based on other etiologies.

Aphasia Profile

The aphasia profile (the predominant language symptomatology) represents yet another critical factor in recovery. Some aphasic defects are relatively easy to overcome, whereas others are considerably more resistant to improvement. Ano-

Table 20.2. Influence of Etiology on Aphasia Recovery

ETIOLOGY	MOST FREQUENT AGE	TYPE OF EFFECT	PROGNOSIS
Head Trauma			
Closed	Young	Global brain damage	Aphasia is associated with general cognitive impairments (amnesia, attentional defects, personality changes, etc.). Prognosis for the language disorder is good. Mild anomia and verbal memory defects are the most common long-term residual deficits.
Open	Young	Focal brain damage in addition to global effect	A notable, often focal, aphasia plus general cognitive deficits can be seen. The prognosis of the aphasia varies but is relatively good.
Vascular Accident			
Hemorrhage	Middle	Mass effect	If the patient survives, once the bleeding disappears or the blood is drained, the prognosis for language recovery is good.
Occlusion	Late	Focal effect (infarction)	Limited, dependent on size of the infarction and the patient's age.
Tumor			
Extracerebral	Middle	Mass effect (brain compression)	Good recovery of language functions.
Intracerebral	Middle	Focal and mass effect	Usually poor, dependent on the degree of malignancy and the amount of involvement of the language area.

mia can be considered a residual of aphasia that follows recovery. Broca aphasia-Type I, extrasylvian motor aphasia, and conduction aphasia tend to improve toward a status of anomic aphasia (Damasio, 1981; Kertesz, Harlock, and Coates, 1979; Mazzochi and Vignolo, 1979). Wernicke aphasia may recover along two paths: (1) better auditory comprehension (Wernicke aphasia-Type II) and improvement in phonemic accuracy and repetition (i.e., toward anomic aphasia); (2) better comprehension but poor repetition (i.e., toward conduction aphasia) (Alexander and Benson, 1991; Lecours, Lhermitte, and Bryans, 1983). Broca aphasia also improves in several ways (Masdeu and O'Hara, 1983); in some cases, sentence length and syntax improves along with normalization of articulation, phonemic production, and repetition (i.e., to extrasylvian motor aphasia and then to anomic aphasia). In other cases, sentence length and syntax recovers without improved articulation, phonemic production, and repetition (i.e., to a conduction aphasia).

It has been observed that poor comprehension generally has a better prognosis for recovery than poor fluency (Lomas and Kertesz, 1978; Mazzoni et al., 1992; Prins, Snow, and Wagenaar, 1978). It is likely that multiple brain systems contribute to the organization of meaning in spoken words (comprehension), including some operant through the right hemisphere (Gazzaniga and Sperry, 1967). Fluency, on the other hand, apparently requires a specific set of facilitating systems that are activated through the left frontal operculum and relatively fixed projecting pathways (Naeser et al., 1989; Rubens, 1977). Fewer and more-dedicated brain regions apparently contribute to the motor aspects of language production; more widespread and varied brain areas are active in the comprehension of spoken language.

Some aspects of aphasia only emerge following partial recovery. Thus, classic Broca aphasia (Broca aphasia-Type II) is most frequently seen as a late stage following an originally more severe aphasia (Mohr et al., 1978), and deep dyslexia is almost exclusively reported in the late recovery stages of a severe aphasia (Friedman and Perlman, 1982; Marin, 1980).

Temporal Factors

It has long been recognized that acute injuries to the nervous system produce more severe deficits than slowly developing abnormalities, a point strongly supported by studies of recovery after brain damage (Stein, 1989). Monakow (1914) proposed the principle of *diaschisis* to explain the pronounced effects of sudden brain damage. He suggested that acute damage to the nervous system deprives both the surrounding and more distant but functionally connected areas from innervation and produces sudden, basically total inactivation. Diaschisis, the distant effect on neuronal tissues that can follow acute brain damage, has been used to explain decreased neuronal activation in areas distant from known brain lesions (e.g., unilateral cerebellar hypometabolism following infarct of the contralateral cortex [Metter et al., 1984]). It has also been proposed that rerouting of neuronal activity could be expected after acute brain damage and that the effect of diaschisis decreases with time. Diaschisis can be viewed as one more factor responsible for late recovery of language, particularly following a cerebrovascular accident.

In contrast to the scenario following acute damage, slowly developing damage to the brain (such as caused by a tumor) allows ongoing readaptation to the pathological condition, a continuous readjustment. A patient with a tumor that grows slowly over several years has had, in one sense, several years of retraining and recovery.

Time from Onset

Although there is some evidence and many claims implying that one difference affecting the degree of recovery from aphasia is the time elapsed between the onset of aphasia and the beginning of aphasia therapy (Butfield and Zangwill, 1946; Darley, 1975a; Vignolo, 1964), this contention remains unproved and controversial.

Longitudinal studies of aphasia recovery usually begin measurement about one month after onset and follow outcome for 6 to 12 months (Kertesz and McCabe, 1977; Pashek and Holland, 1988; Vignolo, 1964). The greatest recovery occurs within the first two to three months with lesser improvement observed in the following months. Pashek and Holland (1988) noted that the greatest improvement actually occurred during the first one to two weeks after onset, and by three months the clinical status of most aphasics approximated, in a significant degree, that to be expected permanently. In a lengthy longitudinal study, Hanson, Metter and Riege (1989) observed that language scores in aphasia patients increased during the first year, became stable in the second year, and either remained level or declined in the third and fourth years post-onset.

Individual aspects of language can improve to different degrees. Comprehension of spoken language continues to improve for considerable periods and some severe nonfluent aphasics slowly increase their supply of short utterances. Minor improvements can be observed for two to three years post-onset, insufficient to alter the aphasia profile but considerably aiding the communication burden of patients and families (Alexander and Benson, 1991).

One major problem hindering scientific investigation is the lack of data on the natural course of recovery from aphasia. Most accumulated data, of necessity, omits control results (i.e., the recovery patterns of untreated aphasia). Spontaneous improvement represents an unmeasured portion of the improvement occurring with early aphasia therapy. If therapy is not initiated for many months after onset and the aphasia has remained severe, the prognosis for significant improvement with aphasia therapy is limited. Based on this observation, most aphasia therapists believe that starting therapy early, at least within the first few months, is highly desirable. There is no convincing proof, however, that commencing aphasia therapy in the first week or even the first month is crucial for producing maximum language improvement.

Treatment

Although the importance of early aphasia therapy remains controversial, there is widespread agreement that the final outcome of language recovery does depend on the implementation of active treatment measures. The duration and appropriateness of treatment can be crucial factors in aphasia recovery (Basso, 1989).

Five clinical questions determine treatment decisions: (1) who to treat, (2) when to treat, (3) what treatment to use, (4) how often to treat, and (5) when to stop treatment (Alexander and Benson, 1991). A number of texts review these problems (Darley, 1975ab; Helm-Estabrooks and Albert, 1991; Rosenbek, Kent, and LaPointe, 1989; Schuell, Jenkins, and Jimenez-Pabon, 1964; Shewan and Kertesz, 1984).

Despite almost universal agreement among language therapists of the value of therapy for aphasics, there is little acceptable proof of this conviction (Weniger and Sarno, 1990). Formal studies are hampered by the universal idiosyncracy of the individual patients in such factors as age, gender, language lateralization, educational level, underlying health, etiology of the brain injury, location and size of lesion, and the capability of family members and other social support structures. Studies are further hampered by the almost equally universal lack of consistency in therapy techniques among language therapists and by the single, most crucial limitation to establishing any firm statistical data—the ethical impossibility of establishing a matched nontherapy group. Most studies of the efficacy of aphasia therapy use either patient-as-his-own-control or a hypothetical outcome for untreated aphasia as comparisons. Neither is statistically satisfactory.

Despite the lack of firm, scientifically acceptable evidence, a plethora of well-defined clinical observations demonstrate that aphasia therapy is effective. Several studies in which aphasia therapy of various types was presented to selected patients (Basso, Capitani, and Vignolo, 1979; Wertz et al., 1981, 1986) have demonstrated that aphasia does provide positive results. Although these studies suffered obvious statistical and scientific design problems, the results were robust (see Chapter 21). Language therapy must certainly be ranked as a significant factor in the outcome of aphasia.

21

Management and Rehabilitation
of Aphasia

· ·

To one who has lived in a foreign-language environment, the feeling of solitude and isolation that the aphasic patient faces is easy to appreciate. Conversely, speaking to a foreign-language user in one's own environment demands special consideration; grammar must be simple, pronunciation clear, and redundancy is required. Both practical experience and common sense are needed to communicate across languages. Errors made and difficulties endured when trying to learn a second language parallel, to some degree, the problems an aphasic patient encounters in rehabilitation of language use.

Language Rehabilitation

During the past few decades formal language rehabilitation programs have become widely available. Most individuals with speech and language difficulties, including those with aphasia, receive formal diagnostic evaluations and many attend remedial therapy programs. The widespread availability of aphasia therapy is a consequence of several factors: (1) language therapy has attained a respectable professional status with a growing scientific basis and the potential for much creativity; (2) the neurophysiological mechanisms of recovery after nervous-system injury are better understood; (3) enhanced understanding of the brain organization for language has facilitated the development of new remedial procedures; (4)

home computers and other technical devices that are now widely available have been programmed for language rehabilitation.

Basic Factors

Language therapy has several goals: (1) to maintain the patient's verbal activity; (2) to gradually increase the level of difficulty in retraining and relearning language; (3) to provide the patient with successful strategies to communicate; (4) to encourage the patient to continue rehabilitation efforts outside the professional program. In addition, language therapy provides psychological support and may play an important psychotherapeutic role (see Chapter 19).

One critical step in aphasia rehabilitation is to train the patient's family members to maximize communication. They must be encouraged to involve the patient as much as possible in verbal activities and everyday conversations. The family must learn to deal with the aphasic patient when his understanding and/or verbal output are severely limited. Keeping the patient verbally active in his own environment represents a key step toward language improvement, one that requires active participation by close relatives and friends. Family therapy or counseling may be advisable (Wahrborg, 1989).

Most language therapists want to start treatment as soon as possible but delay does not appear to be detrimental. In fact, a number of studies have demonstrated that there was no adverse consequence to long-term outcome when therapy was delayed up to six months (Basso, 1989; Basso, Capitani, and Vignolo, 1979; Wepman, 1973; Wertz et al., 1981, 1986). Delay in initiation of language therapy until the patient is medically and neurologically stable is warranted.

Therapy is usually implemented for a limited period of time (often two to three months) after which treatment techniques are stopped and goals reconsidered. It is not advisable to stop therapy abruptly, however. Some patients undergo an emotional breakdown when therapy is discontinued. Ideally, the aphasic patient should be treated three to five times weekly; later, particularly in situations with strong family interaction, one to two sessions per week may be sufficient, and eventually follow-up sessions spaced every one to two months will suffice.

The responsibility for providing ongoing language therapy should be directed, as much as possible, toward the family and the patient. Useful language exercises should be formulated and presented by the therapist. A plan for ongoing language activities outside the therapy unit should be developed and maintained, monitored by periodic follow-up sessions with the therapist.

Many factors influence the final outcome of language therapy, making outcome prediction difficult (Lehman, DeLateur and Fowler, 1975). Based on review of the pertinent literature plus his own considerable experience in aphasia therapy, Darley (1975a) reported nine factors that influence the outcome of aphasia therapy:

1. Intensive language therapy exerts a positive effect on recovery from aphasia
2. The effects are maximal if language therapy is started early and is maintained
3. The younger the patient, the more hopeful the outcome
4. Underlying etiology affects the outcome of aphasia therapy to a significant degree
5. The milder the language loss, the better the outcome
6. Better results can be expected if the patient is relatively free of complicating associated disorders
7. The patient's motivation, insight, and other personal factors influence the outcome
8. No single factor exerts such a strong negative influence that it precludes a trial of therapy
9. Aphasia therapy not only produces language improvement but simultaneously affects the patient's attitude, morale, and other significant social factors.

Effectiveness of Aphasia Therapy

Whether language therapy is truly helpful has been difficult to prove and the value of formal language rehabilitation has been extensively discussed (Benson, 1979b; Wertz et al, 1981, 1986) and even questioned in the aphasia literature (Weniger and Sarno, 1990). In large part the controversy revolves around the inherent difficulty in separating the improvement based on spontaneous recovery from that gained from formal treatment.

Group Studies

Several attempts have been made to test the effectiveness of language therapy. In one pioneer study, the outcome with and without aphasia therapy was studied in a more-or-less controlled manner (Basso, Capitani, and Vignolo, 1979; Basso, Faglioni, and Vignolo, 1975). Results from this study showed clear evidence that, as a group, aphasic patients who underwent formal therapy at any stage attained better residual language performance than those who received no formal therapy. From a relatively large pool of 271 aphasics, one experimental group received aphasia therapy for at least five months while the remainder had no formal therapy. A language test was administered before the start of therapy and at the end of a six-month period; an obvious, measurable degree of improvement was required before success could be claimed. Many more of the treated patients attained a significant improvement in language competency. The number of patients was sufficiently great that such variables as education, social status, severity and location of pathology, and type of aphasia were randomly equated. Inclusion in the treatment or nontreatment group was environmentally determined, however, based on whether the patient was able to travel to the therapy center two times per week. The lack of randomization of treatment/nontreatment may well have biased the results, particularly because the older and more infirm subjects tended not to travel. Although the studies by Basso and colleagues have technical deficiencies (for the epidemiologist and the statistician), the number of individuals studied is sufficiently large and the results are so conclusive that they command respect.

In a smaller study, aphasic patients in Veterans Administration medical centers in the United States were offered various types of language treatment and, not surprisingly, those patients receiving the most intensive rehabilitation measures showed the best levels of recovery (Wertz et al., 1986). The many variables under investigation and the smaller number of subjects included in the study produced less robust outcomes, but, again, the trend clearly indicated that language therapy was an effective tool for aphasia.

Hagen (1973) demonstrated that extended, intensive therapy in a small, heterogenous group of aphasics produced improvement in several aspects of language when results were compared to a similar group of aphasic patients receiving no treatment. Shewan and Kertesz (1984) compared the effects of language treatment on recovery, using three different language treatments in a sample of one hundred patients. In this study, two treatment modalities provided by trained speech-language pathologists were efficacious, and a third method, provided by trained nonprofessionals, approached statistical significance. Additional studies have stressed the importance of involving the aphasic patient in an active therapeutic program (Goodglass, 1987).

Single-Case Studies
To overcome group analysis difficulties, single-case analysis of the effectiveness of aphasia therapy has been proposed (Coltheart, 1983a; Pring, 1986). For single-case studies a significant caveat concerns use of any inferential statistical procedure that assumes that independent replication is necessary. Rigorous statistical procedures have been devised for single-case-study outcomes (Willmes, 1990) and some specific treatment effects have been inferred.

It is generally accepted that a significant proportion of recovery in aphasia occurs spontaneously (see Chapter 20), based on recovery of underlying neurophysiological processes abetted by the compensatory strategies developed by the patient and family members. The importance of providing directed language therapy to the aphasic patient, even in cases of chronic and severe aphasia, has come to be accepted, however. All aphasic patients deserve consideration for language treatment and most deserve a trial of therapy (Benson, 1979a).

Long-Term Considerations

The value of rehabilitation efforts will vary considerably depending on individual conditions. Patients with progressive disorders (e.g., Alzheimer's disease) respond poorly; in patients with chronic remitting diseases such as multiple sclerosis, compensatory therapy may or may not prove useful. Patients will not benefit from language therapy if rapid neurological deterioration (e.g., inoperable glioblastoma) is likely to outpace any treatment effect or if severely impaired attention (delirium) precludes proper interaction (Alexander and Benson, 1991). Language therapy is not only time consuming but intensely demanding; practical considerations (e.g., age and physical status of the patient, availability of a qualified therapist) often limit the use of therapy.

Aphasia Therapy Methodology

Only since World War II have systematic language rehabilitation procedures for aphasia been developed and extensively practiced. In this period, however, many techniques, some differing greatly, have been introduced, utilized, and refined. Only a few of the more widely practiced systems will be presented here. Therapy techniques for specific speech and language disorders, such as for improving articulation (Ribaucourt-Ducarne, 1986; Rosenbek et al., 1973), for expanding syntax (Jones, 1986), for increasing naming (Deloche, Dordain, and Kremin, 1993; Howard et al., 1985), for decreasing perseveration (Helm-Estabrooks, Emery, and Albert, 1987) and for improving reading (De Partz, 1986; Moyer, 1979), have been developed; some have proved useful for selected aphasia problems. A small sample of these will also be presented.

Stimulus-Facilitation Technique

Wepman (1951, 1953) and Schuell, Jenkins, and Jimenez-Pabon (1964) proposed a series of therapy principles that are still widely used for aphasia rehabilitation. Wepman emphasized the need to stimulate language function to improve the aphasic patient's language performance. In this process, the role of the therapist is to verbally stimulate the patient. Schuell also emphasized the importance of adequate stimulation but stressed controlling the rate, the complexity, and even the loudness of language presentation to the patient. In both Wepman's and Schuell's techniques, one language modality was used to stimulate another; it was found that use of topics that were of interest to the patient was beneficial. Thus, a specially planned program, presented in an encouraging atmosphere and containing personally relevant verbal stimulation with increasing levels of difficulty for the patient, provides optimum language rehabilitation. Wepman (1951) emphasized three approaches to language therapy: (1) *stimulation,* an organized presentation of stimuli sufficient to procure a reaction; (2) *facilitation,* repeated practice to increase the patient's efficiency in language tasks as they are accomplished; and (3) *motivation,* encouragement for the patient to continue the therapy process. These three approaches represent the bulk of traditional aphasia therapy, and techniques based on these three are still used by most language therapists.

Programmed Learning Techniques

Following the introduction of programmed learning techniques in education, programmed therapy was attempted as a technique for aphasia retraining. The original premise that a single, well-designed language program could be used for most, if not all, aphasics was rapidly disproved. The language disorder of each aphasic patient is unique, and an individually designed program is needed for each session, an impossibly time-consuming, labor-intensive, and expensive situation. Nonetheless, principles of programmed learning, particularly repeated practice on the same set of tasks until a consistently successful performance is obtained and then advancing to a more difficult level, are now utilized by most aphasia therapists.

LaPointe (1977) developed a therapy program that he called Base-10 Programmed Stimulation. The commanding feature of this program is that when a response is achieved to a predetermined consistency level, the stimulus is changed and the patient practices with a new stimulus until the desired level is again reached. The program is based on the hypothesis that language breaks down in reverse order to its acquisition.

Shewan (1988; Shewan and Bandur, 1986) developed a rehabilitation approach based on current learning theories with a number of operant conditioning paradigms. Her Language-Oriented Treatment (LOT) for aphasia departs from the view that aphasia represents a loss of language or represents impaired access to an otherwise normal language system; rather, specific aspects of the language system (e.g., phonological, semantic, syntactic), or some combination, are impaired. Because language is impaired, not lost, the goal is not considered reeducation. LOT presents a multimodal programmed treatment based on operant conditioning.

Deblocking

Weigl (1961, 1968) promoted a formal technique called deblocking, emphasizing the use of intact (or less damaged) language channels to compensate for and actually improve the operation of malfunctioning channels (i.e., presenting the patient with the printed word simultaneously with the spoken word, when the patient understands better through one channel than through the other). When a word or utterance is produced by the patient, the likelihood of it being produced later increases. Thus, a patient with naming difficulties, if successful at reading a name aloud, will have a better chance to use that name in conversation.

Functional System Reorganization

Luria and Tsvetkova (Luria, 1963; Tsvetkova, 1973), introduced a series of procedures for aphasia rehabilitation. Their thesis contended that reorganization of the damaged functional system is required after brain damage. Each disorder calls for a unique rehabilitation program based on analysis of the underlying deficit; rearrangement of basic language processes may be required. Better-preserved levels of language can be used as the base point from which to achieve the communication goal. For instance, in motor aphasia, automatized and emotional language are better preserved than directed, repetitive, and propositional language. The better-preserved levels of language are used increasingly by the aphasic patient.

In the system advocated by Luria and Tsvetkova, language rehabilitation usually begins with the actualization of language: the patient is encouraged to produce as much language as possible. When an utterance has been produced, the likelihood of it being produced again increases. In motor aphasia, some sounds and/or words can be obtained from recurring emotional and automatic language. They consider it inadvisable to focus on single words in the patient with Broca aphasia; rather, words should be used in grammatical relationships to combat agrammatism, one of the most persistent deficits of Broca aphasia. With the patient's increased verbal mastery at initial levels, movement to more complex language levels becomes possible.

Luria assumed that in every aphasia syndrome some specific aspect or aspects of language processing are impaired while others are unimpaired; the fundamental deficit must be overcome by exploiting the patient's preserved abilities. For example, patients with dynamic (extrasylvian motor) aphasia have difficulty producing the sequence of an utterance. If an external support is provided (e.g., the patient touches or is guided to touch a sequence of three blocks while pronouncing a sequence of words such as "the boy walks"), his language production may be improved. The external support may eventually be eliminated. Similarly, some patients with naming difficulties suffer a disintegration of semantic relationships for words; classification tasks directed toward reorganization of the semantic fields may prove useful.

The rehabilitation principles proposed by Luria and Tsvetkova have proved successful and have been incorporated into other rehabilitation programs (Beyn and Skokhor-Trotskaya, 1966; Goodglass, 1987).

Melodic Intonation Therapy

One successful innovation in aphasia therapy has been Melodic Intonation Therapy (MIT) (Sparks, Helm, and Albert, 1974). In this technique aphasic patients are taught to tap out the rhythm of a spoken phrase as the phrase is intoned by the therapist, and then, while maintaining the rhythmic pattern, the patient also attempts to intone the phrase. As the patient's intonation becomes successful the therapist gradually withdraws from the exercise and the patient can eventually cease rhythm tapping while continuing intonation. Results with MIT have proved dramatically successful in properly selected patients and the technique has gained worldwide use (Benson et al, 1994). MIT has proved useful, however, for only a single, limited type of language disorder—that featuring severe verbal output limitations including poor verbal agility and poor repetition but with relatively preserved comprehension and poor repetition (Helm-Estabrooks and Albert, 1991). MIT is not a successful therapy for Wernicke aphasia or for any of the extrasylvian language disturbances (Helm, 1978).

Sign Language

Another approach to language therapy attempts substitution by other means of communication. Early studies describing the teaching of sign language to aphasic patients report only limited success (Chen, 1971; Eagleson, Vaughn, and Knudson, 1970). One reason suggested for the routine failure of sign language techniques recognizes that aphasia is often associated with dominant-limb paresis and is further contaminated by nondominant-limb apraxia (See Chapter 17). Coelho and Duffy (1990), however, reported the acquisition of signing by two aphasic subjects despite clearly demonstrated limb apraxia and suggested that limb apraxia did not necessarily impede acquisition of sign/gestures by aphasic patients. They suggested that the severity of the language disorder was the crucial factor.

Most sign languages (there are a number of varieties) demand language competency, and the ability to use signs suffers accordingly in patients with aphasia. One attempt to overcome the language disorder has been through use of Amerind (American Indian), a general communication system, not a language, that can be learned by many aphasics who fail the more complex sign languages (Skelly et al., 1974). Efforts to develop a one-hand version of Amerind signing have proved beneficial. Communication through signing appears to act as a channel for language stimulation (deblocking) and has proved valuable as an introduction to more traditional aphasia therapy. Even if the aphasic patient fails in traditional therapy, the learning of a means of communication, even a limited one, increases his ability to interrelate (Anderson et al., 1992).

Visual Symbol Communication Systems

Initial successes in teaching a visual symbol system for communication to chimpanzees (Gardner and Gardner, 1969; Premack, 1971) stimulated attempts to devise a similar system for use in patients with global aphasia. The results were not striking (Gardner et al., 1976; Glass, Gazzaniga, and Premack, 1973; Kraat, 1990) but were sufficiently encouraging to warrant continued effort (Baker et al., 1976; Weniger and Sarno, 1990).

An early visual symbol communication system, Visual Communication (VIC) (Gardner et al., 1976), utilized individual 3-by-5-inch cards, each with a single nonverbal symbol. Through demonstration, each card was equated to an object, a person, or an action; as "vocabulary" was learned by the patient, modestly complicated combinations could be used by the therapist to communicate with the patient, or vice versa. Independent (non-VIC) language testing demonstrated improved function (both comprehension and naming) in patients receiving VIC (Gardner et al., 1976). Based on this "carryover," a therapy program was designed, starting with presentation of objects and actions as depicted on cards or by mime and leading to the patient's intonation of the appropriate words (Helm and Benson, 1978). Steele and colleagues (1989, 1992) further refined this system with the aid of a computer (Computer-Aided Visual Communication [C-VIC] system). In this technique the computer displays a menu with different categories of objects, and, following a hierarchical access path, the patient can select interjections, animate nouns, verbs, prepositions, modifiers, and common names; special symbols mark the type of phrase used (statement, question, negative, affirmative, command). With practice, the patient selects the symbols and arranges them. Several impaired aphasic patients exceeded their ability to communicate in natural language after training with this computer-based system; although the gains were limited, the results were sufficient to warrant additional studies of the technique.

The success observed with visual symbol systems indicates that many patients with reduced language skills retain some capability to use language (Weniger and Sarno, 1990). Kraat (1990) points out that although the complexities of language and cognitive deficits associated with aphasia will continue to challenge rehabilitation efforts, alternative communication systems may enhance the level of communication competence that an individual with aphasia can achieve. Visual symbol systems remain a meaningful but still limited tool for aphasia therapy.

One variety of aphasia, global aphasia, has consistently proven difficult to treat (Baker et al., 1976; Godfrey and Douglass, 1959; Sarno, Silverman, and Sands, 1970). The VIC system appears to aid some patients with global aphasia.

Collins (1986) developed a multitechnique program specifically for global aphasia. In this program Visual Action Therapy (Helm-Estabrooks et al., 1982; Helm-Estabrooks and Albert, 1991), Blissymbols (pictographs) (Horner and La-Pointe, 1979), PACE (Prompting Aphasics' Communicative Effectiveness—Davis and Wilcox, 1985), formal training in gestural communication, and other similar nonverbal programs were utilized. The results of this and other trial programs (Johannsen-Horbach et al., 1985) have been variable, however; failure or limited improvement was common but the number of positive results reported (Collins, 1986) coupled with severe disability produced by global aphasia is sufficient to encourage ongoing research in this area.

Computers in Aphasia Rehabilitation

Starting in the early 1970s and increasing during the 1980s and 1990s, considerable interest and effort have been invested in the use of computerized programs for aphasia rehabilitation (Bracy, 1983; Bruckert et al., 1989; Guyard, Masson, and Quiniou, 1990; Katz, 1986, 1990; Seron et al., 1980). The computer itself does not provide a specific rehabilitation procedure but can act as an additional avenue for retraining efforts. With appropriate programming, computers can provide a useful aid, particularly when directed at specific and limited disorders of language (Kraat, 1990) such as naming difficulties (Bruce and Howard, 1987; Colby et al., 1981; Deloche, Dordain, and Kremin, 1993). Computers can play a dual role in language rehabilitation: (1) they can provide a technical aid to control stimulus presentation, to monitor the patient's improvement, and to objectively follow the improvement; (2) they can provide a technique for improving performance in selected language functions such as a cueing system for word-finding problems. A variety of computer-based language therapy programs are commercially available (Katz, 1986); all have the limitation of a fixed program that may or may not be appropriate for an individual patient's problem.

The use of computers as adjuncts to language therapy and cognitive rehabilitation has been criticized. Robertson (1990) points out that, although some specific disorders of language may improve with computer training, there is no evidence of its general effectiveness in aphasia therapy. Even more critical, the therapist who depends on or stresses the mechanical approach of a preset program may fail to explore, or may actually disguise, other equal or even more promising approaches. Results to date suggest that computerized language programs are capable of producing some beneficial language practice effects but even this limited effect has been difficult to prove (Loverso, Prescott, and Selinger, 1992).

Summary

Traditional language therapy is sufficiently broad that it can be molded to meet most aphasia problems, but this breadth limits the available venues. Strikingly different approaches to aphasia therapy are currently being reported and additional innovations can be anticipated. At present, however, specific, problem-directed therapy is available for only a few language deficits and their use is not imperative. Melodic Intonation Therapy, the best-known and most rigidly exact language therapy technique, has proved effective for only a limited and strictly designated group of aphasic patients. It appears probable that the successful innovations in language therapy in the future will be those designed for similarly restricted language disturbances. Thus, a specific variety of aphasia (e.g., Broca aphasia) or specific linguistic defect (e.g., semantic anomia) will warrant use of a specific therapy mode. Aphasia therapy then, just as now, will consist of many remarkably disparate approaches molded into a program to benefit the individual patient.

References

Achiron A, Ziv I, Djaldetti R, Goldberg H, Kuritzky A, Melamed E. Aphasia in multiple sclerosis: Clinical and radiological correlations. Neurology 42:2195–2197, 1992.

Adams JH, Graham DI, Gennarelli TA. Contemporary neuropathological considerations regarding brain damage in head injury. In DP Becker, JT Povlishock (eds), Central Nervous System Trauma, Status Report. Bethesda, MD: National Institutes of Health, 1985, pp 65–77.

Adams RD, Victor M. Principles of Neurology. New York: McGraw-Hill, 1977.

Adams RD, Victor M. Principles of Neurology, 3d Ed. New York: McGraw-Hill, 1985.

Adams RD, Victor M. Principles of Neurology, 4th Ed. New York: McGraw-Hill, 1989.

Adler A. Course and outcome of visual agnosia. Journal of Nervous and Mental Disease 3:41–50, 1950.

Ajax ET. Dyslexia without agraphia. Archives of Neurology 17:645–652, 1967.

Akelaitis AJ. Studies of the corpus callosum. II: The higher visual functions in each homonymous field following complete section of the corpus callosum. Archives of Neurology and Psychiatry 45:788–796, 1941.

Akelaitis AJ. Studies on the corpus callosum. VII: Study of language functions (tactile and visual lexia and graphia) unilaterally following section of the corpus callosum. Journal of Neuropathology and Experimental Neurology 2:226–262, 1943.

Akelaitis AJ. A study of gnosis, praxis and language following section of the corpus callosum. Journal of Neurosurgery 1:94–102, 1944.

Alajouanine T. Verbal realization in aphasia. Brain 79:1–25, 1956.

Alajouanine T, Lhermitte F. Acquired aphasia in children. Brain 88:653–662, 1965.

Alajouanine TH, Lhermitte F, Ribaucourt-Ducarne B. Les alexies agnosiques et aphasiques. In T Alajouanine (ed), Les Grandes Activités du Lobe Occipital. Paris: Masson, 1960, pp 235–260.

Alajouanine T, Ombredane A, Durand M. Le Syndrome de la Desintegration Phonetique dans l'Aphasie. Paris: Masson, 1939.

Albert ML. Auditory sequencing and left cerebral dominance for language. Neuropsychologia 10:245–248, 1972.

Albert ML, Bear D. Time to understand: A case study of word deafness with reference to the role of time in auditory comprehension. Brain 97:383–394, 1974.

Albert ML, Feldman RG, Willis AL. The "subcortical" dementia of progressive supranuclear palsy. Journal of Neurology, Neurosurgery, and Psychiatry 37:121–130, 1974.

Albert ML, Goodglass H, Helm NA, Rubens AB, Alexander MP. Clinical Aspects of Dysphasia. New York: Springer-Verlag, 1981.

Albert ML, Obler LK. The Bilingual Brain. New York: Academic Press, 1978.

Albert ML, Sparks R, von Stockert T, Sax D. A case of auditory agnosia: Linguistic and non-linguistic processing. Cortex 8:427–443, 1972.

Albert MS. Cognitive function. In MS Albert, MB Moss (eds), Geriatric Neuropsychology. New York: Guilford, 1988, pp 33–53.

Alexander GE, DeLong MR, Strick PL. Parallel organization of functionally segregated circuits linking basal ganglia and cortex. Annual Review of Neuroscience 9:357–381, 1986.

Alexander MP, Benson DF. The aphasias and related disturbances. In RJ Joynt (ed), Clinical Neurology, Vol 1. Philadelphia: Lippincott, 1991 (Chap 10).

Alexander MP, Benson DF, Stuss DT. Frontal lobes and language. Brain and Language 37:656–691, 1989.

Alexander MP, Fischetta MR, Fischer RS. Crossed aphasia can be mirror image or anomalous: Case reports, review and hypothesis. Brain 112:953–973, 1989.

Alexander MP, Friedman RB, Loverson F, Fischer RS. Lesion localization in phonological agraphia. Brain and Language 43:83–95, 1992.

Alexander MP, Hiltbrunner B, Fischer RS. Distributed anatomy of transcortical sensory aphasia. Archives of Neurology 46:885–892, 1989.

Alexander MP, LoVerme SR Jr. Aphasia after left hemispheric intracerebral hemorrhage. Neurology 30:1193–1202, 1980.

Alexander MP, Naeser MA, Palumbo CL. Correlations of subcortical CT lesion sites and aphasia profiles. Brain 110:961–991, 1987.

Alexander MP, Naeser MA, Palumbo CL. Broca's area aphasias: Aphasias after lesions including the frontal operculum. Neurology 40:353–362, 1990.

Alexander MP, Schmitt MA. The aphasia syndrome in the left anterior cerebral artery territory. Archives of Neurology 37:97–100, 1980.

Allen DA, Rapin I, Wiznitzer M. Communication disorders of preschool children: The physician's responsibility. Developmental and Behavioral Pediatrics 9:164–170, 1988.

Altshuler LL, Cummings JL, Mills MJ Jr. Mutism: Review, differential diagnosis and report of 22 cases. American Journal of Psychiatry 143:1409–1414, 1986.

Anderson SW, Damasio AR, Damasio A. Troubled letters but not numbers: Domain specific cognitive impairments following focal damage in the frontal cortex. Brain 113:749–766, 1990.

Anderson SW, Damasio H, Damasio AR, Klima E, Bellugi U, Brandt JP. Acquisition of signs from American sign language in hearing individuals following left hemisphere damage in aphasia. Neuropsychologia 30:329–340, 1992.

Andrews G, Quinn PT, Sorby WA. Stuttering: An investigation into cerebral dominance for speech. Journal of Neurology, Neurosurgery, and Psychiatry 35:414–418, 1972.

Annett M. A classification of hand preference by association analysis. British Journal of Psychology 61:303–321, 1970.

Antell SE, Keating D. Perception of numerical invariance by neonates. Child Development 54:695–701, 1983.

Appell J, Kertesz A, Fisman M. A study of language functioning in Alzheimer dementia. Brain and Language 17:73–91, 1982.

Aram DM, Ekelman BL, Rose DF, Whitaker HA. Verbal and cognitive sequelae following unilateral lesions acquired in early childhood. Journal of Clinical and Experimental Neuropsychology 7:55–78, 1983.

Arbib M, Caplan D. Neurolinguistics must be computational. The Behavioral and Brain Sciences 2:449–483, 1979.

Arbib MA, Caplan D, Marshall JC. Neurolinguistics in historical perspective. In MA Arbib, D Caplan, JC Marshall (eds), Neural Models of Language Processes. New York: Academic Press, 1982, pp 5–24.

Ardila A. Las Afasias. Bogota, Colombia: Instituto Neurologico de Colombia, 1981.

Ardila A. Neglicencia unilateral derecha. Neurologia en Colombia 7:209–214, 1983.

Ardila A. Neurolinguistica: Mecanismos cerebrales de la actividad verbal. Mexico City: Trillas, 1984a.

Ardila A. Right hemisphere participation in language. In A Ardila, F Ostrosky (eds), The Right Hemisphere: Neurology and Neuropsychology. London: Gordon and Breach 1984b, pp 99–108.

Ardila A. Aphasia for Morse code. A comment on Wyler and Ray. Brain and Language 30:363–366, 1987.

Ardila A. On the origins of calculation abilities. Behavioural Neurology 6:89–98, 1993.

Ardila A, Ardila O, Bryden MP, Ostrosky F, Rosselli M, Steenhuis R. Effects of cultural background and education on handedness. Neuropsychologia 27:893–897, 1989a.

Ardila A, Lopez MV. Transcortical motor aphasia: One or two aphasias? Brain and Language 22:350–353, 1984.

Ardila A, Lopez MV. Severe stuttering associated with right hemisphere damage. Brain and Language 27:239–246, 1986.

Ardila A, Lopez MV. Paroxysmal aphasias. Epilepsia 29:630–634, 1988.

Ardila A, Lopez MV, Montanes P. Afasia amnesica: Implicationes para la psicologia cognoscitiva. XIX Interamerican Congress of Psychology, Quito, Ecuador, June 1983.

Ardila A, Lopez MV, Solano E. Semantic aphasia reconsidered. In A Ardila, F Ostrosky (eds), Brain Organization of Language and Cognitive Processes. New York: Plenum, 1989b, pp 177–193.

Ardila A, Montanes P, Caro C, Delgado R, Buckingham HW. Phonological transformations in Spanish-speaking aphasics. Journal of Psycholinguistic Research 18:163–180, 1989c.

Ardila A, Rosselli M. La vejez: Neuropsicologia del fenomeno del envejecimiento. Medellin, Colombia: Prensa Creativa, 1986.

Ardila A, Rosselli M. Consideraciones acerca de la lectoescritura: Un punto de vista neuropsicologico. In A Ardila, F Ostrosky (eds), Lenguage oral y escrito. Mexico City: Trillas, 1988a, pp 274–308.

Ardila A, Rosselli M. Effects of educational level on linguistic abilities. Eighth Annual Meeting, National Academy of Neuropsychology, Orlando, Florida, February, 1988b.

Ardila A, Rosselli M. Neuropsychological characteristics of normal aging. Developmental Neuropsychology 5:307–320, 1989.

Ardila A, Rosselli M. Acalculias. Behavioral Neurology 3:39–48, 1990a.

Ardila A, Rosselli M. Conduction aphasia and verbal apraxia. Journal of Neurolinguistics 5:1–14, 1990b.

Ardila A, Rosselli M. Spatial agraphia. Brain and Cognition 22:75–95, 1993a.

Ardila A, Rosselli M. Language deviations in aphasia: A frequency analysis. Brain and Language 44:165–180, 1993b.

Ardila A, Rosselli M. Spatial alexia. International Journal of Neuroscience 76:49–59, 1994.

Ardila A, Rosselli M, Ardila O. Foreign accent: An aphasic epiphenomenon? Aphasiology 2:493–499, 1988.

Ardila A, Rosselli M, Pinzon O. Alexia and agraphia in Spanish speakers: CAT correlations and interlinguistic analysis. In A Ardila, F Ostrosky-Solis (eds), Brain Organization of Language and Cognitive Processes. New York: Plenum, 1989d, pp 147–175.

Ardila A, Rosselli M, Puente P. Neuropsychological Evaluation of the Spanish-Speaker. New York: Plenum, 1994.

Ardila A, Sanchez E. Neuropsychological symptoms in the migraine syndrome. Cephalalgia 8:67–70, 1988.

Arendt H. The Life of the Mind. New York: Harcourt Brace Jovanovich, 1978.

Arseni C, Constantinovici A, Iliescu D, Dobrata I, Gagea A. Considerations on post-traumatic aphasia in peacetime. Psychiatria, Neurologia et Neurochirurgie 73:105–115, 1970.

Assal G, Chopins G, Zander E. Isolated writing disorders in a patient with stenosis of the left internal carotid artery. Cortex 6:241–248, 1970.

Assal G, Favre C, Regli F. Aphasia as a first sign of dementia. In J Wertheimer, M Marois (eds), Senile Dementia: Outlook for the Future. New York: Alan R. Liss, 1984, pp 279–282.

Assayama T. Über die Aphasie bei Japanern. Deutsche Archiv für Klinische Medizin 113:523–594, 1914.

Atoynatan TH. Elective mutism: Involvement of the mother in the treatment of the child. Child Psychiatry and Human Development 17:15–27, 1986.

Au R, Albert ML, Obler LK. Language in normal aging: Linguistic and neuropsychological factors. Journal of Neurolinguistics 4:347–365, 1989.

Auerbach SH, Alexander MP. Pure agraphia and unilateral optic ataxia associated with a left superior parietal lobule lesion. Journal of Neurology, Neurosurgery, and Psychiatry 44:430–432, 1981.

Auerbach SH, Alland T, Naeser M, Alexander MP, Albert ML. Pure word deafness: Analysis of a case with bilateral lesions and a defect at the prephonemic level. Brain 105:271–300, 1982.

Ausman JI, French LA, Baker AB. Intracranial neoplasms. In AB Baker, LH Baker (eds), Clinical Neurology, Vol. 1. Philadelphia: Harper & Row, 1981 (Chap. 9).

Avila R. Cuestionario para el estudio linguistico de las afasias. Mexico City: Colegio de Mexico, 1976.

Azcoaga J. Las funciones corticales superiores en el hombre y su desarrollo en el nino. Buenos Aires: Cruz de Sur, 1984.

Bachman, DL, Albert ML. Auditory comprehension in aphasia. In F Boller, J Grafman, G Rizzolatti, H Goodglass (eds), Handbook of Neuropsychology, Vol 1. Amsterdam: Elsevier, 1988, pp 281–306.

Baddeley A. Working memory. Science 255:556–559, 1992.

Baker E, Berry T, Gardner H, Zurif E, Davis L, Veroff A. Can linguistic competence be dissociated from natural language functions? Nature 2:609–619, 1976.

Balota DA, Duchek JM. Semantic priming effects, lexical repetition effects, and contextual disambiguation effects in healthy aged individuals and individuals with senile dementia of the Alzheimer type. Brain and Language 40:181–201, 1991.

Bandera L, Della Sala S, Laiacona M, Luzzatti C, Spinnler H. Generative associative learning in dementia of Alzheimer's type. Neuropsychologia 29:291–304, 1991.

Barrett AM. A case of pure word-deafness with autopsy. Journal of Nervous and Mental Disease 37:73–92, 1910.

Barton M, Maruszewski M, Urrea D. Variation of stimulus context and its effect on word-finding ability in aphasics. Cortex 5:351–365, 1969.

Basser LS. Hemiplegia of early onset and the faculty of speech with special reference to the effects of hemispherectomy. Brain 85:427–460, 1962.

Basso A. Therapy of aphasia. In F Boller, J Grafman (eds), Handbook of Neuropsychology, Vol 2. Amsterdam: Elsevier, 1989, pp. 67–82.

Basso A. Prognostic factors in aphasia. Aphasiology 6:337–348, 1992.

Basso A, Capitani E, Laiacona M. Progressive language impairment without dementia: A case with isolated category specific semantic defect. Journal of Neurology,Neurosurgery, and Psychiatry 51:1201–1207, 1988.

Basso A, Capitani E, Vignolo LA. Influence of rehabilitation on language skills in aphasic patients. Archives of Neurology 36:190–196, 1979.

Basso A, Della Sala S, Farabola M. Aphasia arising from purely deep lesions. Cortex 23:29–44, 1987.

Basso A, De Renzi E, Faglioni P. Neuropsychological evidence for the existence of cerebral areas critical to the performance of intelligence tasks. Brain 96:715–728, 1973.

Basso A, Faglioni P, Vignolo LA. Etude contrôlée de la reéducation du langage dans l'aphasie: Comparaison entre aphasiques traités et non-traités. Revue Neurologique 131:607–614, 1975.

Basso A, Farabola M, Grassi MP, Laiacona M, Zanobio ME. Aphasia in left handers. Comparison of aphasia profiles and language recovery in non-right-handed and matched right-handed patients. Brain and Language 38:233–252, 1990.

Bastian HC. On the various forms of loss of speech in cerebral diseases. British and Foreign Medical-Chirurgical Revue 43:209, 470, 1869.

Bastian HC. On different kinds of aphasia. British Medical Journal 2:931–936, 985–990, 1887.

Bastian HC. Aphasia and Other Speech Defects. London: H. K. Lewis, 1898.

Bates E, Friederici A, Wulfeck B. Comprehension in aphasia: A cross-linguistic study. Brain and Language 32:19–67, 1987.

Bates E, Friederici A, Wulfeck B, Juarez LA. On the preservation of word-order in aphasia: Cross-linguistic evidence. Brain and Language 33:232–265, 1988.

Baxter DM, Warrington EK. Neglect dysgraphia. Journal of Neurology, Neurosurgery, and Psychiatry 46:1073–1078, 1983.

Baxter DM, Warrington EK. Category specific phonological dysgraphia. Neuropsychologia 23:653–666, 1985.

Baxter DM, Warrington EK. Ideational agraphia: A single case study. Journal of Neurology, Neurosurgery, and Psychiatry 49:369–374, 1986.

Bay E. Aphasia and non-verbal disorders of language. Brain 85:411–426, 1962.

Bay E. Principles of classification and their influence on our concepts of aphasia. In AVS De Reuck, M O'Connor (eds), Disorders of Language. Boston: Little, Brown, 1964, pp 122–139.

Bayles KA. Language function in senile dementia. Brain and Language 16:265–280, 1982.

Bayles KA, Boone DR. The potential of language tasks for identifying senile dementia. Journal of Speech and Hearing Disorders 47:210–217, 1982.

Bayles KA, Kaszniak AW. Communication and Cognition in Normal Aging and Dementia. Boston: Little, Brown, 1987.

Bayles KA, Tomoeda, CK. Confrontation naming impairment in dementia. Brain and Language 19:98–114, 1983.

Bayles KA, Tomoeda CK, Boone DR. A view of age-related changes in language function. Developmental Neuropsychology 1:231–264, 1985.

Bear DM, Fedio P. Quantitative analysis of interictal behavior in temporal lobe epilepsy. Archives of Neurology 34:454–467, 1977.

Beasley DS, Davis GA (eds). Aging: Communication Processes and Disorders. New York: Grune and Stratton, 1981.

Beauvois MF, Derouesne J. Phonological alexia: Three dissociations. Journal of Neurology, Neurosurgery, and Psychiatry 42:1115–1124, 1979.

Beauvois MF, Derouesne J. Lexical or orthgraphic agraphia. Brain 104:21–49, 1981.

Beauvois MF, Saillant B, Meininger V, Lhermitte F. Bilateral tactile aphasia: A tacto-verbal dysfunction. Brain 101:381–402, 1978.

Behrmann M, Bub D. Surface dyslexia and dysgraphia: Dual routes, single lexicon. Cognitive Neuropsychology 9:209–252, 1992.

Behrmann M, Moscovitch M, Black SE, Mozer M. Perceptual and conceptual mechanisms in neglect dyslexia: Two contrasting studies. Brain 113:1163–1183, 1990.

Bell DS. Speech functions of the thalamus inferred from the effects of thalamotomy. Brain 91:619–638, 1968.

Bellugi U, Poizner H, Klima ES. Brain organization for language: Clues from sign aphasia. Human Neurobiology 2:155–170, 1983.

Benbow CP. Sex differences in mathematical reasoning ability in intellectually talented preadolescents: Their nature, effects and possible causes. Behavioral and Brain Sciences 11:169–232, 1988.

Benjamin B. Phonological performance in gerontological speech. Journal of Psycholinguistic Research 11:159–167, 1981.

Benson DF. Fluency in aphasia: Correlation with radioactive scan localization. Cortex 3:373–394, 1967.

Benson DF. Psychiatric aspects of aphasia. British Journal of Psychiatry 123:555–566, 1973.

Benson DF. Disorders of verbal expression. In DF Benson, D Blumer (eds), Psychiatric Aspects of Neurologic Disease. New York: Grune and Stratton, 1975, pp 121–135.

Benson DF. Alexia. In JT Guthrie (ed), Aspects of Reading Acquisition. Proceedings of 5th Annual Hyman Blumberg Symposium on Research in Early Childhood Education. Baltimore: Johns Hopkins University Press, 1976, pp 7–36.

Benson DF. The third alexia. Archives of Neurology 34:327–331, 1977.

Benson DF. Amnesia. Southern Medical Journal 71:1221–1227, 1978.

Benson DF. Aphasia, Alexia, and Agraphia. New York: Churchill Livingstone, 1979a.

Benson DF. Aphasia rehabilitation. Archives of Neurology 36:187–189, 1979b.

Benson DF. Neurologic correlates of anomia. In Whitaker H, Whitaker HA (eds), Studies in Neurolinguistics, Vol. 4. New York: Academic Press, 1979c, pp 293–328.

Benson DF. Psychiatric problems in aphasia. In MT Sarno, O Hook (eds), Aphasia: Assessment and Treatment. New York: Masson, 1980, pp 192–201.

Benson DF. Alexia and the neuroanatomical basis of reading. In MC Wittrock, FJ Pirozzolo (eds), Neuropsychological and Cognitive Processes in Reading. New York: Academic Press, 1981, pp 69–72.

Benson DF. The alexias: A guide to the neural basis of reading. In HS Kirshner, F Freemon (eds), The Neurology of Aphasia. Amsterdam: Swets, 1982, pp 139–161.

Benson DF. Subcortical dementia: A clinical approach. Advances in Neurology 38:185–194, 1983.

Benson DF. The neurology of human emotion. Bulletin of Clinical Neurosciences 49:23–42, 1984.

Benson DF. Alexia. In JAM Frederiks (ed), Handbook of Clinical Neurology, 2d Ed, Vol 45: Clinical Neuropsychology. Amsterdam: Elsevier, 1985a, pp 433–455.

Benson DF. Language in the left hemisphere. In DF Benson, E Zaidel (eds), The Dual Brain: Hemispheric Specialization in Humans. New York: Guilford Press, 1985b, pp 193–203.

Benson DF. Anomia in aphasia. Aphasiology 2:229–236, 1988a.

Benson DF. Classical syndromes of aphasia. In F Boller, J Grafman, G Rizzolatti, H Goodglass (eds). Handbook of Neuropsychology, Vol 1. Amsterdam: Elsevier, 1988b, pp 267–280.

Benson DF. The Geschwind syndrome. In DB Smith, D Treiman, M Trimble (eds), Advances in Neurology, Vol 55: Neurobehavioral Problems in Epilepsy. New York: Raven Press, 1990, pp 411–421.

Benson DF. Neuropsychiatric aspects of aphasia and related language impairments. In SC Yudofsky, RE Hales (eds), Textbook of Neuropsychiatry, 2d Ed. Washington, DC: American Psychiatric Press, 1992, pp 311–327.

Benson DF. The Neurology of Thinking. New York: Oxford University Press, 1994.

Benson DF, Ardila A. Depression in aphasia. In SE Starkstein, RG Robinson (eds), Depression in Neurological Diseases. Baltimore: John Hopkins University Press, 1993, pp 152–164.

Benson DF, Blumer D (eds). Psychiatric Aspects of Neurologic Disease. New York: Grune and Stratton, 1975.

Benson DF, Brayton-Gerratt S, Dobkin BH, Gonzalez-Rothi LJ, Helm-Estabrooks N, Kertesz A (Expert Panel). Assessment: Melodic Intonation Therapy. Report of the Therapeutics and Technology Assessment Subcommittee of the American Academy of Neurology 44:566–568, 1994.

Benson DF, Brown J, Tomlinson EB. Varieties of alexia. Neurology 21:951–957, 1971.

Benson DF, Cummings JL. Agraphia. In JAM Frederiks (ed), Handbook of Clinical Neurology, 2d Ed, Vol 45: Clinical Neuropsychology. Amsterdam: Elsevier, 1985, pp 457–472.

Benson DF, Cummings JL, Tsai SY. Angular gyrus syndrome simulating Alzheimer's disease. Archives of Neurology 39:616–620, 1982.

Benson DF, Davis RJ, Snyder BD. Posterior cortical atrophy. Archives of Neurology 45:789–793, 1988.

Benson DF, Denckla MB. Verbal paraphasia as a source of calculation disturbance. Archives of Neurology 21:96–102, 1969.

Benson DF, Geschwind N. The alexias. In PJ Vinken, GW Bruyn (eds), Handbook of Clinical Neurology, Vol 4. Amsterdam: North-Holland, 1969, pp 112–140.

Benson DF, Geschwind N. The aphasias and related disturbances. In AB Baker, LH Baker (eds), Clinical Neurology, Vol 1. New York: Harper and Row, 1971 (Chap 8).

Benson DF, Geschwind N. Psychiatric conditions associated with focal lesions of the central nervous system. In S Arieti, M Reiser (eds), American Handbook of Psychiatry, Vol 4. New York: Basic Books, 1975, pp 208–243.

Benson DF, Geschwind N. The aphasias and related disturbances. In AB Baker, LH

Baker (eds), Clinical Neurology, Vol 1. New York: Harper and Row, 1976 (Chap 8).

Benson DF, Geschwind N. Aphasia and related disorders: A Clinical Approach. In AB Baker, RJ Joynt (eds), Clinical Neurology, Vol 1. Philadelphia: Harper and Row, 1985 (Chap 10).

Benson DF, McDaniel KD. Memory disorders. In WG Bradley, RB Daroff, GM Fenichel, CD Marsden (eds), Neurology in Clinical Practice, Vol 2. Boston: Butterworth-Heinemann, 1991, pp 1389–1406.

Benson DF, Patten DH. The use of radioactive isotopes in the localization of aphasia-producing lesions. Cortex 3:258–271, 1967.

Benson DF, Segarra J, Albert M. Visual agnosia-prosopagnosia. A clinicopathologic correlation. Archives of Neurology 30:307–310, 1974.

Benson DF, Sheremata WA, Bouchard R, Segarra JM, Price D, Geschwind N. Conduction aphasia. Archives of Neurology 28:339–346, 1973.

Benson DF, Tomlinson EB. Hemiplegic syndrome of the posterior cerebral artery. Stroke 2:559–564, 1971.

Benson DF, Weir WF. Acalculia: Acquired anarithmetria. Cortex 8:465–472, 1972.

Benson DF, Zaias BW. Progressive aphasia: A case with postmortem correlation. Neuropsychiatry, Neuropsychology, and Behavioral Neurology 4:215–223, 1991.

Benton AL. Right-Left Discrimination and Finger Localization: Development and Pathology. New York: Hoeber-Harper, 1959.

Benton AL. The fiction of the "Gerstmann syndrome." Journal of Neurology, Neurosurgery, and Psychiatry 24:176–181, 1961.

Benton AL. Contributions to aphasia before Broca. Cortex 1:314–327, 1964.

Benton AL. Constructional apraxia and the minor hemisphere. Confinia Neurologica 29:1–16, 1967.

Benton AL. Differential behavioral effects in frontal lobe disease. Neuropsychologia 6:53–60, 1968.

Benton AL. Reflections on the Gerstmann syndrome. Brain and Language 4:45–62, 1977.

Benton AL. Gertsmann's syndrome. Archives of Neurology 49:445–447, 1991.

Benton AL, Eslinger P, Damasio A. Normative observations on neuropsychological test performance in old age. Journal of Clinical Neuropsychology 3:33–42, 1981.

Benton AL, Hamsher K. Multilingual Aphasia Examination. Iowa City: University of Iowa, 1976.

Benton AL, Hamsher KS. Multilingual Aphasia Examination, Rev Ed. Iowa City: University of Iowa, 1978.

Benton AL, Joynt RJ. Early descriptions of aphasia. Archives of Neurology 3:205–222, 1960.

Berger H. Über Rechenstorungen bei Herderkraunkungen des Grosshirns. Archiv für Psychiatrie und Nervenkrankheiten 78:236–263, 1926.

Berndt RS. Category-specific deficits in aphasia. Aphasiology 2:237–240, 1988a.

Berndt RS. Repetition in aphasia: Implications for models of language processing. In F Boller, J Grafman, G Rizzolatti, H Goodglass (eds), Handbook of Neuropsychology, Vol 1. Amsterdam: Elsevier, 1988b, pp 347–366.

Berndt RS, Caramazza A. A redefinition of the syndrome of Broca's aphasia: Implications for a neuropsychological model of language. Applied Psycholinguistics 1:225–278, 1980.

Berndt RS, Caramazza A. Syntactic aspects of aphasia. In MT Sarno (ed), Acquired Aphasia. New York: Academic Press, 1981, pp 157–181.

Bever TG, Chiarello RJ. Cerebral dominance in musicians and non-musicians. Science 185:537–539, 1974.

Beyn ES, Shokhor-Trotskaya MK. The preventive method of speech rehabilitation in aphasia. Cortex 2:96–108, 1966.

Bindman E, Tibbetts RW. Writer's cramp: A rational approach to treatment? British Journal of Psychiatry 131:143–148, 1977.

Bisiach E, Luzzatti C. Unilateral neglect of representational space. Cortex 14:129–133, 1978.

Bisiach E, Perani D, Vallar G, Berti A. Unilateral neglect: Personal and extra-personal. Neuropsychologia 24:759–767, 1986.

Bisiach E, Vallar G. Hemineglect in humans. In F Boller, J Grafman, G Rizzolatti, H Goodglass (eds), Handbook of Neuropsychology, Vol 1. Amsterdam: Elsevier, 1988, pp 196–222.

Bloodstein O. A Handbook of Stuttering. Chicago: National Easterseal Society, 1981.

Blumer D, Benson DF. Psychiatric manifestations of epilepsy. In DF Benson, D Blumer (eds), Psychiatric Aspects of Neurologic Disease, Vol 2. New York: Grune and Stratton, 1982, pp. 25–47.

Blumstein SE. A Phonological Investigation of Aphasic Speech. The Hague: Mouton, 1973.

Blumstein S. Phonological aspects of aphasia. In MT Sarno (ed), Acquired Aphasia. New York: Academic Press, 1981, pp 129–155.

Bogen JE. The other side of the brain. I: Dysgraphia and dyscopia following cerebral commissurotomy. Bulletin of the Los Angeles Neurological Society 34:73–105, 1969.

Bogen JE. Mental duality of the intact brain. Bulletin of Clinical Neurosciences 51:3–29, 1986.

Bogen JE, Bogen GM. The other side of the brain. III: The corpus callosum and creativity. Bulletin of the Los Angeles Neurological Society 34:191–220, 1969.

Bogen JE, Bogen GM. Wernicke's region: Where is it? Annals of the New York Academy of Sciences 280:834–843, 1976.

Bogousslavsky J, Regli F. Unilateral watershed infarcts. Neurology 36:373–377, 1986.

Bogousslavsky J, Regli F, Assal G. The syndrome of unilateral tuberothalamic artery territory infarction. Stroke 17:434–441, 1986.

Bogousslavsky J, Regli F, Assal G. Acute transcortical mixed aphasia. Brain 111:631–641, 1988.

Bogousslavsky J, Regli F, Uske A. Thalamic infarcts: Clinical syndromes, etiology and prognosis. Neurology 38:837–848, 1988.

Boller F. Johann Baptist Schmidt. Archives of Neurology 34:306–307, 1977.

Boller F, Albert ML, LeMay M, Kertesz A. Enlargement of the sylvian aqueduct: A sequel of head injuries. Journal of Neurology, Neurosurgery, and Psychiatry 35:463–467, 1972.

Boller F, Grafman J. Acalculia: Historical development and current significance. Brain and Cognition 2:205–223, 1983.

Boller F, Grafman J. Acalculia. In JAM Frederiks (ed), Handbook of Clinical Neurology, Vol 45: Clinical Neuropsychology. Amsterdam: Elsevier, 1985, pp 473–482.

Boller F, Vignolo LA. Latent sensory aphasia in hemisphere damaged patients: An experimental study with the Token Test. Brain 89:815–831, 1966.

von Bonin G, Bailey P. The Neocortex of *Macaca mulatta*. Urbana: University of Illinois Press, 1947.

Bonvicini G. Die storungen der Lautsprache bei Temporallappenlasionen. In A Marburg (ed), Handbuch der Neurologie des Ohres, Vol 2. Vienna and Berlin: Urban and Schwarzenberg, 1929, pp 1570–1868.

Borod JC, Goodglass H, Kaplan E. Normative data on the Boston Diagnostic Aphasia Examination and the Boston Naming Test. Journal of Clinical Neuropsychology 2:209–215, 1980.

Botez MI. Parietal lobe syndromes. In JAM Frederiks (ed), Handbook of Clinical neurology, Vol 45: Clinical Neuropsychology. Amsterdam: Elsevier, 1985, pp 63–85.

Botez MI, Barbeau A. Role of subcortical structures, and particularly of the thalamus, in the mechanism of speech and language. International Journal of Neurology 8:300–320, 1971.

Botwinick J. Aging and Behavior. New York: Springer, 1978.

Botwinick J, Storandt M. Vocabulary ability in later life. The Journal of Genetic Psychology 125:303–308, 1974.

Bouillaud J-B. Recherches cliniques propres à de'montrer que la perte de la parole correspond à la lésion des lobules antérieurs du cerveau et à confirmer l'opinion de M. Gall sur la siège de l'organe du langage articulé. Archives Générale de Medicine 8:25–45, 1825.

Boyle M, Canter GJ. Neuropsychological analysis of a typewriting disturbance following cerebral damage. Brain and Language 30:147–164, 1987.

Bracy OL. Computer based cognitive rehabilitation. Cognitive Rehabilitation 1:7–8, 1983.

Bradshaw JL, Nettleton NC. The nature of the hemispheric specialization in man. Behavioral and Brain Sciences 4:51–91, 1981.

Brain R. Visual disorientation with special reference to the lesions of the right cerebral hemisphere. Brain 64:244–272, 1941.

Brain R. Speech and handedness. Lancet 2:837–842, 1945.

Brain R. Speech Disorders: Aphasia, Apraxia and Agnosia. London: Butterworth, 1961.

Brais B. The third left frontal convolution plays no role in language: Pierre Marie and the Paris debate on aphasia (1906–1908). Neurology 42:690–695, 1992.

Brierley JB. The neuropathology of amnesic states. In CWM Whitty, OL Zangwill (eds), Amnesia. New York: Appleton-Century-Crofts, 1966, pp 150–180.

Brinkman C. Supplementary motor area of the monkey's cerebral cortex: Short and long term deficits after ablation and the effects of subsequent callosal section. Journal of Neuroscience 4:918–929, 1984.

Broca P. Perte de la parole. Ramollisement chronique et destruction partielle du lobe anterieur gauche du cerveau. Bulletins-Société Anthropologie (Paris) 2:235–238, 1861a.

Broca P. Remarques sur le siège de la faculté du langage articulé, suivies d'une observation d'aphémie. Bulletins-Société Anatomique (Paris) 2:330–357, 1861b.

Broca P. Localisation des functions cerebrales. Siège du langage articulé. Bulletins-Société Anthropologie (Paris) 4:200, 1863.

Broca P. Sur la faculté du langage articulé. Bulletins-Société Anthropologie (Paris) 6:337–393, 1865.

Brodmann K. Beitrage zur histologischen Lokalisation der grosshirnrinde. VI: Die Cortexgleiderung der Menschen. Journal of Psychologie und Neurologie 10:231–246, 1908.

Brodmann K. Neue Ergebnisse über die vergleichende histologische Lokalisation der gross-hirnrinde mit besenderer Berücksichtigung des Stirnhirns. Anatomisch Anzweig (Suppl) 41:157–216, 1912.

Brookshire RH. Subject description and generality of results in experiments with aphasic adults. Journal of Speech and Hearing Disorders 48:342–346, 1983.

Brown JR. A model for central and peripheral behavior in aphasia. Paper delivered at Annual Meeting, Academy of Aphasia, Rochester, Minnesota, October, 1968.

Brown JW. Aphasia, Apraxia, and Agnosia. Springfield, IL: Thomas, 1972.

Brown JW. Language, cognition and the thalamus. Confinia Neurologica 36:33–60, 1974.

Brown JW. The problem of repetition: A study of "conduction" aphasia and the "isolation" syndrome. Cortex 11:37–52, 1975a.

Brown JW. On the neural organization of language: Thalamic and cortical relationships. Brain and Language 2:18–30, 1975b.

Brown JW (ed). Jargonaphasia. New York: Academic Press, 1981.

Brown JW, Leader B, Blum C. Hemiplegic writing in severe aphasia. Brain and Language 19:204–215, 1983.

Brown P, Cathala F, Gajdusek DC, Castaigne P. Creutzfeldt-Jakob disease: Clinical analysis of consecutive series of 230 neuropathologically verified cases. Annals of Neurology 20:597–602, 1986.

Bruce C, Howard D. Computer-generated phonemic cues: An effective aid for naming in aphasia. British Journal of Disorders of Communication 3:279–300, 1987.

Bruckert R, Gonon MH, Michel F, Bez M. The use of computer driven videodisc for the assessment and rehabilitation of aphasia. Aphasiology 5:473–478, 1989.

Bruhn JL, Farah MJ. The relation between spatial attention and reading: Evidence from the neglect syndrome. Cognitive Neuropsychology 8:59–74, 1991.

Brust JCM. Stroke: Diagnostic, anatomical, and physiological considerations. In ER Kandel, JH Schwartz (eds), Principles of Neural Science, 2d Ed. New York: Elsevier, 1985, pp 853–862.

Bryden MP. Ear preferences in auditory perception. Journal of Experimental Psychology 65:103–105, 1963.

Bryden MP. Laterality: Functional Asymmetry in the Intact Brain. New York: Academic Press, 1982.

Bryden MP. Cerebral specialization: Clinical and experimental assessment. In F Boller, J Grafman (eds), Handbook of Neuropsychology, Vol 1. Amsterdam: Elsevier, 1988, pp 143–159.

Bub DN, Black S, Howell J. Word recognition and orthographic context effects in a letter-by-letter reader. Brain and Language 36:357–376, 1989.

Bub DN, Cancelliere A, Kertesz A. Whole-word and analytic translation of spelling to sound in a non-semantic reader. In KE Patterson, JC Marshall, M Coltheart (eds), Surface Dyslexia. London: Lawrence Erlbaum Associates, 1985, pp 15–34.

Bub DN, Chertkow H. Agraphia. In F Boller, J Grafman, G Rizzolatti, H Goodglass. Handbook of Neuropsychology, Vol 1. Amsterdam: Elsevier, 1988, pp 393–414.

Bub DN, Kertesz A. Evidence for lexicographic processing in a patient with preserved written over oral single word naming. Brain 105:697–711, 1982a.

Bub D, Kertesz A. Deep agraphia. Brain and Language 17:146–165, 1982b.

Buchwald L. Aphasia in progressive multifocal leukodystrophy. (Personal communication, 1978).

Buckingham HW. Linguistic aspects of lexical retrieval disturbances in the posterior fluent aphasias. In H Whitaker, HA Whitaker (eds), Studies in Neurolinguistics, Vol 4. New York: Academic Press, 1979a, pp 147–184.

Buckingham HW. Explanations in apraxia with consequences for the concept of apraxia of speech. Brain and Language 8:202–226 1979b.

Buckingham HW. Lexical and semantic aspects of aphasia. In MT Sarno (ed), Acquired Aphasia. New York: Academic Press, 1981a, pp 183–214.

Buckingham HW. Where do neologisms come from? In J Brown (ed), Jargonaphasia. New York: Academic Press, 1981b, pp 39–61.

Buckingham HW. Mechanisms underlying aphasic transformations. In A Ardila, F Ostrosky (eds), Brain Organization of Language and Cognitive Processes. New York: Plenum, 1989, pp 123–145.

Buckingham HW, Kertesz A. Neologistic Jargon Aphasia. Amsterdam: Swets & Zeitlinger, 1976.

Buckingham HW, Yule G. Phonemic false evaluation: Clinical and theoretical aspects. Journal of Clinical Linguistics and Phonetics 1:113–125, 1987.

Burt C. The evidence for the concept of intelligence. British Journal of Educational Psychology 25:158–177, 1955.

Butfield E, Zangwill OL. Re-education in aphasia: A review of 20 cases. Journal of Neurology, Neurosurgery, and Psychiatry 9:75–79, 1946.

Butters N, Sax D, Montgomery K, Tarlow S. Comparison of the neuropsychological deficits associated with early and advanced Huntington's disease. Archives of Neurology 35:585–589, 1978.

Bychowski Z. Ueber die Restitution nach einem Schadelschuss verlorenen Umgangssprache bei einem Polyglotten. Monatsschrift für Psychiatrie und Neurologie 45:184–201, 1919.

Caine ED, Fisher JM. Dementia in Huntington's disease. In JAM Frederiks (ed), Handbook of Clinical Neurology, Vol 46: Neurobehavioral Disorders. Amsterdam: Elsevier, 1985, pp 305–310.

Cairo-Valcarcel E. Neuropsicologia. La Habana: Editorial Universidad de la Habana, Havana 1985.

Cambier J, Elghozi D, Signoret JL, Henin D. Contributions of the right hemisphere to language in aphasic patients. Disappearance of this language after a right-sided lesion. Revue Neurologique 139:55–63, 1983.

Cameron RF, Currier RD, Haerer AF. Aphasia and literacy. British Journal of Communication Disorders 6:161–163, 1971.

Campbell JK, Caselli RJ. Headache and other craniofacial pain. In WG Bradley, RB Daroff, GM Fenichel, CD Marsden (eds), Neurology in Clinical Practice. Boston: Butterworth-Heinemann, 1991, pp 1507–1548.

Canter G. Observations on neurogenic stuttering: A contribution to differential diagnosis. British Journal of Disordered Communication 6:139–143, 1971.

Canter GJ, Trost J, Burns M. Contrasting speech patterns in apraxia of speech and phonemic paraphasia. Brain and Language 24:204–222, 1985.

Caplan D. Neurolinguistics and Linguistic Aphasiology. Cambridge: Cambridge University Press, 1987.

Caplan D. Language Structure, Processing and Disorders. Cambridge, MA: MIT Press, 1992.

Caplan D. Toward a psycholinguistic approach to acquired neurogenic language disorders. American Journal of Speech and Language Pathology 3:59–83, 1993.

Caplan D, Hildebrandt N. Disorders of Syntactic Comprehension. Cambridge, MA: MIT, Bradford Press, 1988.

Caplan DM, Vanier M, Baker C. A case study of reproduction conduction aphasia. I: Word production. Cognitive Neuropsychology 3:99–128, 1986.

Caplan L. An investigation of some aspects of stuttering-like speech in adult dysphasic patients. Journal of the South African Speech and Hearing Association 19:52–66, 1972.

Cappa SF, Cavallotti G, Guidotti M, Papagno C, Vignolo LA. Subcortical aphasia: Two clinical-CT scan correlation studies. Cortex 19:227–241, 1983.

Cappa SF, Guidotti M, Papagno C, Vignolo LA. Speechlessness with occasional vocalizations after bilateral opercular lesions: A case study. Aphasiology 1:35–39, 1987.

Cappa SF, Papagno C, Vallar G, Vignolo LA. Aphasia does not always follow left thalamic haemorrhage: A study of five negative cases. Cortex 22:639–647, 1986.

Cappa SF, Vallar G. The role of the left and right hemispheres in recovery from aphasia. Aphasiology 6:359–372, 1992.

Cappa SF, Vignolo LA. "Transcortical" features of aphasia following left thalamic hemorrhage. Cortex 15:121–130, 1979.

Caramazza A. The logic of neuropsychological research and the problem of patient classification in aphasia. Brain and Language 21:9–20, 1984.

Caramazza A. On drawing inferences about the structure of normal cognitive systems from the analysis of patterns in impaired performance: The case for single patient studies. Brain and Cognition 5:41–66, 1986.

Caramazza A, Basili AG, Koller JJ. An investigation of repetition and language processing in a case of conduction aphasia. Brain and Language 14:235–271, 1981.

Caramazza A, Berndt R, Basili AM. The selective impairment of phonological processing. Brain and Language 18:18–74, 1986.

Caramazza A, McCloskey M. Dissociations of calculation processes. In G Deloche, X Seron (eds), Mathematical Disabilities: A Cognitive Neuropsychological Perspective, Hillsdale, NJ: Lawrence Erlbaum Associates, 1987, pp 221–234.

Caramazza A, Micelli G, Silveri MC, Laudanna A. Reading mechanisms and the organization of the lexicon: Evidence from acquired dyslexia. Cognitive Neuropsychology 2:81–114, 1985.

Carter RL, Satz P, Hohenegger M. Aphasia and speech organization in children. Science 218:797–799, 1982.

Carter RL, Satz P, Hohenegger M. On the statistical estimation of speech organization distribution from aphasia data. Biometrics 40:937–946, 1984.

Caselli RJ, Ivnik RJ, Duffy JR. Associative anomia: Dissociating words and their definitions. Mayo Clinic Proceedings 66:783–791, 1991.

Castro-Caldas A, Confraria A. Age and type of crossed aphasia in dextrals due to stroke. Brain and Language 23:126–133, 1984.

Cauty A. Taxonomie, syntaxe et économie des numerations parlées. Amerindia 9:111–146, 1984.

Cerella J, Fozard JL. Lexical access and age. Developmental Psychology 20:235–243, 1984.

Cermak LS. Human Memory and Amnesia. Hillsdale, NJ: Lawrence Erlbaum Associates, 1982.

Cermak LS, O'Connor MC. The anterograde and retrograde retrieval ability of a patient with amnesia due to encephalitis. Neuropsychologia 21:213–234, 1983.

Chapman LF, Wolff HG. The cerebral hemispheres and the highest integrative functions of man. Archives of Neurology 1:357–424, 1959.

Charcot JM. Lectures on the Diseases of the Nervous System, Vol. 1. London: New Sydenham Society, 1877.

Charcot JM. Clinical Lectures on Diseases of the Nervous System, Vol. 3. London: New Sydenham Society, 1889.

Chedru F, Geschwind N. Disorders of higher cortical functions in acute confusional states. Cortex 8:395–411, 1972.

Chen LCY. Manual communication by combined alphabet and gestures. Archives of Physical Medicine and Rehabilitation 52:381–384, 1971.

Childe VG. Man Makes Himself. London: Pitman, 1936.

Chomsky N. Syntactic Structures. The Hague: Mouton, 1957.

Chomsky N. Language and Mind. New York: Harcourt Brace Jovanovich, 1968.

Chomsky N. Language and Mind, Enlarged Edition. New York: Harcourt Brace Jovanovich, 1972.

Chomsky N. Rules and Representations. New York: Columbia University Press, 1980.

Ciemins VA. Localized thalamic hemorrhage: A cause of aphasia. Neurology 20:776–782, 1970.

Coelho CA, Duffy RJ. Sign acquisition in two aphasic subjects with limb apraxia. Aphasiology 4:1–8, 1990.

Cohen DJ, Volkmar FR, Paul R. Issues in the classification of pervasive developmental disorders. Journal of the American Academy of Child Psychiatry 25:158–161, 1986.

Cohen L, Dehaene S. Neglect dyslexia for numbers? A case report. Cognitive Neuropsychology 8:39–58, 1991.

Cohen MS, Bookheimer SY. Localization of brain function with magnetic resonance imaging. Trends in Neuroscience 17:258–277, 1994.

Cohn R. Dyscalculia. Archives of Neurology 4:301–307, 1961.

Colby K, Christinaz D, Parkinson R, Grahma S, Krapf C. A word-finding computer program with a dynamic lexical-semantic memory for patients with anomia using an intelligent speech prosthesis. Brain and Language 14:272–281, 1981.

Cole M. The anatomical basis of aphasia as seen by Pierre Marie. Cortex 4:172–183, 1968.

Collins M. Diagnosis and Treatment of Global Aphasia. San Diego: College-Hill Press, 1986.

Coltheart M. Deep dyslexia: A review of the syndrome. In M Coltheart, KE Patterson, JC Marshall (eds), Deep Dyslexia. London: Routledge and Kegan Paul, 1980a, pp 22–47.

Coltheart M. Reading, phonological recording and deep dyslexia. In M Coltheart, K Patterson, J Marshall (eds), Deep Dyslexia. London: Routledge and Kegan Paul, 1980b, pp 197–226.

Coltheart M. Aphasia therapy research: A single-case study approach. In C Code, DJ Muller (eds), Aphasia Therapy. London: Edward Arnold, 1983a, pp 193–202.

Coltheart M. The right hemisphere and disorders of reading. In A Young (ed), Functions of the Right Cerebral Hemisphere. London: Academic Press, 1983b, pp 171–201.

Coltheart M, Masterson J, Byng S, Prior M, Riddoch J. Surface dyslexia. Quarterly Journal of Experimental Psychology 35A:469–495, 1983.

Coltheart M, Patterson K, Marshall JC (eds). Deep Dyslexia. London: Routledge and Kegan Paul, 1980.

Conrad K. New problems of aphasia. Brain 77:491–509, 1954.

Corballis MC. The Lopsided Ape. New York: Oxford University Press, 1991.

Corso J. Sensory processes and age effects in normal adults. Journal of Gerontology 26:90–105, 1971.

Coslett HB, Brashear HR, Heilman KM. Pure word deafness after bilateral primary auditory cortex infarcts. Neurology 34:347–352, 1984.

Coslett HB, Gonzalez-Rothi LJ, Heilman KM. Reading dissociation of the lexical and phonologic mechanisms. Brain and Language 24:20–35, 1985.

Coslett HB, Gonzalez-Rothi LJ, Valenstein E, Heilman KM. Dissociations of writing and praxis: Two cases in point. Brain and Language 28:357–369, 1986.

Coslett HB, Roeltgen DP, Gonzalez-Rothi L, Heilman KM. Transcortical sensory aphasia: Evidence for subtypes. Brain and Language 32:362–378, 1987.

Coslett HB, Saffran EM. Evidence for preserved reading in "pure alexia." Brain 112:327–359, 1989.

Costello A, Warrington E. The dissociation of visuospatial neglect and neglect dyslexia. Journal of Neurology, Neurosurgery, and Psychiatry 50:1110–1116, 1987.

Craenhals A, Raison-Van Ruymbeke AM, Rectem D, Seron X, Laterre EC. Is slowly progressive aphasia actually a new clinical entity? Aphasiology 4:485–510, 1990.

Craik FIM. Age differences in remembering. In LR Squire, N Butters (eds), Neuropsychology of Memory. New York: Guilford Press, 1984, pp 3–12.

Crary MA, Heilman KM. Letter imagery deficits in a case of pure apraxic agraphia. Brain and Language 34:147–156, 1988.

Crisp AH, Modolfsky H. A psychosomatic study of writer's cramp. British Journal of Psychiatry 111:841–858, 1965.

Critchley M. The anterior cerebral artery and its syndromes. Brain 53:120–165, 1930.

Critchley M. "Aphasia" in a partial deaf-mute. Brain 61:163–169, 1938.

Critchley M. Articulatory defects in aphasia. Journal of Laryngology and Otolaryngology 66:1–17, 1952.

Critchley M. The Parietal Lobes. London: Edward Arnold, 1953.

Critchley M. Premorbid literacy and pattern of subsequent aphasia. Proceedings of the Royal Society of Medicine 49:335–336, 1956.

Critchley M. The neurology of psychotic speech. British Journal of Psychiatry 110:353–364, 1964.

Critchley M. The enigma of the Gerstmann's syndrome. Brain 89:183–198, 1966.

Critchley M. Testamentary capacity in aphasia. In Critchley M, Aphasiology. London: Edward Arnold, 1970a, pp 288–295.

Critchley M. Non-articulate modalities of speech and their disorders. In M Critchley (ed), Aphasiology. London: Edward Arnold Ltd., 1970a, pp 325–347.

Critchley M. Preface to Traumatic Aphasia by A. R. Luria. New York: Basic Books, 1970b.

Critchley M. Specific developmental dyslexia. In JAM Frederiks (ed), Handbook of Clinical Neurology, Vol 46: Neurobehavioral Disorders. Amsterdam: Elsevier, 1985, pp 105–121.

Croisile B, Laurent B, Michel D, Trillet M. Pure agraphia after deep left hemisphere haematoma. Journal of Neurology, Neurosurgery, and Psychiatry 53:263–265, 1990.

Crosby EC, Humphrey E, Lauer EW. Correlative Anatomy of the Nervous System. New York: Macmillan, 1962.

Cross JA, Ozanne AE. Acquired childhood aphasia: Assessment and treatment. In BE Burdoch (ed), Acquired Neurological Speech/Language Disorders in Childhood. London: Taylor and Francis, 1990, pp 66–123.

Crosson B. Subcortical functions in language: A working model. Brain and Language 25:257–292, 1985.

Crosson B, Parker JC, Kim AK, Warren RL, Kepes JJ, Tully R. A case of thalamic aphasia with postmortem verification. Brain and Language 29:301–314, 1986.

Crystal HA, Horoupian DS, Katzman R, Jotkowitz S. Biopsy-proved Alzheimer disease presenting as a right parietal lobe syndrome. Annals of Neurology 12:186–188, 1982.

Culton GL. Spontaneous recovery from aphasia. Journal of Speech and Hearing Research 18:825–832, 1969.

Cummings JL. Hemispheric asymmetries in visual-perceptual and visual-spatial function. In Benson DF, Zaidel E (eds), The Dual Brain: Hemispheric Specialization in Humans. New York: Guilford Press, 1985a, pp 233–246.

Cummings JL. Clinical Neuropsychiatry. Orlando, FL: Grune and Stratton, 1985b.

Cummings JL, Benson DF. Dementia: A Clinical Approach. Boston: Butterworth, 1983.

Cummings JL, Benson DF. Subcortical dementia: Review of an emerging concept. Archives of Neurology 41:874–879, 1984.

Cummings JL, Benson DF. Dementia of the Alzheimer type: An inventory of diagnostic clinical features. Journal of the American Geriatrics Society 34:12–19, 1986.

Cummings JL, Benson DF. Speech and language alterations in dementia syndromes. In A Ardila, F Ostrosky (eds), Brain Organization of Language and Cognitive Processes. New York: Plenum, 1989, pp 107–120.

Cummings JL, Benson DF. Subcortical mechanisms and human thought. In Cummings JL (ed), Subcortical Dementia. New York: Oxford University Press, 1990, pp 251–259.

Cummings JL, Benson DF. Dementia: A Clinical Approach, 2d Ed. Boston: Butterworth-Heinemann, 1992.

Cummings JL, Benson DF, Hill MA, Read S. Aphasia in dementia of the Alzheimer type. Neurology 35:394–397, 1985.

Cummings JL, Benson DF, LoVerme S Jr. Reversible dementia: Illustrative cases, definition, and review. JAMA 243:2434–2439, 1980.

Cummings JL, Benson DF, Walsh MJ, Levine H. Left to right transfer of language dominance: A case study. Neurology 29:1547–1550, 1979.

Cummings JL, Darkins A, Mendez M, Hill MA, Benson DF. Alzheimer's disease and Parkinson's disease: Comparison of speech and language alterations. Neurology 38:680–684, 1988.

Cutting J. A study of anosognosia. Journal of Neurology, Neurosurgery, and Psychiatry 41:548–555, 1978.

Dahmen W, Hartje W, Bussing A, Strum W. Disorders of calculation in aphasic patients: Spatial and verbal components. Neuropsychologia 20:145–153, 1982.

Damasio AR. Disorders of complex visual processing: Agnosias, achromatopsia, Balint's syndrome and related difficulties of orientation and construction. In Mesulam M-M (ed), Principles of Behavioral Neurology. Philadelphia: Davis, 1985, pp 259–288.

Damasio A, Castro-Caldas A, Grosso JT, Ferro JM. Brain specialization for language does not depend on literacy. Archives of Neurology 33:300–301, 1976.

Damasio A, Damasio H. The anatomic basis of pure alexia. Neurology 33:1573–1583, 1983.

Damasio A, Damasio H. Hemianopsia, hemiachromatopsia, and the mechanisms of alexia. Cortex 22:161–170, 1986.

Damasio AR, Damasio H, Rizzo M, Varney N, Gersh F. Aphasia with non-hemorrhagic lesions in the basal ganglia and internal capsule. Archives of Neurology 39:15–20, 1982.

Damasio AR, Damasio H, Van Hoesen GW. Prosopagnosia: Anatomic basis and behavioral mechanisms. Neurology 32:331–341, 1982.

Damasio AR, Kassel NF. Transcortical motor aphasia in relation to lesions of the supplementary motor area. Paper presented at Annual Meeting, American Academy of Neurology, Los Angeles, April, 1978.

Damasio AR, Van Hoesen GW. Emotional disorders associated with focal lesions of the limbic frontal lobe. In Heilman KM, Satz P (eds), Neuropsychology of Human Emotion. New York: Guilford, 1983, pp 85–110.

Damasio AR, Van Hoesen GW, Damasio H. The role of the supplementary motor area in speech production and language processing. Paper presented at the 18th Annual Meeting, Academy of Aphasia, South Yarmouth, MA, October, 1980.

Damasio H. Cerebral localization of the aphasias. In MT Sarno (ed), Acquired Aphasia. New York: Academic Press, 1981, pp 27–50.

Damasio H. Neuroimaging contributions to the understanding of aphasia. In H Goodglass, AR Damasio (eds), Handbook of Neuropsychology, Vol 2. Amsterdam: Elsevier, 1989, pp 3–46.

Damasio H, Damasio A. The anatomical basis of conduction aphasia. Brain 103:337–350, 1980.

Damasio H, Damasio AR. Lesion Analysis in Neuropsychology. New York: Oxford University Press, 1989.

Darley FL. Apraxia of speech: 101 years of terminological confusion. Paper presented at Annual Meeting, American Speech and Hearing Association, 1968.

Darley FL. Aphasia. Philadelphia: Saunders, 1975a.

Darley FL. Treatment of acquired aphasia. In WJ Friedlander (ed), Advances in Neurology, Vol 7: Current Reviews of Higher Nervous System Dysfunction. New York: Raven Press, 1975b, pp 111–145.

Darley FL, Aronson AE, Brown JR. Differential diagnostic patterns of dysarthria. Journal of Speech and Hearing Research 12:246–269, 1969.

Darley FL, Aronson AE, Brown JR. Motor Speech Disorders. Philadelphia: Saunders, 1975.

Davidson GM. The syndrome of Capgras. Psychiatric Quarterly 15:513–521, 1941.

Davis GA, Wilcox MJ. Adult Aphasia Rehabilitation: Applied Pragmatics. San Diego: College-Hill Press, 1985.

Davis H, Albert M, Barron RW. Detection of number or numerousness by human infants. Science 228:1222, 1985 (letter).

Dax M. Lésions de la moitié gauche de l'encéphale coincidant l'oubli des signes de la pensée. (Paper presented in Montpellier, 1836.) Gazette hebdomadaire de Médecine et de Chiurgie 33:259, 1865.

Deal J, Cannito MP. Acquired neurologic dysfluency. In D Vogel, MP Cannito (eds), Treating Disordered Motor Speech Control. Austin, TX: Pro-Ed, 1991, pp 217–239.

Dejerine J. Sur un cas de cécité verbale avec agraphie, suivi d'autopsie. Memoires-Société Biologie 3:197–201, 1891.

Dejerine J. Contribution à l'étude anatomo-pathologique et clinique des differentes variétés de cécité verbale. Memoires-Société Biologie 4:61–90, 1892.

Dejerine J. Semiologie des affections du systeme nerveaux. Paris: Masson, 1914.

Dejerine J, Mirallie C. Sur les altérations de la lecture mentale chez les aphasiques moteurs corticaux. C.R. Society Biology 47:523–527, 1895.

Dejerine J, Roussy G. La syndrome thalamique. Revue Neurologique 14:521–532, 1906.

Deloche G, Andreewsky E, Desi M. Surface dyslexia: A case report and some theoretical implications to reading models. Brain and Language 15:12–31, 1982.

Deloche G, Dordain M, Kremin H. Rehabilitation of confrontation naming in aphasia: Relation between oral and written modalities. Aphasiology 7:201–216, 1993.

Deloche G, Seron X. From three to 3: A differential analysis of skills in transcoding quantities between patients with Broca's and Wernicke's aphasia. Brain 105:719–733, 1982.

Deloche G, Seron X. Some linguistic aspects of acalculia. In FC Rose (ed), Advances in Neurology, Vol 42: Progress in Aphasiology. New York: Raven Press, 1984, pp 215–222.

Deloche G, Seron X. Numerical transcoding: A general production model. In G Deloche, X Seron (eds), Mathematical Disabilities: A Cognitive Neuropsychological Perspective. Hillsdale, NJ: Lawrence Erlbaum Associates, 1987, pp 137–170.

Dennett DC. Toward a cognitive theory of consciousness. In DC Dennett, Brainstorms. Brighton, England: Harvester Press, 1986, pp 149–173.

Dennis M, Kohn B. Comprehension of syntax in infantile hemiplegics after cerebral hemidecortication: Left hemisphere superiority. Brain and Language 2:472–482, 1975.

Denny-Brown D, Banker BQ. Amorphosynthesis from left parietal lesion. Archives of Neurology and Psychiatry 71:302–313, 1954.

Denny-Brown D, Meyer JS, Horenstein S. The significance of perceptual rivalry resulting from a parietal lesion. Brain 75:433–471, 1952.

De Partz MP. Reeducation of a deep dyslexia patient: Rationale of the method and results. Cognitive Neuropsychology 3:149–177, 1986.

De Renzi E. Disorders of spatial orientation. In JAM Frederiks (ed), Handbook of Clinical Neurology, Vol 45: Clinical Neuropsychology. Amsterdam: Elsevier, 1985, pp 405–422.

De Renzi E. Slowly progressive visual agnosia or apraxia without dementia. Cortex 22:171–180, 1986.

De Renzi E, Faglioni P. Normative data and screening power of a shortened version of the Token Test. Cortex 14:41–49, 1978.

De Renzi E, Faglioni P, Scotti G. Hemispheric contribution to exploration of space through the visual and tactile modality. Cortex 6:191–203, 1970.

De Renzi E, Pieczuro A, Vignolo LA. Oral apraxia and aphasia. Cortex 2:50–73, 1966.

De Renzi E, Vignolo LA. The Token Test: A sensitive test to detect receptive disturbances in aphasics. Brain 85:665–678, 1962.

Derouesne J, Beauvois MF. The "phonemic" stage in the non-lexical reading process: Evidence from a case of phonological alexia. In KE Patterson, JC Marshall, M Coltheart (eds), Surface Dyslexia. London: Lawrence Erlbaum Associates, 1985, pp 399–457.

Devinsky O. Behavioral Neurology: 100 Maxims. St. Louis: Mosby, 1992.

Diesenfeldt HFA. Semantic impairment in senile dementia of the Alzheimer type. Aphasiology 3:41–54, 1989.

Dodrill CB, Troupin AS. Psychotropic effects of carbamazepine in epilepsy: A doubleblind comparison with phenytoin. Neurology 27:1023–1028, 1977.

Douglass E, Richardson JC. Aphasia in a congenital deaf mute. Brain 82:68–80, 1959.

Dubois J, Hécaen H, Angelergues R, Maufras du Chatelier A, Marcie P. Etude neurolinguistique de l'aphasie de conduction. Neuropsychologia 2:9–44, 1964.

Dubois J, Hécaen H, Angelergues R, Maufras du Chatelier A, Marcie P. Neurolinguistic study of conduction aphasia. In H Goodglass, S Blumstein (eds), Psycholinguistics and Aphasia. Baltimore: Johns Hopkins University Press, 1973, pp 9–44.

Dubois J, Hécaen H, Marcie P. L'agraphie "pure." Neuropsychologia 7:271–286, 1969.

Duffy JR, Petersen RC. Primary progressive aphasia. Aphasiology 6:1–16, 1992.

Dunn LM. Expanded Manual for the Peabody Individual Achievement Test. Circle Pines, MN: American Guidance Service, 1965a.

Dunn LM. Expanded Manual for the Peabody Picture Vocabulary Test. Minneapolis: American Guidance Service, 1965b.

Eagleson HM, Vaughn GR, Knudson AB. Hand signals for dysphasia. Archives of Physical Medicine and Rehabilitation 51:111–113, 1970.

Edelman GM. The Remembered Present. New York: Basic Books, 1989.

Efron R. The Decline and Fall of Hemispheric Specialization. Hillsdale, NJ: Lawrence Erlbaum Associates, 1990.

Eisenson J. Examining for Aphasia. New York: Psychological Corp., 1954.

Elliott FA. Violence: The neurological contribution: An overview. Archives of Neurology 49:595–603, 1992.

Ellis AW. Spelling and writing (and reading and speaking). In AW Ellis (ed), Normality and Pathology in Cognitive Functions. London: Academic Press, 1982.

Ellis AW. Normal writing processes and peripheral acquired dysgraphias. Language and Cognitive Processes 3:99–127, 1988.

Ellis AW, Flude BM, Young AW. "Neglect dyslexia" and the early visual processing of letters in words and nonwords. Cognitive Neuropsychology 4:439–464, 1987.

Ellis AW, Young AW, Flude BM. "Afferent dysgraphia" in a patient and in normal subjects. Cognitive Neuropsychology 4:465–486, 1987.

Emery OB. Language and aging. Experimental Aging Research 11:3–60, 1985.

Engel J Jr. Seizures and Epilepsy. Philadelphia: Davis, 1989.

Erkulvrawratr S. Alexia and left homonymous hemianopsia in a non-right-hander. Archives of Neurology 3:549–552, 1978.

Exner S. Untersuchungen über die lokalisation der Functionen in der Grosshirnrinde des Menschen. W. Braumuller: Vienna, 1881.

Eysenck M. Age differences in incidental learning. Developmental Psychology 10:936–941, 1974.

Farah MJ. Visual Agnosia. Cambridge, MA: MIT Press, 1990.

Farah M, Wallace MA. Pure alexia as a visual impairment: A reconsideration. Cognitive Neuropsychology 8:313–334, 1991.

Farmakides MN, Boone DR. Speech problems of patients with multiple sclerosis. Journal of Speech and Hearing Disorders. 25:385–390, 1960.

Farmer A. Stuttering repetitions in aphasic and nonaphasic brain damaged adults. Cortex 11:391–396, 1975.

Fedio P, Van Buren JM. Memory and perceptual deficits during electrical stimulation in the left and right thalamus and parietal subcortex. Brain and Language 2:78–100, 1975.

Feinberg TE, Gonzalez-Rothi LJ, Heilman KM. Multimodal agnosia after unilateral left hemisphere lesion. Neurology 36:864–867, 1986.

Ferro JM, Botelho MH. Alexia for arithmetical signs: A cause of disturbed calculation. Cortex 16:175–180, 1980.

Finger S, LeVere LE, Almli CR, Stein DG (eds). Brain Recovery: Theoretical and Controversial Issues. New York: Plenum, 1988.

Fisher CM. The anatomy and pathology of the cerebral vasculature. In JS Meyer (ed), Modern Concepts of Cerebrovascular Disease. New York: Spectrum, 1975, pp 1–41.

Fisher CM. Thalamic pure sensory stroke: A pathologic study. Neurology 28:1141–1144, 1978.

Flor-Henry P. Psychosis and temporal lobe epilepsy. Epilepsia 10:363–395, 1969.

Flourens P. Researches Expérimentalis sur les Propriétés et les fonctions du Systéme Nerveux dans les animaux vertébrés. Paris: Bailliere, 1824.

Flourens P (trans Charles De Lucena Meigs). Phrenology Examined. Philadelphia: Hogan and Thompson, 1846.

Fodor JA. The Language of Thought. Cambridge, MA: Harvard University Press, 1975.

Fodor JA. The Modularity of Mind. Cambridge, MA: MIT Press, 1983.

Foerster O. Motorische Felder und bahnen. Sensible corticale Felder. In O Bumke, O Foerster (eds), Handbuch der Neurologie, Vol 6. Berlin: Julius Springer, 1936, pp 1–488.

Folstein MF, Breitner JCS. Language disorder predicts familial Alzheimer's disease. Johns Hopkins Medical Journal 149:145–147, 1981.

Folstein MF, Folstein SE, McHugh PR. "Mini-Mental State": A practical method for grading the mental state for the clinician. Journal of Psychiatric Research 12:189–198, 1975.

Folstein MF, Maiberger R, McHugh PR. Mood disorder as a specific complication of stroke. Journal of Neurology, Neurosurgery, and Psychiatry 40:1018–1020, 1977.

Fox C. Vocabulary ability in latter maturity. Journal of Educational Psychology 38:482–492, 1947.

Frederichs JAM (ed). Clinical neuropsychology. In PJ Vinken, GW Bruyn, and HL Klawans (eds), Handbook of Clinical Neurology, Vol. 46. Amsterdam, Elsevier, 1985.

Frederiks JAM. Disorders of the body schema. In JAM Frederiks (ed), Handbook of Clinical Neurology, Vol 45: Clinical Neuropsychology. Amsterdam: Elsevier, 1985, pp 373–404.

Freedman M, Alexander MP, Naeser MA. The anatomical basis of transcortical motor aphasia. Neurology 34:409–417, 1984.

Freud S (trans E Stengl). On Aphasia. New York: International Universities Press, 1891/1953.

Freund CS. Ueber optische Aphasie und Seelenblindheit. Archiv für Psychiatrie und Nervenkhrankheit 20:276–297, 1888.

Friedland J. Assessment of language in aphasia: An examination of hemiplegic writing. Aphasiology 4:241–258, 1990.

Friedland RP, Weinstein EA. Hemi-inattention and hemisphere specialization: Introduction and historical review. In EA Weinstein, RP Friedland (eds), Advances in Neurology, Vol 18: Hemi-inattention and Hemisphere Specialization. New York: Raven Press, 1977, pp 1–21.

Friedman RB. Mechanisms of reading and spelling in a case of alexia without agraphia. Neuropsychologia 20:533–545, 1982.

Friedman RB. Acquired alexia. In F Boller, J Grafman, G Rizzolatti, H Goodglass (eds), Handbook of Neuropsychology, Vol 1. Amsterdam: Elsevier, 1988, pp 377–392.

Friedman RB, Albert ML. Alexia. In KM Heilman, E Valenstein (eds), Clinical Neuropsychology, 2d Ed. New York: Oxford University Press, 1985, pp 49–73.

Friedman RB, Alexander MP. Pictures, images and pure alexia: A case study. Cognitive Neuropsychology 1:9–23, 1984.

Friedman RB, Hadley JA. Letter-by-letter surface alexia. Cognitive Neuropsychology 9:185–208, 1992.

Friedman RB, Perlman MP. On the underlying causes of semantic paralexias in a patient with deep dyslexia. Neuropsychologia 20:559–568, 1982.

Fromkin VA. Implications of hemispheric differences for linguistics. In DF Benson, E Zaidel (eds), The Dual Brain: Hemispheric Specialization in Humans. New York: Guilford Press, 1985, pp 319–327.

Funnell E. Phonological processes in reading: New evidence from acquired dyslexia. British Journal of Psychology 74:159–180, 1983.

Fuster JM. The Prefrontal Cortex: Anatomy, Physiology, and Neuropsychology of the Frontal Lobe. New York: Raven Press, 1980.

Fuster JM. The Prefrontal Cortex: Anatomy, Physiology, and Neuropsychology of the Frontal Lobe, 2d Ed. New York: Raven Press, 1989.

Gainotti G. Constructional apraxia. In JAM Frederiks (ed), Handbook of Neurology, Vol 45: Clinical Neuropsychology. Amsterdam: Elsevier, 1985, pp 491–506.

Gainotti G. The status of semantic-lexical structures in anomia. Aphasiology 1:449–461, 1987.

Gainotti G, Carlomagno S, Craca A, Silveri MC. Disorders in classificatory activity in aphasia. Brain and Language 28:181–195, 1986.

Gainotti G, Parlato E, Monteleone D, Carlomagno S. Verbal memory disorders in Alzheimer's disease and multi-infarct dementia. Journal of Neurolinguistics 4:327–346, 1989.

Gainotti G, Silveri MC, Villa G, Miceli G. Anomia with and without lexical comprehension disorders. Brain and language 29:18–33, 1986.

Galaburda AM, Kemper TL. Cytoarchitectonic abnormalities in developmental dyslexia: A case study. Annals of Neurology 6:94–100, 1979.

Gall F, Spurzheim G. Anatomie et Physiologie du Système nerveux en général et du Cerveau en particulier avec des Observations sur la Possibilité de Reconnoître Plusiers Dispositions intellectuelles et morales de l'Homme et des Animaux par la Configuration de leurs Têtes, 4 Vols. Paris: F. Schoell, 1810–1819.

Gao S, Benson DF. Aphasia after stroke in native Chinese speakers. Aphasiology 4:31–43, 1990.

Gardner H. The contribution of operativity to naming capacity in aphasic patients. Neuropsychologia 11:213–220, 1973.

Gardner H. The Mind's New Science. New York: Basic Books, 1985.

Gardner H, Zurif E, Berry T, Baker E. Visual communication in aphasia. Neuropsychologia 14:275–292, 1976.

Gardner RA, Gardner B. Teaching sign-language to a chimpanzee. Science 165:664–672, 1969.

Gates A, Bradshaw JL. Music perception and cerebral asymmetries. Cortex 39:390–401, 1977.

Gazzaniga MS. The Bisected Brain. New York: Appleton-Century-Crofts, 1970.

Gazzaniga MS, Glass AA, Sarno MT, Posner JB. Pure word deafness and hemispheric dynamics: A case history. Cortex 9:136–143, 1973.

Gazzaniga MS, Sperry RW. Language after section of the cerebral commissures. Brain 90:131–148, 1967.

Gelman R, Meck E. Preschoolers' counting: Principles before skill. Cognition 13:343–359, 1983.

Gerstmann J. Zur symptomatologie der hirnlasionen im Übergangsgebiet der unteren parietal und mittleren occipitalwindung. Nervenarzt 3:691–695, 1931.

Gerstmann J. The syndrome of finger agnosia, disorientation for right and left, agraphia and acalculia. Archives of Neurology and Psychiatry 44:398–408, 1940.

Geschwind N. The anatomy of acquired disorders of reading. In J Money (ed), Reading Disability: Progress and Research Needs in Dyslexia. Baltimore: Johns Hopkins University Press, 1962, pp 115–129.

Geschwind N. Disconnexion syndromes in animals and man. Brain 88:237–294, 585–644, 1965.

Geschwind N. The apraxias. In EW Strauss, RM Griffith (eds), Phenomenology of Will and Action. Pittsburgh: Duquesne University Press, 1967a, pp 91–102.

Geschwind N. The varieties of naming errors. Cortex 3:97–112, 1967b.

Geschwind N. Wernicke's contribution to the study of aphasia. Cortex 3:449–463, 1967c.

Geschwind N. Late changes in the nervous system: An overview in plasticity and recovery of function in the central nervous system. In D Stein, J Rosen, N Butters (eds), Plasticity and Recovery of Function in the Central Nervous System. New York: Academic Press, 1974, pp 467–508.

Geschwind N. Mechanisms of change after brain lesions. In R Nottebohm (ed), Annals of the New York Academy of Sciences, Vol 457: Hope for a New Neurology. New York: Academy of Sciences, 1985, pp 1–11.

Geschwind N, Damasio AR. Apraxia. In JAM Frederiks (ed), Handbook of Clinical Neurology, 2d. Ed., Vol 45: Clinical Neuropsychology. Amsterdam: Elsevier, 1985, pp 422–432.

Geschwind N, Fusillo M. Color naming defects in association with alexia. Archives of Neurology 15:137–146, 1966.

Geschwind N, Kaplan EF. A human cerebral deconnection syndrome. Neurology 12:675–685, 1962.

Geschwind N, Quadfasel FA, Segarra J. Isolation of the speech area. Neuropsychologia 6:327–340, 1968.

Gilbert AN, Wysocki CJ. Hand preference and age in the United States. Neuropsychologia 30:601–608, 1992.

Gilbert J, Leveer R. Patterns of memory decline. Journal of Gerontology 26:70–75, 1971.

Glass AV, Gazzaniga MS, Premack D. Artificial language training in global aphasias. Neuropsychologia 11:95–103, 1973.

Gloning I, Gloning K. Aphasia in polyglots: Contributions to the dynamics of language disintegration as well as to the question of the localization of these impairments. In M Paradis (ed), Readings on Aphasia in Bilinguals and Polyglots. Montreal: Marcel Didier, 1965/1983, pp 681–716.

Gloning I, Gloning K, Haub C, Quatember R. Comparison of verbal behavior in right-handed and non-right-handed patients with anatomically verified lesions of one hemisphere. Cortex 5:43–52, 1969.

Gloning I, Gloning K, Hoff H. Aphasia: A clinical syndrome. In L Halpern (ed.), Problems of Dynamic Neurology. Jerusalem: Hebrew University, 1963, pp 63–70.

Gloning I, Gloning K, Seitelberger F, Tschabitscher H. Ein Fall von reiner Wortblindheit mit Obduktionsbefund. Wiener Zeitschrift für Nervenheilkunde 12:194–215, 1955.

Gloning K. Handedness and aphasia. Neuropsychologia 15:355–358, 1977.

Godfrey C, Douglass E. The recovery process in aphasia. Canadian Medical Association Journal 80:618–624, 1959.

Goldberg E, Costa LD. Hemispheric differences in relationship to the acquisition and use of descriptive systems. Brain and Language 14:144–173, 1981.

Goldberg G. Supplementary motor area structure and function: Review and hypotheses. The Behavioral and Brain Sciences 8:567–616, 1985.

Goldman-Rakic PS. Cellular and circuit basis of working memory in prefrontal cortex of nonhuman primates. In HBM Uylings, CG Van Eden, JPC De Bruin, MA Corner, MGP Feenstra (eds), Progress in Brain Research, Vol 85. Amsterdam: Elsevier, 1990, pp 325–336.

Goldstein FC, Green J, Presley R, Green RC. Dysnomia in Alzheimer disease: An evaluation of neurobehavioral subtypes. Brain and Language 43:308–323, 1992.

Goldstein K. Die Transkortikalen Aphasien. Jena, Germany: Gustav Fischer, 1917.

Goldstein K. Das wesen der amnestischen Aphasie. Schweizer Archiv für Neurologie und Psychiatrie 15:163–175, 1924.

Goldstein K. Language and Language Disturbances. New York: Grune and Stratton, 1948.

Goldstein M. Auditory agnosia for speech (pure word deafness): A historical review with current implications. Brain and Language 1:195–204, 1974.

Goldstein MN, Brown M, Hollander J. Auditory agnosia and cortical deafness: Analysis of a case with three years follow-up. Brain and Language 2:324–332, 1975.

Goldstein M, Joynt R, Goldblatt D. Word blindness. Neurology 21:873–876, 1971.

Gonzalez-Rothi LJ. Transcortical aphasias. In LL LaPointe (ed), Aphasia and Related Neurogenic Language Disorders. New York: Thieme, 1990, pp 78–95.

Goodglass H. Naming disorders in aphasia and aging. In LK Obler, ML Albert (eds), Language and Communication in the Elderly: Clinical, Therapeutic, and Experimental Issues. Lexington, MA: Lexington Books, 1980, pp 37–45.

Goodglass H. Neurolinguistic principles and aphasia therapy. In M Meier, A Benton, L Diller (eds), Neuropsychological Rehabilitation. New York: Plenum, 1987, pp 315–326.

Goodglass H. Understanding Aphasia. San Diego: Academic Press, 1993.

Goodglass H, Baker E. Semantic field, naming and auditory comprehension in aphasia. Brain and Language 3:359–374, 1976.

Goodglass H, Barton MI, Kaplan E. Sensory modality and object-naming in aphasia. Journal of Speech and Hearing Research 11:488–496, 1968.

Goodglass H, Berko J. Agrammatism and inflectional morphology in English. Journal of Speech and Hearing Research 3:257–267, 1960.

Goodglass H, Geschwind N. Language disturbance (aphasia). In EC Carterette, MP Friedman (eds), Handbook of Perception, Vol. 7: Language and Speech. New York: Academic Press, 1976, pp 389–428.

Goodglass H, Gleason JB, Bernholtz NA, Hyde MR. Some linguistic structures in the speech of a Broca's aphasic. Cortex 8:191–212, 1972.

Goodglass H, Kaplan E. The Assessment of Aphasia and Related Disorders. Philadelphia: Lea and Febiger, 1972.

Goodglass H, Kaplan E. The Assessment of Aphasia and Related Disorders, 2d Ed. Philadelphia: Lea and Febiger, 1983.

Goodglass H, Klein B, Carey P, Jones K. Specific semantic word categories in aphasia. Cortex 2:74–89, 1966.

Goodglass H, Quadfasel F. Language laterality in left handed aphasics. Brain 77:521–548, 1954.

Goodglass H, Quadfasel F, Timberlake W. Phrase length and the type and severity of aphasia. Cortex 1:133–153, 1964.

Gorelick PB, Hier DB, Benevento L, Levitt S, Tan W. Aphasia after left thalamic infarction. Archives of Neurology 41:1296–1298, 1984.

Gorman DG, Benson DF, Vogel DG, Vinters HV. Creutzfeldt-Jakob disease in a pathologist. Neurology 42:463, 1992 (letter).

Gott PS, Saul RE. Agenesis of the corpus callosum: Limits of functional compensation. Neurology 28:1272–1279, 1978.

Gould R, Miller BL, Goldberg MA, Benson DF. The validity of hysterical signs and symptoms. Journal of Nervous and Mental Disease 174:593–597, 1986.

Gould SJ. The Mismeasure of Man. New York: Norton, 1981.

Graff-Radford NR, Damasio AR, Hyman BT, Hart MN, Tranel D, Damasio H, Van Hoesen SW, Rezai K. Progressive aphasia in a patient with Pick's disease: A neuropsychological, radiologic, and anatomical study. Neurology 40:620–626, 1990.

Graff-Radford NR, Eslinger PJ, Damasio AR, Yamada T. Nonhemorrhagic infarction of the thalamus: Behavioral, anatomic and physiologic correlates. Neurology 34:14–23, 1985.

Grafman J. Acalculia. In F Boller, J Grafman (eds), Handbook of Neuropsychology, Vol I. Amsterdam: Elsevier, 1988, pp 415–431.

Grafman J, Passafiume D, Faglioni P, Boller F. Calculation disturbances in adults with focal hemisphere damage. Cortex 18:37–49, 1982.

Graham L. Wernicke's aphasia. In LL LaPointe (ed), Aphasia and Related Neurogenic Language Disorders. New York: Thieme, 1990, pp 38–53.

Gratiolet LP. Mémoire sur les plis cérébraux de l'homme et des primates. Paris: Bertrand, 1854.

Green E. Phonological and grammatical aspects of jargon in an aphasic patient. Language and Speech 12:103–118, 1969.

Green E, Howes D. Conduction aphasia. In H Whitaker, HA Whitaker (eds), Studies in Neurolinguistics, Vol 3. New York: Academic Press, 1977, pp 123–156.

Green J, Morris JC, Sandson J, McKeel DW, Miller JW. Progressive aphasia: A precursor of global dementia? Neurology 40:423–429, 1990.

Greenblatt SH. Alexia without agraphia or hemianopsia. Brain 96:307–316, 1973.

Greenblatt SH. Subangular alexia without agraphia or hemianopsia. Brain and Language 3:229–245, 1976.

Greenblatt SH. Neurosurgery and the anatomy of reading: A practical review. Neurosurgery 1:6–15, 1977.

Greenblatt SH. Localization of lesions in alexia. In A Kertesz (ed), Localization in Neuropsychology. New York: Academic Press, 1983, pp 324–356.

Grewel F. The acalculias. In PJ Vinken, GW Bruyn (eds), Handbook of Clinical Neurology, Vol 4. Amsterdam: North-Holland, 1960, pp 181–196.

Grober E, Perecman E, Kellar L, Brown JW. Lexical knowledge in anterior and posterior aphasics. Brain and Language 10:318–330, 1980.

Grossi D, Fragassi NA, Orsini A, De Falco LA, Sepe O. Residual reading capability in a patient with alexia without agraphia. Brain and Language 23:337–348, 1984.

Groswasser Z, Korn C, Groswasser-Reider I, Solzi P. Mutism associated with buccofacial apraxia and bihemispheric lesions. Brain and Language 34:157–168, 1988.

Grotta JC. Acute stroke management: Diagnosis (Part I). Stroke Clinical Updates 3:17–20, 1993.

Grüsser O-J, Landis T. Visual Agnosias and Other Disturbances of Visual Perception and Cognition. London: Macmillan, 1991.

Guttman E. Aphasia in children. Brain 65:205–219, 1942.

Guyard H, Masson V, Quiniou R. Computer-based aphasia treatment meets artificial intelligence. Aphasiology 6:599–614, 1990.

Hagen, C. Communication abilities in hemiplegia: Effect of speech therapy. Archives of Physical Medicine and Rehabilitation 54:454–463, 1973.

Halpern H, Darley FL, Brown JR. Differential language and neurological characteristics in cerebral involvement. Journal of Speech and Hearing Disorders 38:162–173, 1973.

Halta T. Recognition of Japanese Kanji in the right and left visual fields. Neuropsychologia 15:685–688, 1977.

Hamsher K. Intelligence and aphasia. In MT Sarno (ed), Acquired Aphasia. New York: Academic Press, 1981, pp 327–359.

Hanson WR, Metter EJ, Riege EH. The course of chronic aphasia. Aphasiology 3:19–29, 1989.

Harris LJ. Cultural influences on handedness: Historical and contemporary theory and evidence. In S Coren (ed), Left-handedness: Behavioral Implications and Anomalies. Amsterdam: North-Holland, 1990, pp 195–258.

Hart J, Berndt RS, Caramazza A. Category-specific naming deficit following cerebral infarction. Nature 316:439–440, 1985.

Hatfield MF. Visual and phonological factors in acquired agraphia. Neuropsychologia 23:13–29, 1985.

Hatfield FM, Patterson K. Phonological spelling. Quarterly Journal of Experimental Psychology 35:451–458, 1983.

Haymaker W, Schiller F. Founders of Neurology. Springfield, IL: Charles C Thomas, 1953.

Head H. Aphasia and Kindred Disorders, 2 Vol. London: Cambridge University Press, 1926.

Healey JM, Liederman J, Geschwind N. Handedness is not a unilateral trait. Cortex 22:33–54, 1986.

Heath PD, Kennedy P, Kapur N. Slowly progressive aphasia without generalized dementia. Archives of Neurology 13:687–688, 1983.

Heaton RK, Nelson LM, Thompson DS, Burks JS, Franklin GM. Neuropsychological findings in relapsing-remitting and chronic-progressive multiple sclerosis. Journal of Consulting Clinical Psychology 53:103–110, 1985.

Hécaen H. Clinical symptomatology in right and left hemisphere lesions. In VB Mountcastle (ed), Interhemispheric Relations and Cerebral Dominance. Baltimore: Johns Hopkins University Press, 1962, pp 215–243.

Hécaen H. Essai de dissociation du syndrome de l'aphasie sensorielle. Revue Neurologique 120:229–231, 1969.

Hécaen H. Introduction à la Neuropsychologie. Paris: Larousse, 1972.

Hécaen H. Acquired aphasia in children and the ontogenesis of hemispheric functional specialization. Brain and Language 3:114–134, 1976.

Hécaen H. Acquired aphasia in children: Revisited. Neuropsychologia 21:581–587, 1983.

Hécaen H, de Ajuriaguerra J. Le troubles mentaux au cours du tumeurs intracraniennes. Paris: Masson, 1956.

Hécaen H, Albert ML. Human Neuropsychology. New York: Wiley, 1978.

Hécaen H, Angelergues R. Etude anatomo-clinique de 280 cas de lesions cerebraux. Encephale 6:533–562, 1961.

Hécaen H, Angelergues R. Localization of symptoms in aphasia. In AVS DeReuck, M O'Connor (eds), Disorders of Language. Boston: Little, Brown, 1964, pp 223–246.

Hécaen H, Angelergues R. Pathologie du Langage. Paris: Larousse, 1965.

Hécaen H, Angelergues R, Douzenis JA. Les agraphies. Neuropsychologia 1:179–208, 1963.

Hécaen H, Angelergues T, Houiller S. Les variétés cliniques des acalculies au cours des lésions retrorolandiques. Revue Neurologique 105:85–103, 1961.

Hécaen H, Dell MB, Roger A. L'aphasie de conduction. L'Encephale 2:170–195, 1955.

Hécaen H, Marcie P. Disorders of written language following right hemisphere lesions: Spatial dysgraphia. In SJ Dimond, JG Beaumont (eds), Hemispheric Function in the Human Brain. London: Elek Science, 1974, pp 345–366.

Hécaen H, Penfield W, Bertrand C, Malmo R. The syndrome of apractagnosia due to lesions of the minor cerebral hemisphere. Archives of Neurology and Psychiatry 75:400–434, 1956.

Hécaen H, Sauguet J. Cerebral dominance in left-handed subjects. Cortex 7:19–48, 1971.

Hedderly F. Phrenology: A Study of Mind. London: Fowler, 1970.

Heilman KM. Ideational apraxia: A re-definition. Brain 96:861–864, 1973.

Heilman KM. Neglect and related syndromes. In KM Heilman, E Valenstein (eds), Clinical Neuropsychology. New York: Oxford University Press, 1979, pp 268–307.

Heilman KM, Gonzalez-Rothi LJ. Apraxia. In KM Heilman, E Valenstein (eds), Clinical Neuropsychology, 3d ed. New York: Oxford University Press, 1993, pp 141–164.

Heilman KM, Safran A, Geschwind N. Closed head trauma and aphasia. Journal of Neurology, Neurosurgery, and Psychiatry 34:265–269, 1971.

Heilman KM, Scholes R. The nature of comprehension errors in Broca's, conduction and Wernicke's aphasics. Cortex 12:258–265, 1978.

Heilman KM, Tucker DM, Valenstein E. A case of mixed transcortical aphasia with intact naming. Brain 99:415–426, 1976.

Heilman KM, Valenstein E. Auditory neglect in man. Archives of Neurology 26:32–35, 1972.

Heilman KM, Valenstein E. Mechanisms underlying hemispatial neglect. Annals of Neurology 5:166–170, 1979.

Heilman KM, Valenstein E (eds). Clinical Neuropsychology, 3d Ed. New York: Oxford University Press, 1993.

Heilman KM, Valenstein E, Watson RT. Behavioral aspects of neurologic disease: Attentional, intentional and emotional disorders. In AB Baker, RJ Joynt (eds), Clinical Neurology. Philadelphia: Harper and Row, 1985a (Chap 22).

Heilman KM, Valenstein E, Watson RT. The neglect syndrome. In JAM Frederiks (ed), Handbook of Clinical Neurology, 2d Ed., Vol 45: Clinical Neuropsychology. Amsterdam: Elsevier, 1985b, pp 153–183.

Heilman KM, Watson RT, Valenstein E. Neglect and related disorders. In KM Heilman, E Valenstein (eds), Clinical Neuropsychology, 2d Ed. New York: Oxford University Press, 1985c, pp 243–293.

Heimburger RF, Demyer W, Reitan RM. Implications of Gerstmann's syndrome. Journal of Neurology, Neurosurgery, and Psychiatry 27:53–57, 1961.

Helm NA. Criteria for selecting aphasic patients for melodic intonation therapy. Paper presented at Annual Meeting, AAAS, Washington, DC, February, 1978.

Helm N, Benson DF. Visual action therapy for global aphasia. Paper presented at Annual Meeting, Academy of Aphasia, Chicago, Illinois, October, 1978.

Helm NA, Butler RB, Benson DF. Acquired stuttering. Neurology 28:1159–1165, 1978.

Helm-Estabrooks N, Albert ML. Manual of Aphasia Therapy. Austin, TX: Pro-Ed, 1991.

Helm-Estabrooks N, Emery P, Albert ML. Treatment of aphasic perseveration (TAP) program: A new approach to aphasia therapy. Archives of Neurology 44:1253–1255, 1987.

Helm-Estabrooks N, Fitzpatrick PM, Barresi B. Visual action therapy for global aphasia. Journal of Speech and Hearing Disorders 47:385–389, 1982.

Henderson VW. Speech fluency in crossed aphasia. Brain 100:1–8, 1983.

Henderson VW. Jules Dejerine and the third alexia. Archives of Neurology 41:430–432, 1984.

Henderson VW. Anatomy of the posterior pathways in reading: A reassessment. Brain and Language 29:119–133, 1986.

Henderson VW. Alalia, aphemia and aphasia. Archives of Neurology 47:85–88, 1990.

Henderson VW, Friedman RB, Teng EL, Weiner JM. Left hemisphere pathways in reading: Inferences from pure alexia without hemianopia. Neurology 35:962–966, 1985.

Henschen SE. Klinische und Anatomische Beitrage zur Pathologie des Gehirns. Stockholm: Almquist and Wiksell, 1922.

Henschen SE. Clinical and anatomical contributions on brain pathology. Archives of Neurology and Psychiatry 13:226–249, 1925.

Henschen SE. On the function of the right hemisphere of the brain in relation to the left hemisphere in speech, music and calculation. Brain 49:110–123, 1926.

Hier DB, Davis KR, Richardson EP, Mohr JP. Hypertensive putaminal hemorrhage. Annals of Neurology 1:152–159, 1977.

Hier DB, Hagenlocker K, Shindler AG. Language disintegration in dementia: Effects of etiology and severity. Brain and Language 25:117–133, 1985.

Hier DB, Mogil SI, Rubin NP, Komros BR. Semantic aphasia: A neglected entity. Brain and Language 10:120–131, 1980.

Hier DB, Mohr JP. Incongruous oral and written naming: Evidence for a subdivision of the syndromes of Wernicke aphasia. Brain and Language 4:115–126, 1977.

Hillis AE, Caramazza A. The effects of attentional deficits on reading and spelling. In A Caramazza (ed), Cognitive Neuropsychology and Neurolinguistics. Hillsdale, NJ, Lawrence Erlbaum Associates, 1990, pp 211–275.

Hinshelwood J. Letter-, Word- and Mind-Blindness. London: H. K. Lewis, 1900.

Hitch G, Cundick J, Haughey M, Pugh R, Wright H. Aspects of counting in children's arithmetics. In JA Sloboda, D Rogers (eds), Cognitive Processes in Mathematics. Oxford: Clarendon Press, 1987, pp 26–41.

Holland AL. Communicative Abilities in Daily Living. Baltimore: University Park Press, 1980.

Holland AL, McBurney DH, Moossy J, Reinmuth OM. The dissolution of language in Pick's disease with neurofibrillary tangles: A case study. Brain and Language 24:36–58, 1985.

Holman BL, Hill TC. Perfusion imaging with single-photon emission computed tomography. In JH Wood (ed), Cerebral Blood Flow: Physiologic and Clinical Aspects. New York: McGraw-Hill, 1987, pp 243–258.

Holmes G. Disturbances of vision by cerebral lesions. British Journal of Ophthalmology 2:353–384, 1918.

Holmes G. Mental symptoms associated with cerebral tumours. Proceedings of the Royal Society of Medicine 24:997–1008, 1931.

Hoops R, Lebrun Y (eds) Intelligence and Aphasia. Amsterdam: Swets & Zeitlinger, 1974.

Horner J, LaPointe LI. Evaluation of learning potential of a severe aphasic adult through analysis of five performance variables. In R Brookshire (ed), Proceedings of the Conference on Clinical Aphasiology. Minneapolis: BRK Publishers, 1979.

Horner J, Massey EW. Progressive dysfluency associated with right hemisphere disease. Brain and Language 18:71–85, 1983.

Howard D, Patterson K, Franklin S, Orchard-Lisse V, Morton J. Treatment of word retrieval deficits in aphasia: A comparison of two therapy methods. Brain 108:817–829, 1985.

Howard D, Patterson K, Wise R, Brown RD, Friston K, Weiller C, Frackowiak R. The cortical location of the lexicons: Positron emission tomography evidence. Brain 115:1769–1782, 1992.

Howes D. Application of the word-frequency concept to aphasia. In AVS DeReuck, M O'Connor (eds), Disorders of Language. Boston: Little, Brown, 1964, pp 47–78.

Howes D, Boller F. Comparison of lesion size in radioisotope brain scan with actual pathology at post-mortem (Personal communication, 1978).

Howes D, Geschwind N. Quantitative studies of aphasic language. In D McK Rioch, EA Weinstein (eds), Disorders of Communication (Proceedings of the Association for Research in Nervous and Mental Disease, Vol 42). Baltimore: Williams and Wilkins, 1964, pp 229–244.

Huber SJ, Shuttleworth EC, Freidenberg DL. Neuropsychological differences between the dementias of Alzheimer's disease and Parkinson's disease. Archives of Neurology 46:1287–1291, 1989.

Huber W, Poeck K, Willmes K. The Aachen Aphasia Test. In FC Rosen (ed), Advances in Neurology, Vol 42: Progress in Aphasiology. New York: Raven Press, 1984, pp 291–304.

Huber W, Stachowiak FJ, Poeck K, Kerschensteiner M. Die Wernicke's aphasie. Journal of Neurology 210:77–97, 1975.

Huff FJ, Collins C, Corkin S, Rosen TJ. Equivalent forms of the Boston Naming Test. Journal of Clinical and Experimental Neuropsychology 8:556–562, 1986.

Humphrey G. Thinking: An Introduction to Experimental Psychology. New York: Wiley, 1951.

Ingvar DH, Schwartz MD. Blood flow patterns induced in the dominant hemisphere by speech and reading. Brain 97:274–288, 1974.

Isserlin M. Die pathologische Physiologie der Sprache. Ergebnisse der Physiologie 29:129–149, 1929.

Isserlin M. Die pathologische Physiologie der Sprache. Ergebnisse der Physiologie 33:1–102, 1931.

Isserlin M. Die pathologische Physiologie der Sprache. Ergebnisse der Physiologie 34:1065–1144, 1932.

Iwata M. Neural mechanisms of reading and writing in the Japanese language. Functional Neurology 1:43–52, 1986.

Jackson JH. Clinical remarks on cases of defects of expression (by words, writing, signs, etc.) in diseases of the nervous system. Lancet 1:604–605, 1864.

Jackson JH. Reprints of some of Hughlings Jackson's papers on affections of speech. Brain 38:28–190, 1915.

Jackson JH (ed J Taylor). Selected Writings. London: Hodder and Stoughton, 1932.

Jackson M, Warrington EK. Arithmetic skills in patients with unilateral cerebral lesions. Cortex 22:611–622, 1986.

Jakobson R. Two aspects of language and two types of aphasic disturbance. In Jakobson R, Halle M (eds), Fundamentals of Language. The Hague: Mouton, 1956, pp 55–87.

Jakobson R. Towards a linguistic typology of aphasic impairments. In AVS DeReuck, M O'Connor (eds), Disorders of Language. Boston: Little, Brown, 1964, pp 21–46.

Jakobson R, Halle M. Fundamentals of Language. The Hague: Mouton, 1956.

Jambor KL. Cognitive functioning in multiple sclerosis. British Journal of Psychiatry 115:765–775, 1969.

James W. The Principles of Psychology. New York: Henry Holt, 1890/1983.

Joanette Y. Aphasia in left-handers and crossed aphasia. In H Goodglass, AR Damasio (eds), Handbook of Neuropsychology, Vol 2. Amsterdam: Elsevier, 1989, pp 173–184.

Johannsen-Horbach H, Cegla B, Mager U, Schempp B, Wallesch CW. Treatment of chronic global aphasia with nonverbal communication system. Brain and Language 24:74–82, 1985.

Jones GV. Deep dyslexia, imageability, and ease of predication. Brain and Language 24:1–19, 1985.

Jones GV. Building the foundations for sentence production in non-fluent aphasia. British Journal of Communication Disorders 21:63–82, 1986.

Jones RK. Observations on stammering after localized cerebral injury. Journal of Neurology, Neurosurgery, and Psychiatry 29:192–195, 1966.

Kahn HJ, Whitaker HA. Acalculia: An historical review of localization. Brain and Cognition 17:102–115, 1991.

Kaplan E. The process approach to neuropsychological assessment of psychiatric patients. Journal of Neuropsychiatry and Clinical Neuroscience 2:72–87, 1990.

Kaplan E, Goodglass H. Aphasia-related disorders. In MT Sarno (ed), Acquired Aphasia. New York: Academic Press, 1981, pp 303–325.

Kaplan EF, Goodglass H, Weintraub S. The Boston Naming Test. Philadelphia: Lea and Febiger, 1978.

Karanth P, Rangamani GN. Crossed aphasia in multilinguals. Brain and Language 34:169–180, 1988.

Karis R, Horenstein S. Localization of speech parameters by brain scan. Neurology 26:3:226–231, 1976.

Katz JJ. Semantic Theory. New York: Harper and Row, 1972.

Katz RB, Goodglass H. Deep dysphasia: Analysis of a rare form of repetition disorder. Brain and Language 39:153–185, 1990.

Katz RC. Aphasia Treatment and Microcomputers. San Diego: College-Hill Press, 1986.

Katz RC. Intelligent computerized treatment or artificial aphasia therapy? Aphasiology 6:621–624, 1990.

Katzman R, Karasu TB. The differential diagnosis of dementia. In WS Fields (ed), Neurological and Sensory Disorders in the Elderly. New York: Grune and Stratton, 1975, pp. 103–134.

Kaufer DI, Benson DF. Neuropsychiatric manifestations of global auditory agnosia. Neurology 44 (Suppl 2):A400, 1994 (Abstract).

Kay J, Hanley R. Simultaneous form perception and serial letter recognition in a case of letter-by-letter reading. Cognitive Neuropsychology 8:249–275, 1991.

Kay J, Lesser R. The nature of phonological processing in oral reading: Evidence from surface dyslexia. Quarterly Journal of Experimental Psychology 37A:39–81, 1986.

Kean ML (ed). Agrammatism. New York: Academic Press, 1985.

Kearns KP. Broca's aphasia. In LL La Pointe (ed), Aphasia and Related Neurogenic Disorders. New York: Thieme, 1990, pp 1–37.

Kelly JP. Anatomy of the central visual pathways. In ER Kandel, JH Schwartz (eds), Principles of Neural Science, 2d Ed. New York: Elsevier, 1985, pp 356–365.

Kempler D, Curtiss S, Jackson C. Syntactic preservation in Alzheimer's disease. Journal of Speech and Hearing Research 30:343–350, 1987.

Kempler D, Metter EJ, Jackson CA, Hanson WR, Riege WH, Mazziotta JC, Phelps ME. Disconnection and cerebral metabolism: The case of conduction aphasia. Archives of Neurology 45:275–279, 1988.

Kempler D, Metter EJ, Riege WH, Jackson CA, Benson DF, Hanson WR. Slowly progressive aphasia: Three cases with language, memory, CT and PET data. Journal of Neurology, Neurosurgery, and Psychiatry 53:987–993, 1990.

Kennard M. Alterations in response to visual stimuli following lesions of the frontal lobe in monkeys. Archives of Neurology and Psychiatry 41:1153–1165, 1939.

Kernohan JW, Sayre GP. Tumors of the Central Nervous System. Washington, DC: Armed Forces Institute of Pathology, 1952.

Kertesz A. Aphasia and Associated Disorders. New York: Grune and Stratton, 1979.

Kertesz A. The Western Aphasia Battery. New York: Grune and Stratton, 1982.

Kertesz A (ed). Localization in Neuropsychology. New York: Academic Press, 1983.

Kertesz A. Aphasia. In PJ Vinken, GW Bruyn, HL Klawans (eds), Handbook of Clinical Neurology, Vol 45: Clinical Neuropsychology. Amsterdam: Elsevier, 1985, pp 287–331.

Kertesz A. Recovery of language disorders: Homologous contralateral or connected ipsilateral compensation? In S Finger, TE LeVere, CR Almli, DG Stein (eds), Brain Recovery: Theoretical and Controversial Issues. New York: Plenum, 1988a, pp 307–321.

Kertesz A. What do we learn from recovery from aphasia? In SG Waxman (ed), Advances in Neurology, Vol 47: Functional Recovery in Neurological Diseases. New York: Raven Press, 1988b, pp 277–292.

Kertesz A, Benson DF. Neologistic jargon: A clinico-pathological study. Cortex 6:362–386, 1970.

Kertesz A, Black SE, Nicholson L, Carr T. The sensitivity and specificity of MRI in stroke. Neurology 37:1580–1585, 1987.

Kertesz A, Black SE, Tokar G, Benke T, Carr T, Nicholson L. Periventricular and subcortical hyperintensities on magnetic resonance imaging: "Rims, caps and unidentified bright objects." Archives of Neurology 45:404–408, 1988.

Kertesz A, Harlock W, Coates R. Computer tomographic localization, lesion size and prognosis in aphasia and nonverbal impairment. Brain and Language 8:34–50, 1979.

Kertesz A, Lesk D, McCabe P. Isotope localization of infarcts in aphasia. Archives of Neurology 34:590–601, 1977.

Kertesz A, McCabe P. Recovery patterns and prognosis in aphasia. Brain 100:1–18, 1977.

Kertesz A, Polk M, Carr T. Cognitive and white matter changes on magnetic resonance imaging in dementia. Archives of Neurology 47:387–391, 1990.

Kertesz A, Poole E. The aphasia quotient: The taxonomic approach to measurement of aphasic disability. Canadian Journal of Neurological Science 1:7–16, 1974.

Kertesz A, Sheppard A, MacKenzie R. Localization in transcortical sensory aphasia. Archives of Neurology 39:475–478, 1982.

Kinsbourne M. The minor cerebral hemisphere as a source of aphasic speech. Archives of Neurology 25:202–206, 1971.

Kinsbourne M, Rosenfield DB. Agraphia selective for written spelling. Brain and Language 1:215–226, 1974.

Kinsbourne M, Warrington EK. A study of finger agnosia. Brain 85:47–66, 1962a.

Kinsbourne M, Warrington EK. A variety of reading disability associated with right hemisphere lesions. Journal of Neurology, Neurosurgery, and Psychiatry 25:339–344, 1962b.

Kinsbourne M, Warrington EK. Observations on color agnosia. Journal of Neurology, Neurosurgery, and Psychiatry 27:296–299, 1964.

Kinsbourne M, Warrington EK. A case showing selective impaired oral spelling. Journal of Neurology, Neurosurgery, and Psychiatry 28:563–566, 1965.

Kirshner HS, Tanridag O, Thurman L, Wells CE. Progressive aphasia without dementia: Two cases with focal spongiform degeneration. Annals of Neurology 41:491–496, 1987.

Kirshner HS, Webb WG, Kelly MP. The naming disorder of dementia. Neuropsychologia 22:23–30, 1984.

Kirshner HS, Webb WG, Kelly MP, Wells CE. Language disturbance: An initial symptom of cortical degenerations and dementia. Archives of Neurology 41:491–496, 1984.

Klein A, Starkey PS. The origins and development of numerical cognition: A comparative analysis. In JA Sloboda, D Rogers (eds), Cognitive Processes in Mathematics. Oxford: Clarendon Press, 1987, pp 1–25.

Kleist K. Gehirnpathologie. Leipzig: Barth, 1934a.

Kleist K. Leitungsaphasie (Nachsprechaphasie). In K Bonhoeffer (ed), Handbuch der Artzlichen Erfahrungen im Weltkriege 1914/1918. Leipzig: Barth, 1934b, pp 725–737.

Knopman DS, Rubens AB, Klassen AC, Meyer MW. Regional cerebral blood flow correlates of auditory processing. Archives of Neurology 39:487–493, 1989.

Knopman DS, Rubens AB, Selnes OA, Klassen AC, Meyer MW. Mechanisms of recovery from aphasia: Evidence from serial Xenon-133 cerebral blood flow studies. Annals of Neurology 15:530–535, 1984.

Koffka K. The Principles of Gestalt Psychology. New York: Harcourt Brace Jovanovich, 1935.

Kohn SE. Conduction aphasia. Hillsdale, NJ: Erlbaum and Associates, 1992.

Kohn SE, Goodglass H. Picture naming in aphasia. Brain and Language 24:266–283, 1985.

Kolb B, Whishaw IQ. Fundamentals of Human Neuropsychology. New York: Freeman, 1990.

Kolk HHJ, Van Grunsven MJF, Keyser A. On parallelism between production and comprehension in agrammatism. In ML Kean (ed), Agrammatism. New York: Academic Press, 1985, pp 165–206.

Konorski J. The Integrative Activity of the Brain. Chicago: University of Chicago Press, 1969.

Kontiola P, Laaksonen R, Sulkava R, Erkinjuntti T. Pattern of language impairment is different in Alzheimer's disease and multi-infarct dementia. Brain and Language 38:364–383, 1990.

Kraat AW. Augmentative and alternative communication: Does it have a future in aphasia rehabilitation? Aphasiology 4:321–338, 1990.

Krashen S. Lateralization, language learning and the critical period. Language Learning 23:63–74, 1973.

Krashen S, Harshman R. Lateralization and the critical period. Papers on Phonetics 22:6–12, 1972.

Kremer M, Russell WR, Smyth GE. A mid-brain syndrome following head injury. Journal of Neurology, Neurosurgery, and Psychiatry 10:49–60, 1947.

Kremin H. Naming and its disorders. In F Boller, J Grafman, G Rizzolatti, H Goodglass (eds), Handbook of Neuropsychology, Vol 1. Amsterdam: Elsevier, 1988, pp 307–328.

Kudo T. Aphasics' appreciation of hierarchical semantic categories. Brain and Language 30:33–51, 1987.

Kurtzke JF. Clinical manifestations of multiple sclerosis. In PJ Vinken, GW Bruyn (eds), Handbook of Clinical Neurology, Vol 9. Amsterdam: North-Holland, 1970, pp 161–216.

Kussmaul A. Disturbances of speech. Encyclopedia of Practical Medicine 14:581–875, 1877. New York: Wood (as quoted by Kertesz, 1985).

LaBarge E, Edwards D, Knesevich JW. Performance of normal elderly on the Boston Naming Test. Brain and Language 27:380–384, 1986.

Lambert W, Fillenbaum S. A pilot study of aphasia among bilinguals. Canadian Journal of Psychology 13:28–34, 1959.

Landau WM, Goldstein R, Kleffner FR. Congenital aphasia: a clinico-pathologic study. Neurology 10:915–921, 1960.

Landis T, Regard M, Serrat A. Iconic reading in a case of alexia without agraphia caused by a brain tumor. Brain and Language 11:45–53, 1980.

Langer J. The Origins of Logic: One to Two Years. New York: Academic Press, 1986.

Laplane D, Degos JD. Motor neglect. Journal of Neurology, Neurosurgery, and Psychiatry 46:152–158, 1983.

LaPointe LI. Base-10 programmed stimulation: Task specification scoring and plotting performance in aphasia therapy. Journal of Speech and Hearing Disorders 42:90–105, 1977.

Larsen B, Skinhøj E, Endo H. Localization of basic speech functions as revealed by rCBF measurements in normals and in patients with aphasia. In AS Meyer, M Lechner, M Revich (eds), Cerebral Vascular Disease (8th International Salzburg Conference). Amsterdam: Excerpta Medica, 1977.

Larsen B, Skinhøj E, Lassen NA. Variations in regional cortical blood flow in the right and left hemispheres during automatic speech. Brain 101:193–210, 1978.

Lashley KS. Brain Mechanisms and Intelligence. Chicago: University of Chicago Press, 1929.

Lebrun Y (ed). Intelligence and Aphasia. Amsterdam: Swets & Zeitlinger, 1974.

Lebrun Y. Neurolinguistic models of language and speech. In H Whitaker, HA Whitaker (eds), Studies in Neurolinguistics, Vol 1. New York: Academic Press, 1976, pp 1–30.

Lebrun Y. Disturbances of written language and associated abilities following damage to the right hemisphere. Applied Psycholinguistics 6:231–260, 1985.

Lebrun Y. Unilateral agraphia. Aphasiology 1:317–329, 1987.

Lebrun Y, Rubio S. Reduplications et omissions graphiques chez des patients attients d'une lésion hémisphèrique droite. Neuropsychologia 10:249–251, 1972.

Lecours AR. Dyslexies et dysgraphies: Théorie, formes cliniques et examen (unpublished doctoral dissertation).

Lecours AR, Chain F, Poncet M, Nespoulos J-L. Paris 1908: The hot summer of aphasiology or a season in the life of a chair. Brain and Language 32:105–152, 1992.

Lecours AR, Lhermitte F. Phonemic paraphasias: Linguistic structures and tentative hypotheses. Cortex 5:193–228, 1969.

Lecours AR, Lhermitte F. The "pure form" of the phonetic disintegration syndrome (pure anarthria): Anatomo-clinical report of a historical case. Brain and Language 2:88–113, 1976.

Lecours AR, Lhermitte F, Bryans B. Aphasiology. London: Bailliere-Tindall, 1983.

Lecours AR, Mehler J, Parente MA, Beltrami MC, Canossa de Tolipan L, Cary L, Castro MJ et al. Illiteracy and brain damage. III: A contribution to the study of speech and language disorders in illiterates with unilateral brain damage (initial testing). Neuropsychologia 26:575–589, 1988.

Lecours AR, Rouillon F. Neurolinguistic analysis of jargonaphasia and jargonagraphia. In H Whitaker, HA Whitaker (eds), Studies in Neurolinguistics, Vol 2. New York: Academic Press, 1976, pp 95–144.

Lecours AR, Tainturier M-J, Boeglin J. Classification of aphasia. In FC Rose, R Whurr, MA Wyke (eds), Aphasia. London: Whurr, 1988, pp 3–22.

Lecours AR, Trepagnier C, Naesser CJ, Lavelle-Huynh G. The interaction between linguistics and aphasiology. In AR Lecours, F Lhermitte, B Bryans (eds), Aphasiology. London: Bailliere-Tindall, 1983, pp 292–310.

Lecours AR, Vanier M, Lhermitte F. The thalamus and linguistic function. In AR Lecours, F Lhermitte, B Bryans (eds), Aphasiology. London: Bailliere-Tindall, 1983, pp 141–162.

Lehman JR, DeLateur BJ, Fowler RF Jr. Does rehabilitation affect outcome? Archives of Physical Medicine and Rehabilitation 56:383–389, 1975.

Leischner A. The agraphias. In PJ Vinken, GW Bruyn (eds), Handbook of Clinical Neurology, Vol 4. Amsterdam: North-Holland, 1969, pp 141–180.

Leischner A. Side differences in writing to dictation of aphasics with agraphia: A graphic disconnection syndrome. Brain and Language 18:1–19, 1983.

Lenneberg EH. Biological Foundations of Language. New York: Wiley, 1967.

Lesser R. Linguistic Investigations of Aphasia. London: Edward Arnold, 1978.

Levin HS, Benton AL, Grossman RG. Neurobehavioral Consequences of Closed Head Injury. New York: Oxford University Press, 1982.

Levin HS, Goldstein FC, Williams DH, Eisenberg HM. The contribution of frontal lobe lesions to the neurobehavioral outcome of closed head injury. In HS Levin, HM

Eisenberg, AL Benton (eds), Frontal Lobe Function and Dysfunction. New York: Oxford University Press, 1991, pp 318–338.

Levin HS, Grossman RG. Behavioral sequelae of closed head injury. Archives of Neurology 35:712–719, 1978.

Levin H, Spiers PA. Acalculia. In KM Heilman, E Valenstein (eds), Clinical Neuropsychology, 2d Ed. New York: Oxford University Press, 1985, pp 97–115.

Levine DN, Calvanio R. A study of the visual defect in verbal alexia-simultanagnosia. Brain 101:65–81, 1978.

Levine DN, Calvanio R. Conduction aphasia. In H Kirshner, FR Freemon (eds), Neurolinguistics, Vol 12: The Neurology of Aphasia. Amsterdam: Swets & Zeitlinger, 1982, pp 79–111.

Levine DN, Mohr JP. Language after bilateral cerebral infarction: Role of the minor hemisphere in speech. Neurology 29:927–938, 1979.

Levine DN, Sweet E. Localization of lesions in Broca's motor aphasia. In A Kertesz (ed), Localization in Neuropsychology. New York: Academic Press, 1983, pp 185–208.

Levy J. Psychobiological implications of bilateral asymmetry. In SJ Dimond, JG Beaumont (eds), Hemisphere Function in the Human Brain. London: Elek Science, 1974, pp 121–183.

Levy-Bruhl L. Las Funciones Mentales en las Sociedades Inferiores [Mental Functions in Lower Societies]. Buenos Aires: Lautaro, 1910/1947.

Lezak MD. Neuropsychological Assessment, 3d Ed. New York: Oxford University Press, 1995.

Lhermitte F, Beauvois MF. A visual-speech disconnexion syndrome. Brain 96:695–714, 1973.

Lhermitte F, Chain F, Escourelle R. Etude anatomo-clinique d'un cas de prosopagnosie. Revue Neurologique 126:329–346, 1972.

Lichtheim L. On aphasia. Brain 7:433–484, 1885.

Lieberman A, Benson DF. Control of emotional expression in pseudobulbar palsy. Archives of Neurology 34:717–719, 1977.

Liederman J, Kohn S, Wolf M, Goodglass H. Lexical creativity during instances of word-finding difficulty: Broca's versus Wernicke's aphasia. Brain and Language 20:21–32, 1983.

Liepmann H. Das Krankheitsbild der apraxie ("motorische asymbolie"). Monatsschrift für Psychiatrie und Neurologie 8:15–44, 102–132, 182–197, 1900.

Liepmann H. Das Krankheitsbild der apraxie. Monatsschrift für Psychiatrie und Neurologie 17:289–311, 1905.

Liepmann H, Maas O. Fall von linksseitiger agraphie und apraxie bei rechtsseitiger lahrmung. Journal of Psychiatry and Neurology 10:214–227, 1907.

Liepmann H, Storch E. Ein Fall von reiner Sprachtaubheit. Monatsschrift für Psychiatrie und Neurologie 11:115–120, 1902.

Lipowski ZJ. Acute Confusional States. New York: Oxford University Press, 1990.

Lippa CF, Cohen R, Smith TW, Drachman DA. Primary progressive aphasia with focal neuronal achromasia. Neurology 41:882–886, 1991.

Lishman WA. Split minds: A review of the results of brain bisection in man. British Journal of Hospital Medicine 3:477–484, 1969.

Lishman WA. Organic Psychiatry. Oxford: Blackwell, 1978.

Lishman WA. Organic Psychiatry, 2d Ed. Oxford: Blackwell, 1987.

Lissauer H. Ein Fall von Seelenblindheit nebst einem Beitrage zur Theorie derselben. Archiv für Psychiatrie 21:2–50, 1889.

Liversedge LA, Sylvester JD. Conditioning techniques in the treatment of writer's cramp. Lancet 1:1147–1149, 1955.

Lomas J, Kertesz A. Patterns of spontaneous recovery in aphasic groups: A study of adult stroke patients. Brain and Language 5:388–401, 1978.

Lopera F. Secuelas del daño encefalico en la primera infancia. In M Rosselli, A Ardila (eds), Neuropsicologia Infantil. Medellin, Colombia: Prensa Creativa, 1992, pp 217–233.

Lopera F, Ardila A. Prosopamnesia and visuolimbic disconnection syndrome. Neuropsychology 6:3–12, 1992.

Loverso FL, Prescott TE, Selinger M. Microcomputer treatment applications in aphasiology. Aphasiology 6:155–164, 1992.

Luders H, Lesser RP, Hahn J, Dinner DS, Morris HH, Wylie E, Godoy J. Basal temporal language area. Brain 114:743–754, 1991.

Luria AR. Traumatic Aphasia. The Hague: Mouton, 1947/1970.

Luria AR. Restoration of Functions after Brain Injury. New York: Macmillan, 1963.

Luria AR. Neuropsychology in the local diagnosis of brain damage. Cortex 1:3–18, 1964a.

Luria AR. Factors and forms of aphasia. In AVS De Reuck, M O'Connor (eds), Disorders of Language. Boston: Little, Brown, 1964b, pp 143–161.

Luria AR. Higher Cortical Functions in Man. New York: Basic Books, 1966.

Luria AR. The Working Brain. New York: Basic Books, 1973.

Luria AR. Basic Problems in Neurolinguistics. The Hague: Mouton, 1976a.

Luria AR. Fundamentals of Neurolinguistics. New York: Basic Books, 1976b.

Luria AR. On quasi-aphasic speech disturbances in lesions of the deep structures of the brain. Brain and Language 4:432–459, 1977.

Luria AR, Pribram KH, Homskaya ED. An experimental analysis of the behavioral disturbance produced by a left frontal arachnoidal endothelioma. Neuropsychologia 2:257–280, 1964.

Luria AR, Tsvetkova L. The programming of constructive ability in local brain injuries. Neuropsychologia 2:95–108, 1964.

Luria AR, Tsvetkova L. Towards the mechanisms of "dynamic aphasia." Acta Neurologica et Psychiatrica Belgica 67:1045–1057, 1967.

Luzzatti C, Poeck K. An early description of slowly progressive aphasia. Archives of Neurology 48:228–229, 1991.

Lyman RS, Kwan ST, Chao WH. Left occipito-parietal brain tumor with observations on alexia and agraphia in Chinese and English. Chinese Medical Journal 54:491–516, 1938.

Mandell AM, Alexander MP, Carpenter S. Creutzfeldt-Jakob disease presenting as isolated aphasia. Neurology 39:55–58, 1989.

Marcel AJ. Surface dyslexia and beginning reading: A revised hypothesis of the pronunciation of print and its impairments. In M Coltheart, K Patterson, J Marshall (eds), Deep Dyslexia. London: Routledge and Kegan Paul, 1980, pp 227–258.

Marcie P, Hécaen H. Agraphia: Writing disorders associated with unilateral cerebral disorders. In KM Heilman, E Valenstein (eds), Clinical Neuropsychology. New York: Oxford University Press, 1979, pp 92–127.

Marcie P, Hécaen H, Dubois J, Angelergues R. Les troubles de la réalisation de la parole au cours des lésions de l'hémisphère droit. Neuropsychologia 3:217–247, 1965.

Margolin DI. Cognitive neuropsychology: Resolving enigmas about Wernicke's aphasia and other higher cortical disorders. Archives of Neurology 48:751–765, 1991.

Margolin DI, Binder L. Multiple component agraphia in a patient with atypical cerebral dominance: An error analysis. Brain and Language 24:26–40, 1984.

Marie P. Révision de la question de l'aphasie. Semaine Médicale 26:241–247, 1906a.

Marie P. Révision de la question de l'aphasie. Semaine Médicale 26:493–500, 1906b.

Marie P. Revision de la question de l'aphasie. Semaine Médicale 26:565–571, 1906c.

Marie P, Foix C. Les aphasies de guerre. Revue Neurologique 24:53–87, 1917.

Marin OSM. CAT scans of five deep dyslexic patients. In M Coltheart, K Patterson, JC Marshall (eds), Deep Dyslexia. London: Routledge and Kegan Paul, 1980, pp 407–411.

Marshall J. The effect of aging upon physiological tremor. Journal of Neurology, Neurosurgery, and Psychiatry 24:14–17, 1968.

Marshall JC. On some relationships between acquired and developmental dyslexias. In FH Duffy, N Geschwind (eds), Dyslexia: A Neuroscientific Approach to Clinical Evaluation. Boston: Little, Brown, 1985, pp 55–66.

Marshall JC, Newcombe F. Syntactic and semantic errors in paralexia. Neuropsychologia 4:169–176, 1966.

Marshall JC, Newcombe F. Patterns of paralexias: A psycholinguistic approach. Journal of Psycholinguistic Research 2:175–199, 1973.

Martin AD. Some objections to the term Apraxia of Speech. Journal of Speech and Hearing Disorders 39:53–64, 1974.

Martin JP. Pure word blindness considered as a disturbance of visual space perception. Proceedings of the Royal Society of Medicine 47:293–295, 1954.

Martin RC. Articulatory and phonological deficits in short-term memory and their relation to syntactic processing. Brain and Language 32:159–192, 1987.

Martin RC, Blossom-Stach C. Evidence of syntactic deficits in a fluent aphasic. Brain and Language 28:196–234, 1986.

Maruszewski M. Language Communication and the Brain. The Hague: Mouton, 1975.

Masdeu JC, O'Hara RJ. Motor aphasia unaccompanied by faciobrachial weakness. Neurology 33:519–521, 1983.

Maspes PE. Le syndrome expérimental chez l'homme de la section du splenium corps calleux. Alexie visuelle pure hémianopsique. Revue Neurologique 2:101–113, 1948.

Mateer CA, Polen SB, Ojemann GA, Wyler AR. Cortical localization of finger spelling and oral language: A case study. Brain and Language 17:46–57, 1982.

Matute E. El aprendizaje de la lectoescritura y la especialization hemisferica para el lenguaje. In A Ardila, F Ostrosky (eds), Lenguage oral y escrito. Mexico City: Trillas, 1988, pp 310–338.

Mauguiere F, Desmedt JE. Thalamic pain syndrome of Dejerine-Roussy. Archives of Neurology 45:1312–1320, 1988.

Max W. The economic impact of Alzheimer's disease. Neurology 43 (Suppl 4):S6–S10, 1993.

Mayer-Gross W, Slater E, Roth M. Clinical Psychiatry, 3d Ed. London: Bailliere, Tindall and Cassell, 1969.

Mazziotta JC. Mapping human brain activity in vivo. Western Journal of Medicine 161:273–278, 1994.

Mazziotta JC, Phelps ME. Human neuropsychological imaging studies of local brain metabolism: Strategies and results. In L Sokoloff (ed), Brain Imaging and Brain Function. New York: Raven Press, 1985, pp 121–137.

Mazziotta JC, Phelps ME, Carson RE, Kuhl DE. Tomographic mapping of human cerebral metabolism: Auditory stimulation. Neurology 32:921–937, 1982.

Mazziotta JC, Phelps ME, Halgren E, Carson RE, Huang SC, Bayer J. Hemispheric lateralization and local cerebral metabolic and blood flow responses to physiologic stimuli. Journal of Cerebral Blood Flow and Metabolism 3:S246–S247, 1983.

Mazziotta JC, Valentino D, Pellizzari CA, Chen GT, Bookstein F. Structure-function correlations of the living human brain with MRI and PET: A means of anatomical and functional localization. Clinical Pharmacology 13 (Suppl 2):460–461, 1990.

Mazzochi F, Vignolo LA. Localization of lesions in aphasia: Clinical CT scan correlation in stroke patients. Cortex 15:627–654, 1979.

Mazzoni N, Vista M, Pardossi L, Avila L, Bianchi F, Moretti P. Spontaneous evolution of aphasia after ischemic stroke. Aphasiology 6:387–396, 1992.

McCarthy R, Warrington EK. Phonologiocal reading: Phenomena and paradoxes. Cortex 22:359–380, 1986.

McCloskey M, Aliminosa D, Sokol SM. Facts, rules, and procedures in normal calculation: Evidence from multiple single-patient studies of impaired arithmetic fact retrieval. Brain and Cognition 17:154–203, 1991.

McCloskey M, Caramazza A. Cognitive mechanisms in normal and impaired number processing. In G Deloche, X Seron (eds), Mathematical Disabilities: A Cognitive Neuropsychological Perspective. Hillsdale, NJ: Lawrence Erlbaum Associates, 1987, pp 201–220.

McCloskey M, Caramazza A, Basili A. Cognitive processes in number processing and calculation: Evidence from dyscalculia. Brain and Cognition 4:313–330, 1985.

McCloskey M, Sokol SM, Goodman RA. Cognitive processes in verbal number processing: Inference from the performance of brain-damaged subjects. Journal of Experimental Psychology 115:313–330, 1986.

McFarling D, Rothi LJ, Heilman KM. Transcortical aphasia from ischemic infarcts of the thalamus: A report of two cases. Journal of Neurology, Neurosurgery, and Psychiatry 45:107–112, 1982.

McGlone J. Sex differences in human brain asymmetry: A critical survey. The Behavioral and Brain Sciences 5:215–264, 1980.

McHugh PR, Folstein MF. Psychiatric syndromes of Huntington's chorea: A clinical and phenomenologic study. In DF Benson, D Blumer (eds), Psychiatric Aspects of Neurologic Disease. New York: Grune and Stratton, 1975, pp 267–286.

McKhann G, Drachman D, Folstein M, Katzman R, Price D, Stadlan EM. Clinical diagnosis of Alzheimer's disease: Report of the NINCDS-ADRDA Work Group, Department of Health and Human Services, Task Force on Alzheimer's Disease. Neurology 34:939–944, 1984.

McLennan JE, Nakano K, Tyler HR, Schwab RS. Micrographia in Parkinson's disease. Journal of Neurological Sciences 15:141–152, 1972.

McNamara P, Obler LK, Au R, Durso R, Albert ML. Speech monitoring skills in Alzheimer's disease, Parkinson's disease, and normal aging. Brain and Language 42:38–51, 1992.

McRae DL, Branch CL, Milner B. The occipital horns and cerebral dominance. Neurology 18:95–98, 1968.

Meadows JC. The anatomical basis of prosopagnosia. Journal of Neurology, Neurosurgery, and Psychiatry 37:489–501, 1974.

Mehler MF. Mixed transcortical aphasia in nonfamilial dysphasic dementia. Cortex 24:545–554, 1988.

Mendez MF, Benson DF. Atypical conduction aphasia: A disconnection syndrome. Archives of Neurology 42:886–891, 1985.

Mendez MF, Zander BA. Dementia presenting with aphasia: Clinical characteristics. Journal of Neurology, Neurosurgery, and Psychiatry 54:542–545, 1991.

Menn L, Obler LK. Agrammatic Aphasia: A Cross-Language Narrative Sourcebook. Amsterdam: John Benjamins, 1990.

Merleau-Ponty M. Signs. Evanston, IL: Northwestern University Press, 1964.

Mesulam M-M. A cortical network for directed attention and unilateral neglect. Annals of Neurology 10:309–325, 1981.

Mesulam M-M. Slowly progressive aphasia without generalized dementia. Annals of Neurology 11:592–598, 1982.

Mesulam M-M. Attention, confusional states and neglect. In Mesulam M-M (ed), Principles of Behavioral Neurology. Philadelphia: Davis, 1985, pp 125–168.

Mesulam M-M. Primary progressive aphasia: Differentation from Alzheimer's disease. Annals of Neurology 22:533–534, 1987.

Mesulam M-M. Large scale neurocognitive networks and distributed processing for attention, language and memory. Annals of Neurology 28:597–613, 1990.

Metter EJ. Speech Disorders. New York: Spectrum, 1985.

Metter EJ, Hanson WR, Jackson CA, Kempler D, Van Lancker D, Mazziotta J, Phelps ME. Temporoparietal cortex in aphasia. Archives of Neurology 47:1235–1238, 1990.

Metter EJ, Riege WH, Hanson WR, Canras LR, Phelps ME, Kuhl DE. Correlation of glucose metabolism and structural damage to language function in aphasia. Brain and Language 23:187–207, 1984.

Metter EJ, Riege WH, Hanson WR, Jackson CA, Kempler D, Van Lancker D. Subcortical structures in aphasia: An analysis based on (F-18)-fluorodeoxyglucose positron emission tomography and computed tomography. Archives of Neurology 45:1229–1235, 1988.

Metter EJ, Wasterlain CG, Kuhl DE, Hanson WR, Phelps ME. 18-FDG positron emission computed tomography in a study of aphasia. Annals of Neurology 10:173–183, 1981.

Metz-Lutz M-N, Dahl E. Analysis of word comprehension in a case of pure word deafness. Brain and Language 23:12–28, 1984.

Meyer JS, Sakai F, Nautenu H, Grant P. Normal and abnormal patterns of cerebrovascular reserve tested by 133 Xe inhalation. Archives of Neurology 35:350–359, 1978.

Miceli G, Silveri MC, Villa G, Caramazza A. On the basis for the agrammatic's difficulty in producing main verbs. Cortex 20:207–220, 1984.

Miller GA, Galanter E, Pribram KL. Plans and the Structure of Behavior. New York: Holt, Rinehart and Winston, 1960.

Miller GA, Johnson-Laird PN. Language and Perception. Cambridge, MA: Belknap Press, 1976.

Milner B. Some effects of frontal lobectomy in man. In JM Warren, K Akert (eds), The Frontal Granular Cortex and Behavior. New York: McGraw-Hill, 1964, pp 313–334.

Milner B. Hemispheric specialization: Scope and limits. In FO Schmitt, FG Worden (eds), The Neurosciences Third Study Program. Cambridge, MA: MIT Press, 1974, pp 75–89.

Milner B, Teuber HL. Alteration of perception and memory in man. In L Weiskrantz (ed), Analysis of Behavioral Change. New York: Harper and Row, 1968, pp 268–375.

Modolfsky H. Occupational cramp. Journal of Psychosomatic Research 15:439–444, 1971.

Mohr JP. Rapid amelioration of motor aphasia. Archives of Neurology 28:77–82, 1973.

Mohr JP. Thalamic lesions and syndromes. In A Kertesz (ed), Localization in Neuropsychology. New York: Academic Press, 1983, pp 269–293.

Mohr JP, Pessin MS, Finkelstein S, Funkenstein HH, Duncan GW, Davis KR. Broca's aphasia: Pathologic and clinical aspects. Neurology 28:311–324, 1978.

Mohr JP, Watters WC, Duncan GW. Thalamic hemorrhage and aphasia. Brain and Language 2:3–17, 1975.

Mohs RC, Rosen WG, Greenwald BG, Davis KL. Neuropathologically validated scales for Alzheimer's disease. In T Crook, S Ferris, R Bartus (eds), Assessment in Geriatric Psychopharmacology. New Canaan, CT: Mark Powley, 1983, pp 37–48.

von Monakow C. Die Lokalisation im Grosshirn. Wiesbaden, Germany: Bergmann, 1914.

von Monakow C, Mourque R. Introduction Biologique a l'Étude de la Neurologie et de la Psychiatrie. Paris: Alcan, 1928.

Monrad-Krohn GH. Dysprosody or altered melody of language. Brain 70:405–415, 1947.

Mori E, Yamadori A, Furumoto M. Left precentral gyrus and Broca's aphasia: A clinico-pathological study. Neurology 39:51–54, 1989.

Morton J, Patterson K. A new attempt of an interpretation, or, an attempt at a new interpretation. In M Coltheart, K Patterson, J Marshall (eds), Deep Dyslexia. London: Routledge and Kegan Paul, 1980, pp 91–118.

Motomura N, Yamadori A, Mitani Y. Left thalamic infarction and disturbance of verbal memory: A clinicoanatomical study with a new method of computed tomographic stereotaxic lesion localization. Annals of Neurology 20:671–676, 1986.

Moutier F. L'Aphasie de Broca. Doctoral dissertation, Paris, 1908.

Moyer SB. Rehabilitation of alexia: A case study. Cortex 15: 139–144, 1979.

Murdoch BE. Language disorders in dementia and aphasia syndromes. Aphasiology 2:181–186, 1988.

Murdoch BE, Chenery HJ, Wilks V, Boyle RS. Language disorders in dementia of the Alzheimer type. Brain and Language 31:122–137, 1987.

Nadeau SE. Impaired grammar with normal fluency and phonology: Implications for Broca's aphasia. Brain 111:1111–1137, 1988.

Naeser MA. CT scan lesion size and lesion locus in cortical and subcortical aphasias. In A Kertesz (ed), Localization in Neuropsychology. New York: Academic Press, 1983, pp 63–120.

Naeser MA, Alexander MP, Helm-Estabrooks N, Levine H, Laughlin SA, Geschwind N. Aphasia with predominantly subcortical lesion sites. Archives of Neurology 39:2–14, 1982.

Naeser MA, Hayward RW. Lesion localization in aphasia with cranial computed tomography and the Boston Diagnostic Aphasia Examination. Neurology 28:545–551, 1978.

Naeser MA, Mazurski P, Goodglass H, Peraino M, Laughlin S, Leaper WC. Auditory syntactic comprehension in nine aphasia groups (with CT scan) and children: Differences in degree but not order of difficulty observed. Cortex 23:259–280, 1987.

Naeser MA, Palumbo CL, Helm-Estabrooks N, Stiassny-Eder D, Albert ML. Severe non-fluency in aphasia: Role of the medial subcallosal fasciculus plus other white matter pathways in recovery of spontaneous language. Brain 112:1–38, 1989.

Nauta WJH, Feirtag M. Fundamental Neuroanatomy. New York: Freeman, 1986.

Neumann MA, Cohn R. Incidence of Alzheimer's disease in a large mental hospital. Archives of Neurology and Psychiatry 69:615–636, 1953.

Newcombe F, Marshall JC. Transcoding and lexical stabilization in deep dyslexia. In M Coltheart, K Patterson, JC Marshall (eds), Deep Dyslexia. London: Routledge and Kegan Paul, 1980, pp 176–188.

Newell A, Simon HA. Human Problem Solving. Englewood Cliffs, NJ: Prentice-Hall, 1972.

Nielsen JM. Agnosia, Apraxia and Aphasia: Their Value in Cerebral Localization. New York: Hafner, 1936.

Nielsen JM. The unsolved problems in aphasia. I: Alexia in "motor" aphasia. Bulletin of the Los Angeles Neurological Society 4:114–122, 1938.

Nielsen JM. The unsolved problems in aphasia. II: Alexia resulting from a temporal lesion. Bulletin of the Los Angeles Neurological Society 5:78–84, 1939.

Nielsen JM. The unsolved problems in aphasia. III: Amnesic aphasia. Bulletin of the Los Angeles Neurological Society 5: 78–84, 1940.

Nielsen JM, Friedman AP. The quadrilateral space of Marie. Bulletin of the Los Angeles Neurological Society 7:131–136, 1942.

Nielsen JM, Raney RB. Symptoms following surgical removal of major (left) angular gyrus. Bulletin of the Los Angeles Neurological Society 3:42–46, 1938.

Niemi J, Koivuselka-Sallinen P, Laine M. Lexical deformations are sensitive to morphosyntactic factors in posterior aphasia. Aphasiology 1:53–57, 1987.

Nilipour R, Ashayeri H. Alternating antagonism between two languages with successive recovery of a third in a trilingual patient. Brain and Language 36:23–48, 1989.

Northen B, Hopcutt B, Griffiths H. Progressive aphasia without dementia. Aphasiology 4:55–66, 1990.

Obler LK, Albert ML. Influence of aging on recovery from aphasia in polyglots. Brain and Language 4:460–463, 1977.

Obler LK, Albert ML. Language and aging: A neurobiological analysis. In DS Beasley, GA Davis (eds), Aging: Communication Processes and Disorders. New York: Grune and Stratton, 1981, pp 107–121.

Ogle JW. Aphasia and agraphia in St. George's Hospital. Report of the Medical Research Counsel of St. George's Hospital (London) 2:83–122, 1867.

Ojemann GA. Object naming and recall during and after thalamic stimulation. Brain and Language 2:101–120, 1975.

Ojemann GA. Subcortical language mechanisms. In H Whitaker, HA Whitaker (eds), Studies in Neurolinguistics, Vol 1. New York: Academic Press, 1976, pp 103–138.

Ojemann GA. Brain organization for language from the perspective of electrical stimulation mapping. Behavioral and Brain Sciences 6:189–230, 1983.

Ojemann G, Ward A. Speech representation in ventrolateral thalamus. Brain 94:669–680, 1971.

Oldendorf WH. The Quest for an Image of the Brain. New York: Raven, 1980.

Olmos-Lau N, Ginsberg MD, Geller JB. Aphasia in multiple sclerosis. Neurology 27:623–626, 1977.

Orenstein R. The Psychology of Consciousness. New York: Freeman, 1972.

Orgass B, Hartje W, Kerschensteiner M, Poeck K. Aphasie und nachtsprachliche intelligenz. Nervenarzt 43:623–627, 1972.

Ostrosky-Solis F, Quintanar L, Madrazo I, Drucker-Colin R, Franco R, Leon-Meza V. Neuropsychological effects of brain autograft of adrenal medullary tissue for the treatment of Parkinson's disease. Neurology 38:1442–1450, 1988.

Owens NA. Age and mental abilities: A longitudinal study. Genetic Psychology Monographs 48:3–54, 1953.

Ozanne AE, Murdoch BE. Acquired childhood aphasia: Neuropathology, linguistic characteristics and prognosis. In BE Murdoch (ed), Acquired Neurological Speech/Language Disorders in Childhood. London: Taylor and Francis, 1990, pp 1–65.

Pandya DN, Vignolo LA. Intra- and interhemispheric projections of the precentral, premotor and arcuate areas in the rhesus monkey. Brain Research 26:217–233, 1971.

Panse F, Shimoyama T. Zur Auswirkung Aphasischer Störungen in Japanischen. Archiv für Psychiatrie 193:139–145, 1955.

Papagno C. A case of peripheral dysgraphia. Cognitive Neuropsychology 9:259–270, 1992.

Papanicolaou AC, Moore BD, Deutsch G, Levin HS, Eisenberg HM. Evidence for right-hemisphere involvement in recovery from aphasia. Archives of Neurology 45:1025–1029, 1988.

Paradis M. Bilingualism and aphasia. In H Whitaker, HA Whitaker (eds), Studies in Neurolinguistics, Vol 3. New York: Academic Press, 1977, pp 65–121.

Paradis M. The Assessment of Bilingual Aphasia. Hillsdale, NJ: Lawrence Erlbaum Associates, 1987.

Paradis M. Language lateralization in bilinguals: Enough already! Brain and Language 39:576–586, 1990.

Paradis M. Bilingual aphasia rehabilitation. In M Paradis (ed), Foundations of Aphasia. Oxford: Pergamon Press, 1993, pp 413–419.

Pashek GV, Holland AL. Evolution of aphasia in the first year post onset. Cortex 24:411–423, 1988.

Patterson KE. Phonemic dyslexia: Errors of meaning and the meaning of errors. Quarterly Journal of Experimental Psychology 30:587–601, 1978.

Patterson KE. The relation between reading and phonological coding: Further neuropsychological observations. In AW Ellis (ed), Normality and Pathology in Cognitive Functions. London: Academic Press, 1982, pp 77–111.

Patterson KE, Kay J. Letter-by-letter reading: Psychological description of a neurological syndrome. Quarterly Journal of Experimental Psychology 34A:411–441, 1982.

Patterson KE, Morton J. From orthography to phonology: An attempt at an old interpretation. In KE Patterson, JC Marshall, M Coltheart (eds), Surface Dyslexia. London: Lawrence Erlbaum Associates, 1985, pp 335–359.

Patterson KE, Wilson B. A ROSE is a ROSE or a NOSE: A deficit in initial letter identification. Cognitive Neuropsychology 7:447–477, 1992.

Payne M, Cooper WE. Paralexic errors in Broca's and Wernicke's aphasia. Neuropsychologia 23:571–574, 1985.

Penfield W, Boldrey E. Somatic motor and sensory representation in the cerebral cortex as studied by electrical stimulation. Brain 60:389–443, 1937.

Penfield W, Roberts L. Speech and Brain Mechanisms. Princeton, NJ: Princeton University Press, 1959.

Penn C. Compensation and language recovery in the chronic aphasic patient. Aphasiology 1:235–245, 1987.

Peterson SE, Fox PT, Posner MI, Mintum M, Raichle ME. Positron emission tomographic studies of the cortical anatomy of single word processing. Nature 331:585–589, 1988.

Phelps ME, Huang SC, Hoffman EJ, Selin C, Sokoloff L, Kuhl DE. Tomographic measurement of local cerebral glucose metabolism in humans with (F-18) 2-Fluoro-2-Deoxy-D-glucose: Validation of method. Annals of Neurology 6:371–388, 1979.

Pick A. Die Agrammatischen Sprachstorungen. Berlin: Springer, 1913.

Pick A. Aphasia. Springfield, IL: Charles C. Thomas, 1931/1973.

Piercy M. The effects of cerebral lesions on intellectual function. British Journal of Psychiatry 110:310–352, 1964.

Pillon B, Bakchine S, Lhermitte F. Alexia without agraphia in a left-handed patient with a right occipital lesion. Archives of Neurology 44:1257–1262, 1987.

Pineda D, Ardila A. Lasting mutism associated with buccofacial apraxia. Aphasiology 6:285–292, 1992.

Pitres A. Etude sur l'aphasie chez les polyglottes. Revue Médicin 15:873–899, 1895.

Pizzamiglio L, Mammucari A. Evidence for sex differences in brain organization in recovery in aphasia. Brain and Language 25:313–323, 1985.

Plum F. Dementia: An approaching epidemic. Nature 279:372–373, 1979.

Plum F, Posner JB. Stupor and Coma, 3d Ed. Philadelphia: Davis, 1982.

Poeck K. Stimmung und Krankheitseinsicht bei Aphasien. Archiv für Psychiatrie und Nervenkrankheiten 216:246–254, 1972.

Poeck K, Kerschensteiner M. Analysis of the sequential motor events in oral apraxia. In K Zulch, O Kreutzfeldt, G Gallbraith (eds), Otfried Foerster Symposium. Berlin: Springer, 1975, pp 98–109.

Poeck K, Kerschensteiner M, Hartje W. A qualitative study on language understanding in fluent and non-fluent aphasia. Cortex 8:299–304, 1972.

Poeck K, Luzzatti C. Slowly progressive aphasia in three patients. Brain 111:151–168, 1988.

Poeck K, Orgass B. Gerstmann's syndrome and aphasia. Cortex 2:421–437, 1966.

Poeck K, Orgass B. An experimental investigation of finger agnosia. Neurology 19:501–507, 1969.

Pool JL, Correll JW. Psychiatric symptoms masking brain tumor. Journal of the Medical Society of New Jersey 33:4–9, 1958.

Popper KR, Eccles JC. The Self and Its Brain. New York: Springer, 1977.

Porch B. Porch Index of Communicative Ability. Palo Alto, CA: Consulting Psychologists, 1967.

Powell AL, Cummings JL, Hill MA, Benson DF. Speech and language alterations in multi-infarct dementia. Neurology 38:717–719, 1988.

Premack O. Language in the chimpanzee. Science 172:808–822, 1971.

Price CJ, Humphreys GW. Letter by letter reading? Functional deficits and compensatory strategies. Cognitive Neuropsychology 9:427–457, 1992.

Pring T. Evaluating the effects of speech therapy in aphasics: Developing the single-case methodology. British Journal of Disorders of Communication 21:103–115, 1986.

Prins RS, Snow CE, Wagenaar E. Recovery from aphasia: Spontaneous language versus language comprehension. Brain and Language 6:192–211, 1978.

Puel M, Cordebat D, Demonet JF, Elghozi D, Cambier J, Guiraud-Chaumeil B, Rascol A. La rôle du thalamus dans les aphasies sous-corticales. Revue Neurologique 142:431–440, 1986.

Quadfasel FA. Aspects of the life and work of Kurt Goldstein. Cortex 4:113–124, 1968.

Rao SM. Neuropsychology of multiple sclerosis. Journal of Clinical and Experimental Psychology 8:503–542, 1986.

Rapcsak SZ, Arthur SA, Rubens AB. Lexical agraphia from focal lesion of the left precentral gyrus. Neurology 38:1119–1123, 1988.

Rapcsak SZ, Gonzalez-Rothi L, Heilman KM. Phonological alexia with optic and tactile anomia: A neuropsychological and anatomical study. Brain and Language 31:109–121, 1987.

Rapin I, Allen DA. Developmental language disorders: Nosologic considerations. In V Kirk (ed), Neuropsychology of Language, Reading and Spelling. New York: Academic Press, 1983, pp 155–184.

Rapin I, Allen DA. Communication disorders of early childhood: Attempts at classification. In I Fleshmig, L Stern (eds), Child Development and Learning Behavior. New York: Gustav Fischer-Verlag, 1986, pp 255–263.

Rapp BC, Caramazza A. Spatially determined deficits in letter and word processing. Cognitive Neuropsychology 7:653–689, 1990.

Rasmussen T, Milner B. The role of early brain injury in determining lateralization of cerebral speech functions. Annals of the New York Academy of Sciences 299:355–369, 1977.

Rausch HR. Differences in cognitive function with left and right temporal lobe dysfunction. In DF Benson, E Zaidel (eds), The Dual Brain: Hemispheric Specialization in Humans. New York: Guilford Press, 1985, pp 247–261.

Reed GF. Elective mutism in children: A re-appraisal. Journal of Child Psychology and Psychiatry 4:99–107, 1963.

Regard M, Landis T, Hess K. Preserved stenography reading in a patient with pure alexia. Archives of Neurology 42:400–402, 1985.

Reitan RM, Wolfson D. Halstead-Reitan Neuropsychological Test Battery. Tucson, AZ: Neuropsychology Press, 1985.

Reuter-Lorenz PA, Brunn JL. A prelexical basis for letter-by-letter reading: A case study. Cognitive Neuropsychology 7:1–20, 1990.

Rey GJ, Levin BE, Rodas R, Bowen BC, Nedd K. A longitudinal examination of crossed aphasia. Archives of Neurology 51:95–100, 1994.

Ribaucourt-Ducarne B. Rééducation Sémiologie de l'Aphasie. Paris: Masson, 1986.

Ribot T. Les Maladies de la Mémoire. Paris: Libraire Germer Bailliere, 1883.

Riddoch MJ. Neglect and the peripheral dyslexias. Cognitive Neuropsychology 7:369–389, 1990.

Riddoch MJ, Humphreys GW, Cleton P, Fery P. Interaction of attentional and lexical processes in neglect dyslexia. Cognitive Neuropsychology 7:479–517, 1990.

Riklan M, Cooper IS. Psychometric studies of verbal functions following thalamic lesions in humans. Brain and Language 2:62–73, 1975.

Riklan M, Levita E. Psychological studies of thalamic lesions in humans. Journal of Nervous Mental Disease 150:251–265, 1970.

Ring BA, Waddington MM. Occlusion of small intracranial arteries as a cause of stroke. JAMA 204:303–305, 1968.

Robertson I. Does computerized cognitive rehabilitation work? Aphasiology 4:371–380, 1990.

Robinson RG, Benson DF. Depression in aphasic patients: Frequency, severity, and clinical-pathological correlations. Brain and Language 14:282–291, 1981.

Robinson RG, Chait RM. Emotional correlates of structural brain injury with particular emphasis on post-stroke mood disorders. CRC Critical Review of Clinical Neurobiology 4:285–318, 1985.

Robinson RG, Price TR. Post-stroke depressive disorders: A follow-up study of 103 outpatients. Stroke 13:635–641, 1982.

Robinson RG, Shoemaker WJ, Schlumpf M, Valk T, Bloom FE. Effect of cerebral infarction in rat brain: Effect on catechomalines and behavior. Nature 255:332–334, 1975.

Robinson RG, Szetela B. Mood changes following left hemispheric brain injury. Annals of Neurology 9:447–453, 1981.

Roeltgen D. The neurolinguistics of writing: Anatomy and neurologic correlates. Paper presented at the International Neuropsychological Society, Mexico City, February 1983.

Roeltgen D. Agraphia. In KM Heilman, E Valenstein (eds), Clinical Neuropsychology, 2d Ed. New York: Oxford University Press, 1985, pp 75–96.

Roeltgen DP. Agraphia. In KM Heilman, E Valenstein (eds), Clinical Neuropsychology, 2d Ed. New York: Oxford University Press, 1993: 63–89.

Roeltgen D, Heilman KM. Apractic agraphia in a patient with normal praxis. Brain and Language 18:35–46, 1983.

Roeltgen D, Heilman KM. Lexical agraphia. Brain 107:811–827, 1984.

Roeltgen D, Sevush S, Heilman KM. Phonological agraphia, writing by the lexical-semantic route. Neurology 33:755–765, 1983.

Romanul FCA. Examination of the brain and spinal cord. In CG Tedeschi (ed), Neuropathology. Boston: Little, Brown, 1970, pp 131–214.

Romanul FCA, Abramowitz A. Changes in brain and pial vessels in arterial borderzones. Archives of Neurology 11:40–49, 1961.

Rose FC, Symonds CP. Persistent memory defect following encephalitis. Brain 83 (Pt 2):195–212, 1960.

Rosenbek JC, Kent DR, LaPointe LL. Apraxia of speech: An overview and some perspectives. In JC Rosenbek, MR McNeil, AE Aronson (eds), Apraxia of Speech. San Diego: College-Hill Press, 1989, pp 1–28.

Rosenbek JC, Lemme ML, Ahern MB, Harris EH, Wertz RT. A treatment of apraxia of speech in adults. Journal of Speech and Hearing Disorders 38:462–473, 1973.

Rosenbek J, Messert B, Collins M, Wertz RT. Stuttering following brain damage. Brain and Language 6:82–96, 1978.

Rosenfield DB. Stuttering. CRC Critical Review of Clinical Neurobiology 1:117–139, 1984.

Rosenfield DB, Goree JA. Angiographic localization of aphasia. Neurology 25:349, 1975 (Abstract).

Ross ED. The aprosodias: Functional-anatomic organization of the affective components of language in the right hemisphere. Archives of Neurology 38:561–569, 1981.

Ross ED, Mesulam M-M. Dominant language functions of the right hemisphere? Prosody and emotional gesturing. Archives of Neurology 36:144–148, 1979.

Rosselli D, Rosselli M, Penagos B, Ardila A. Huntington's disease in Colombia: A neuropsychological analysis. International Journal of Neuroscience 32:933–942, 1987.

Rosselli M, Ardila A. Calculation deficits in patients with right and left hemisphere damage. Neuropsychologia 27:607–617, 1989.

Rosselli M, Ardila A, Florez A, Castro C. Normative data on the Boston Diagnostic Aphasia Examination in a Spanish speaking population. Journal of Clinical and Experimental Neuropsychology 12:313–322, 1990.

Rosselli M, Ardila A, Rosas P. Neuropsychological assessment in illiterates. II: Language and praxic abilities. Brain and Cognition 12:281–296, 1990.

Rothi LJ, Heilman KM. Transcortical motor aphasia and syntactic comprehension. Paper presented at the 18th Annual Meeting of the Academy of Aphasia, South Yarmouth, MA, October, 1980.

Rothi LJ, McFarling D, Heilman KM. Conduction aphasia, syntactic alexia, and the anatomy of syntactic comprehension. Archives of Neurology 39:272–275, 1982.

Rubens AB. Aphasia with infarction in the territory of the anterior cerebral artery. Cortex 11:239–250, 1975.

Rubens AB. Transcortical motor aphasia. In H Whitaker, HA Whitaker (eds), Studies in Neurolinguistics, Vol 1. New York: Academic Press, 1976, pp 293–304.

Rubens AB. The role of changes within the central nervous system during recovery from aphasia. In M Sullivan, MS Kommers (eds), Rationale for Adult Aphasia Therapy. Lincoln: University of Nebraska Press, 1977, pp 28–43.

Rubens AB, Benson DF. Associative visual agnosia. Archives of Neurology 24:305–315, 1971.

Rubens AB, Kertesz A. The localizations of lesions in transcortical aphasias. In A Kertesz (ed), Localization in Neuropsychology. New York: Academic Press, 1983, pp 245–268.

Ruch F. The differentiative effects of age upon human learning. Journal of Genetic Psychology 11:261–286, 1934.

Russell WR. The neurology of brain wounds. British Journal of Surgery (War Surgery Supplement) 1:250–252, 1947.

Russell WR, Espir MLE. Traumatic Aphasia: A Study of Aphasia in War Wounds of the Brain. London: Oxford University Press, 1961.

Ryalls J, Valdois S, Lecours AR. Paraphasia and jargon. In F Boller, J Grafman, G Rizzolatti, H Goodglass (eds), Handbook of Neuropsychology, Vol 1. Amsterdam: Elsevier, 1988, pp 367–376.

Saffran EM, Marin OSM. Reading without phonology: Evidence from aphasia. Quarterly Journal of Experimental Psychology 29:515–525, 1977.

Sak K, Larsen B, Skinhøj E, Lassen NA. Regional cerebral blood flow in aphasia. Archives of Neurology 35:625–632, 1978.

Salfield DJ. Observations on elective mutism in children. Journal of Mental Science 96:1024–1032, 1950.

Salthouse T, Somberg B. Isolating the age deficit in speeded performance. Journal of Gerontology 37:59–63, 1982.

Samarel A, Wright TL, Sergay S, Tyler HR. Thalamic hemorrhage with speech disorder. Transactions of the American Neurological Association 101:283–285, 1976.

Sampson G. Writing Systems. Stanford, CA: Stanford University Press, 1985.

Samra K, Riklan M, Levita E, Zimmerman J, Waltz JM, Bergmann L, Cooper IS. Language and speech correlates of anatomically verified lesions in thalamic surgery for Parkinsonism. Journal of Speech and Hearing Research 12:510–540, 1969.

Samuels JA, Benson DF. Some aspects of language comprehension in aphasia. Brain and Language 8:275–286, 1979.

Sands E, Sarno MT, Shankweiler D. Long-term assessment of language function in aphasia due to stroke. Archives of Physical Medicine and Rehabilitation 50:203–207, 1969.

Sapin LR, Anderson FH, Pulaski PD. Progressive aphasia without dementia: Further documentation. Annals of Neurology 25:411–413, 1989.

Sarno J. Emotional aspects of aphasia. In MT Sarno (ed), Acquired Aphasia. New York: Academic Press, 1981, pp 465–483.

Sarno JE, Swisher LP, Sarno MT. Aphasia in a congenitally deaf man. Cortex 5:398–414, 1969.

Sarno MT. The Communication Profile: Manual of Directions. New York: University Medical Center, 1969.

Sarno MT. The nature of verbal impairment after closed head injury. Journal of Nervous and Mental Disease 168:685–692, 1980.

Sarno MT. Recovery and rehabilitation in aphasia. In MT Sarno (ed), Acquired Aphasia. New York: Academic Press, 1981, pp 485–529.

Sarno MT, Levita E. Natural course of recovery in severe aphasia. Archives of Physical Medicine and Rehabilitation 52:175–178, 1971.

Sarno MT, Sands E. An objective method for the evaluation of speech therapy in aphasia. Archives of Physical Medicine and Rehabilitation 52:49–54, 1970.

Sarno MT, Silverman M, Sands E. Speech therapy and language recovery in severe aphasia. Journal of Speech and Hearing Research 13:607–623, 1970.

Sasanuma S. Kana and Kanji Processing in Japanese aphasics. Brain and Language 2:369–383, 1975.

Sasanuma S, Fujimura O. Kanji versus Kana processing in alexia with transient agraphia: A case report. Cortex 7:1–18, 1971.

Satz P, Bullard-Bates C. Acquired aphasia in children. In MT Sarno (ed), Acquired Aphasia. New York: Academic Press, 1981, pp 399–426.

Saunders AM, Strittmatter WJ, Schmechel D, St. George-Hyslop PH, Pericak-Vance MA, Joo SH, Rosi BL, Gusella JF, Crapper-MacLachlan DR, Alberts MJ, Hulette C, Crain B, Goldgaber D, Roses AD. Association of apolipoprotein E allele e4 with late-onset familial and sporadic Alzheimer's disease. Neurology 43:1467–1472, 1993.

Schiff HB, Alexander MP, Naeser MA, Galaburda AM. Aphemia. Archives of Neurology 40:720–727, 1983.

Schilder P. Fingeragnosie, fingerapraxie, fingeraphasie. Nervenarzt 4:625–629, 1931.

Schilder P. Psyche Monographs, No. 4: The Image and Appearance of the Human Body: Studies in Constructive Energies of the Psyche. London: Kegan Paul, Trench, Trulner, 1935.

Schiller F. Aphasia studied in patients with missile wounds. Journal of Neurology, Neurosurgery, and Psychiatry 10:183–197, 1947.

Schneider G. Is it really better to have your brain damage early? A revision of the "Kennard Principle." Neuropsychologia 17:557–583, 1979.

Schnider A, Benson DF, Alexander DN, Schnider-Klaus A. Non-verbal environmental sound recognition after unilateral hemispheric stroke. Brain 117:281–287, 1994.

Schuell H. Minnesota Test for the Differential Diagnosis of Aphasia. Minneapolis: University of Minnesota Press, 1955.

Schuell H. A short examination for aphasia. Neurology 7:625–634, 1957.

Schuell H. Differential Diagnosis of Aphasia with the Minnesota Test. Minneapolis: University of Minnesota Press, 1965.

Schuell H. Differential Diagnosis of Aphasia with the Minnesota Test, 2d Ed. Minneapolis: University of Minnesota Press, 1973.

Schuell H, Jenkins JJ, Carroll JB. A factor analysis of the Minnesota Test for the Differential Diagnosis of Aphasia. Journal of Speech and Hearing Research 5:350–369, 1962.

Schuell H, Jenkins JJ, Jimenez-Pabon E. Aphasia in Adults. New York: Harper and Row (Hoeber Medical Division), 1964a.

Schvartzman P, Hornshtein I, Klein E, Yechezkel A, Ziv M, Herman J. Elective mutism in family practice. The Journal of Family Practice 31:319–320, 1990.

Schwab O. Ueber vorubergehende aphasische storungen nach Rindenexzision aus dem linken stirnhirn bei Epileptikern. Deutsche Zeitschrift für Nervenheilkunde 94:177–184, 1926.

Schwartz MF. What the classical aphasia categories can't do for us, and why. Brain and Language 21:3–8, 1984.

Schwartz MF, Linebarger MC, Saffran EM. The status of the syntactic deficit theory of agrammatism. In ML Kean (ed), Agrammatism. New York: Academic Press, 1985, pp 83–124.

Schwartz MF, Saffran EM, Marin OS. The word order problem in agrammatism: Comprehension. Brain and Language 10:249–262, 1980.

Segalowitz SJ, Bryden MP. Individual differences in hemispheric representation of language. In SJ Segalowitz (ed), Language Functions and Brain Organization. New York: Academic Press, 1983, pp 341–372.

Segarra JM. Cerebral vascular disease and behavior. Archives of Neurology 22:408–418, 1970.

Seltzer B, Sherwin I. A comparison of clinical features in early and late onset primary degenerative dementia. Archives of Neurology 40:143–146, 1983.

Semmes J. Hemispheric specialization: A possible clue to mechanism. Neuropsychologia 6:11–26, 1968.

Seron X, Deloche G. The production of counting sequences by aphasics and children: A matter of lexical processing. In G Deloche, X Seron (eds), Mathematical Disabilities: A Cognitive Neuropsychological Perspective, Hillsdale, NJ: Lawrence Erlbaum Associates, 1987, pp 171–200.

Seron X, Deloche G, Moulard G, Rouselle M. A computer-based therapy for the treatment of aphasic subjects with writing disorders. Journal of Speech and Hearing Disorders 45:45–58, 1980.

Shalev RS, Weirtman R, Amir N. Developmental dyscalculia. Cortex 24:555–562, 1988.

Shallice T. Phonological agraphia and lexical route in writing. Brain 104:412–429, 1981.

Shallice T. From Neuropsychology to Mental Structure. New York: Cambridge University Press, 1988.

Shallice T, Saffran EM. Lexical processing in the absence of explicit word identification: Evidence from a letter-by-letter reader. Cognitive Neuropsychology 3:429–458, 1986.

Shallice T, Warrington EK. The possible role of selective attention in acquired dyslexia. Neuropsychologia 15:31–42, 1977.

Shallice T, Warrington EK. Single and multiple component central dyslexia syndrome. In

M Coltheart, KE Patterson, JC Marshall (eds), Deep Dyslexia. London: Routledge and Kegan Paul, 1980, pp 109–145.

Shallice T, Warrington EK, McCarthy R. Reading without semantics. Quarterly Journal of Experimental Psychology 35A:111–138, 1983.

Sheehy MP, Marsden CD. Writer's cramp: A focal dystonia. Brain 105:461–480, 1982.

Shewan CM. The Shewan Spontaneous Language Analysis (SSLA) system for aphasic adult: Description, reliability and validity. Journal of Communication Disorders 21:103–138, 1988.

Shewan CM, Bandur DL. Treatment of Aphasia: A Language Oriented Approach. Boston: College-Hill, 1986.

Shewan CM, Kertesz A. Effects of speech and language treatment on recovery from aphasia. Brain and Language 23:272–299, 1984.

Shuttleworth EC, Huber SJ. A longitudinal study of the naming disorders of dementia of the Alzheimer type. Neuropsychiatry, Neuropsychology, and Behavioral Neurology 4:267–282, 1988.

Shuttleworth EC, Yates AC, Paltan-Ortiz JD. Creutzfeldt-Jakob disease presenting as progressive aphasia. Journal of the National Medical Association 77:649–650, 1985.

Simernitskaya EG. On two forms of writing defect following local brain lesions. In SJ Dimond, JG Beaumont (eds), Hemispheric Function in the Human Brain. London: Elek Science, 1974, pp 335–344.

Simmons NN. Conduction aphasia. In LL LaPointe (ed), Aphasia and Related Neurogenic Language Disorders. New York: Thieme, 1990, pp 54–77.

Singer HD, Low AA. Acalculia: A clinical study. Archives of Neurology and Psychiatry 29:467–498, 1933.

Skelly M, Schinsky L, Smith RW, Fust RS. American Indian sign (Amerind) as a facilitator of verbalization for the oral verbal apraxic. Journal of Speech and Hearing Disorders 39:445–456, 1974.

Skelton MR, Jones S. Nominal dysphasia and the severity of senile dementia. British Journal of Psychiatry 145:168–171, 1984.

Sklar M. Sklar Aphasia Scale. Los Angeles: Western Psychological Services, 1966.

Skyhøj-Olsen T, Bruhn P, Obert RGW. Cortical hypoperfusion as a possible cause of subcortical aphasia. Brain 109:393–410, 1986.

Slande PD, Russell GFM. Developmental dyscalculia: A brief report of four cases. Psychological Medicine 1:292–298, 1971.

Smith A. Speech and other functions after left dominant hemispherectomy. Journal of Neurology, Neurosurgery, and Psychiatry 29:467–471, 1966.

Smith A. Diagnosis, Intelligence and Rehabilitation of Chronic Aphasics: Final Report. Ann Arbor: University of Michigan Press, 1972.

Smith A, Sugar O. Development of above-normal language and intelligence 21 years after left hemispherectomy. Neurology 25:813–818, 1975.

Smith AM, Bourbonnais D, Blanchette G. Interactions between forced grasping and a learned precision grip after ablation of the supplementary motor area. Brain Research 222:395–400, 1981.

Smith SR, Chenery HJ, Murdoch BE. Semantic abilities in dementia of the Alzheimer type. II. Grammatical semantics. Brain and Language 36:533–542, 1989.

Smyth V, Ozanne AE, Woodhouse LM. Communicative disorders in childhood infectious diseases. In BE Murdoch (ed), Acquired Neurological Speech/Language Disorders in Childhood. London: Taylor and Francis, 1990, pp 148–176.

Snowden JS, Neary D, Mann DMA, Goulding PJ, Testa HJ. Progressive language disorder due to lobar atrophy. Annals of Neurology 31:174–183, 1992.

Soh K, Larsen B, Skinhøj E, Lassen NA. Regional cerebral blood flow in aphasia. Archives of Neurology 35:625–632, 1978.

Sommers LM, Pierce RS. Naming and semantic judgements in dementia of the Alzheimer type. Aphasiology 4:573–587, 1990.

Souques A. Quelques cas d'anarthrie de Pierre Marie. Revue Neurologique 2:319–368, 1928.

Sparks R, Helm N, Albert M. Aphasia rehabilitation resulting from melodic intonation therapy. Cortex 10:303–316, 1974.

Speedie L, O'Donnell W, Rabins P, Pearlson G, Poggi M, Rothi L. Language performance deficits in elderly depressed patients. Aphasiology 4:197–206, 1990.

Spellacy FJ, Spreen O. A short form of the Token Test. Cortex 5:390–397, 1969.

Sperry RW. Consciousness, personal identity and the divided brain. In DF Benson, E Zaidel (eds), The Dual Brain: Hemispheric Specialization in Humans. New York: Guilford Press, 1985, pp 11–26.

Spiers PA. Acalculia revisited: Current issues. In G Deloche, X Seron (eds), Mathematical Disabilities: A Cognitive Neuropsychological Perspective. Hillsdale, NJ: Lawrence Erlbaum Associates, 1987, pp 1–25.

Spreen O, Benton AL. Neurosensory Center Comprehensive Examination for Aphasia. Victoria, BC: Neuropsychology Laboratory, University of Victoria, 1969.

Spreen O, Benton AL. Neurosensory Center Comprehensive Examination for Aphasia, Rev. Ed. Victoria, BC: Neuropsychological Laboratory, Department of Psychology, University of Victoria, 1977.

Spreen O, Benton A, Fincham R. Auditory agnosia without aphasia. Archives of Neurology 13:84–92, 1965.

Spreen O, Risser A. Assessment of aphasia. In MT Sarno (ed), Acquired Aphasia. New York: Academic Press, 1981, pp 67–127.

Stark R, Genesee F, Lambert W, Seitz M. Multiple language experience and the development of cerebral asymmetry. In S Segalowitz, F Gruber (eds), Language Development and Neurological Theory. New York: Academic Press, 1977, pp 47–55.

Starkstein SE, Robinson RG. Aphasia and depression. Aphasiology 2:1–20, 1988.

Starkstein SE, Robinson RG. Depression in cerebrovascular disease. In SE Starkstein, RG Robinson (eds), Depression in Neurological Disease. Baltimore: Johns Hopkins University Press, 1993, pp 28–49.

Steele RD, Kleczewska MK, Carlson GS, Weinrich M. Computers in the rehabilitation of chronic, severe aphasia: C-VIC 2.0. Aphasiology 6:185–194, 1992.

Steele RD, Weinrich M, Wertz RT, Kleczewska MK, Carlson GS. Computer based visual communication in aphasia. Neuropsychologia 27:409–426, 1989.

Stein D. Development and plasticity in the central nervous system: Organismic and environmental influences. In A Ardila, F Ostrosky (eds), Brain Organization of Language and Cognitive Processes. New York: Plenum, 1989, pp 229–252.

Stengel E. Loss of spatial orientation, constructional apraxia, and Gerstmann's syndrome. Journal of Mental Science 90:753–760, 1944.

Stengel E. A clinical and psychological study of echo reactions. Journal of Mental Science 93:598–612, 1947.

Storandt M. Age, ability level and method of administering and scoring the WAIS. Journal of Gerontology 32:175–178, 1977.

Strang JD, Rourke BP. Arithmetic disability subtypes: The neurological significance of specific arithmetical impairments in children. In BP Rourke (ed), Neuropsychology of Learning Disabilities: Essentials of Subtype Analysis. New York: Guilford Press, 1985, pp 167–183.

Strub RL, Gardner H. The repetition deficit in conduction aphasia: Amnestic or linguistic? Brain and Language 1:241–256, 1974.

Strub RL, Geschwind N. Gerstmann syndrome without aphasia. Cortex 10:378–387, 1974.

Stuss DT, Benson DF. The Frontal Lobes. New York: Raven Press, 1986.

Subirana A. The prognosis of aphasia in relation to the factor of cerebral dominance and handedness. Brain 81:415–425, 1958.

Sugishita M, Otomo K, Kabe S, Yunoki K. A critical appraisal of neuropsychological correlates of Japanese ideogram (Kanji) and phonogram reading. Brain 115:1563–1586, 1992.

Sussman NM, Gur RC, Gur RF, O'Connor MJ. Mutism as a consequence of callosotomy. Journal of Neurosurgery 59:514–519, 1983.

Suzuki I, Shimizu H, Ishijima B, Tani K, Sugishita M, Adachi N. Aphasic seizure caused by focal epilepsy in the left fusiform gyrus. Neurology 42:2207–2210, 1992.

Sweet EW, Panis W, Levine DN. Crossed Wernicke's aphasia. Neurology 34:475–479, 1984.

Takayama Y, Sugishita M, Akiguchi I, Kimura J. Isolated acalculia due to left parietal lesion. Archives of Neurology 51:286–291, 1994.

Tanridag O, Kirshner H. Aphasia and agraphia in lesions of the posterior internal capsule and putamen. Neurology 35:1797–1801, 1985.

Taylor ML. A measurement of functional communication in aphasia. Archives of Physical Medicine and Rehabilitation 46:101–107, 1968.

Taylor MS. Preliminary findings in a study of age, linguistic evolution and quality of life in recovery from aphasia. Scandinavian Journal of Rehabilitation Medicine 26:43–59, 1992.

Taylor WL. "Cloze Procedure": A new tool for measuring readability. Journalism Quarterly 30:415–433, 1953.

Temple CM. Anomia for animals in a child. Brain 109:1225–1242, 1986.

TenHouten WD. Cerebral-lateralization theory and the sociology of knowledge. In DF Benson, E Zaidel (eds), The Dual Brain: Hemispheric Specialization in Humans. New York: Guilford Press, 1985, pp 341–358.

Terman LM, Merrill MA. Stanford-Binet Intelligence Scale. Manual for the Third Revision, Form L-M. Boston: Houghton-Mifflin, 1973.

Teuber HL. Alteration of perception and memory in man. In L Weiskrantz (ed), Analysis of Behavioral Change. New York: Harper and Row, 1968, pp 268–375.

Tilney F, Morrison JF. Pseudobulbar palsy, clinically and pathologically considered, with clinical report of 5 cases. Journal of Neurology, Neurosurgery, and Psychiatry 39:305–355, 1912.

Tissot R, Constantinidis J, Richard J. Pick's disease. In JAM Frederiks (ed), Handbook of Clinical Neurology, Vol 46: Neurobehavioral Disorders. Amsterdam: Elsevier, 1985, pp 233–246.

Tissot R, Lhermitte F, Ducarne B. Etat intellectuel des aphasiques. Essai d'une nouvelle approche à travers des épreuves perceptives et opératoires. L'Encéphale 52:285–320, 1963.

Tognola G, Vignolo L. Brain lesions associated with oral apraxia in stroke patients. Neuropsychologia 18:257–272, 1980.

Tonkonogy JM. Vascular Aphasia. Cambridge, MA: MIT Press, 1986.

Tonkonogy JM, Goodglass H. Language function, foot of the third frontal gyrus and Rolandic operculum. Archives of Neurology 38:486–490, 1981.

Trescher JH, Ford FR. Colloid cyst of the third ventricle. Archives of Neurology and Psychiatry 37:959–973, 1937.

Trimble MR, Reynolds EH. Neuropsychiatric toxicity of anticonvulsant drugs. In WB Matthews, GH Glaser (eds), Recent Advances in Clinical Neurology, Vol 4. London: Churchill Livingstone, 1984, pp 261–280.

Trousseau A. De l'aphasie, maladie décrite récemment sans le nom impropre d'aphémie. Gazette Hospital (Paris) 37:13, 25, 37, 49, 1864.

Trost J. Apraxic dysfluency in patients with Broca's aphasia. Paper presented at Annual Meeting, American Speech and Hearing Association, Chicago, IL, October, 1971.

Trost JE, Canter GL. Apraxia of speech in patients with Broca's aphasia. Brain and Language 1:63–79, 1974.

Troster AI, Salmon DP, McCullough D, Butters N. A comparison of the category fluency deficits associated with Alzheimer's disease and Huntington's disease. Brain and Language 37:500–512, 1989.

Tsvetkova L. Rehabilitation of Language in Focal Brain Lesions. Moscow: Moscow State University, 1973 (in Russian).

Tyrrell PJ, Warrington EK, Frackowiak RS, Rossor MN. Heterogeneity in progressive aphasia due to focal cortical atrophy: A clinical and PET study. Brain 113:1321–1336, 1990.

Vaid J. Bilingualism and brain lateralization. In SJ Segalowitz (ed), Language Functions and Brain Organization. New York: Academic Press, 1983, pp 315–338.

Vaid J. Language Processing in Bilinguals. Hillsdale, NJ: Lawrence Erlbaum Associates, 1986.

Valenstein ES. Great and Desperate Cures. New York: Basic Books, 1986.

Van Buren JM. The question of thalamic participation in speech mechanisms. Brain and Language 2:31–44, 1975.

Van Buren JM, Burke RC. Alterations in speech and the pulvinar. Brain 92:255–284, 1969.

Van Gorp WG, Mahler MM. Subcortical features of normal aging. In JL Cummings (ed): Subcortical Dementia. New York: Oxford University Press, 1990; 231–250.

Van Gorp WG, Satz P, Kiersch ME, Henry R. Normative data on the Boston Naming Test for a group of normal older adults. Journal of Clinical and Experimental Neuropsychology 8:702–705, 1986.

Vignolo L. Evolution of aphasia and language rehabilitation: A retrospective exploratory study. Cortex 1:344–367, 1964.

Vignolo LA. Auditory agnosia: A review and report of recent evidence. In AL Benton (ed), Contributions to Clinical Neuropsychology. Chicago: Aldine, 1969, pp 172–208.

Vinarskaya EN. Clinical Problems of Aphasia. Moscow: Meditsina, 1971 (in Russian).

Vogt C, Vogt O. Allgemeinere Ergebnisse unserer Hirnforschung. Journal of Psychology and Neurology 25:279–462, 1919.

Vygotsky LS (Trans E Hanfmann, G Vakar). Thought and Language. Cambridge, MA: MIT Press, 1934/1962.

Wagenaar E, Snow C, Prins R. Spontaneous speech of aphasic patients: A psycholinguistic analysis. Brain and Language 2:281–303, 1975.

Wahrborg P. Aphasia and family therapy. Aphasiology 3:479–482, 1989.

Wallach M, Kogan N. Aspects of judgement and decision making: Interrelationships and changes with age. Behavioral Science 6:23–36, 1961.

Wallesch C-W. Two syndromes of aphasia occurring with ischemic lesions involving the left basal ganglia. Brain and Language 25:357–361, 1985.

Wallesch C-W, Kornhuber HH, Brunner RJ, Kunz T, Hollerbach B, Suger G. Lesions of the basal ganglia, thalamus, and deep white matter: Differential effects on language functions. Brain and Language 20:286–304, 1983.

Wallesch C-W, Papagno C. Subcortical aphasia. In FC Rose, R Whurr, MA Wyke (eds). Aphasia. London: Whurr, 1985, pp 256–287.

Walsh K. Neuropsychology: A Clinical Approach. New York: Churchill Livingstone, 1978.

Warach S, Gur RC, Gur RE, Skolnick BE, Obrist WD, Reivich M. Decreases in frontal and parietal lobe regional cerebral blood flow related to habituation. Journal of Cerebral Blood Flow and Metabolism 12:546–555, 1992.

Warrington EK. Constructional apraxia. In PJ Vinken, GW Bruyn (eds), Handbook of Clinical Neurology, Vol. 4: Disorders of Speech, Perception and Symbolic Behavior. Amsterdam: North Holland, 1969; 67–83.

Warrington EK. Neuropsychological studies of verbal semantic systems. Philosophical transactions of the Royal Society of London B 295:411–423, 1981.

Warrington EK. The fractionation of arithmetical skills: A single case study. Quarterly Journal of Experimental Psychology 34A:31–51, 1982.

Warrington EK. Right neglect dyslexia: A single case study. Cognitive Neuropsychology 8:177–191, 1991.

Warrington EK, McCarthy R. Category specific access dysphasia. Brain 106:859–878, 1983.

Warrington EK, Shallice T. The selective impairment of auditory verbal short-term memory. Brain 92:885–896, 1969.

Warrington EK, Shallice T. Word-form dyslexia. Brain 103:99–112, 1980.

Warrington EK, Shallice T. Category specific semantic impairments. Brain 107:829–854, 1984.

Warrington EK, Zangwill OL. A study of dyslexia. Journal of Neurology, Neurosurgery, and Psychiatry 20:208–215, 1957.

Watson JB. Behaviorism. London: Kegan Paul, 1930.

Watson JDG, Frackowiak JV, Woods RP, Mazziotta JC, Shipp S, Zeki S. Area V5 of the human brain: Evidence from a combined study using positron emission tomography and magnetic resonance imaging. Cerebral Cortex 3:79–94, 1993.

Waxman SG, Geschwind N. Hypergraphia in temporal lobe epilepsy. Neurology 24:629–636, 1974.

Webb WG. Acquired dyslexias. In LL LaPointe (ed), Aphasia and Related Neurogenic Language Disorders. New York: Thieme, 1990, pp 130–146.

Wechsler AF. Presenile dementia presenting as aphasia. Journal of Neurology, Neurosurgery, and Psychiatry 40:303–305, 1977.

Wechsler AF, Verity MA, Rosenschein S, Fried I, Scheibel AB. Pick's disease: A clinical, computed tomographic, and histologic study with Golgi inpregnation observations. Archives of Neurology 39:287–290, 1982.

Wechsler D. Intelligence: Definitions, theory and the IQ. In R Cancro (ed), Intelligence: Genetic and Environmental Influences. New York: Grune and Stratton, 1971, pp 50–55.

Wechsler I. Textbook of Clinical Neurology, 7th Ed. Philadelphia: Saunders, 1952.

Weigl E. The phenomenon of temporary deblocking in aphasia. Zeitschrift für Phoniatrie und Kommunikation 14:337–364, 1961.

Weigl E. On the problem of cortical syndromes. In ML Simmel (ed), The Reach of Mind: Essays in Memory of Kurt Goldstein. New York: Springer, 1968, pp 143–160.

Weinstein EA, Friedland RP. Behavioral disorders associated with hemi-inattention. In EA Weinstein, RP Friedland (eds), Advances in Neurology, Vol 18: Hemi-inattention and Hemisphere Specialization. New York: Raven Press, 1977, pp 51–62.

Weinstein EA, Kahn RL. Non-aphasic misnaming (paraphasia) in organic brain disease. Archives of Neurology and Psychiatry 67:72–79, 1952.

Weinstein EA, Keller NJA. Linguistic patterns of misnaming in brain injury. Neuropsychologia 1:79–90, 1973.

Weintraub S, Robin NP, Mesulam M-M. Primary progressive aphasia. Longitudinal courses, neuropsychological profiles, and language features. Archives of Neurology 47:1329–1335, 1990.

Weisenburg TS, McBride KL. Aphasia. New York: Hafner, 1935/1964.

Wells CE. Dementia, 2d Ed. Philadelphia: Davis, 1977.

Weniger D, Sarno MT. The future of aphasia therapy: More than just new wine in old bottles? Aphasiology 4:301–306, 1990.

Wepman JM. Recovery from Aphasia. New York: Ronald, 1951.

Wepman JM. A conceptual model for the processes involved in recovery from aphasia. Journal of Speech and Hearing Disorders 18:4–13, 1953.

Wepman JM. Language Modalities Test for Aphasia. Chicago: Education Industry Service, 1961.

Wepman JM. Aphasia therapy: A new look. Journal of Speech and Hearing Disorders 37:203–214, 1973.

Wepman JM, Jones LV. Five aphasias: A commentary on aphasia as a regressive linguistic problem. In D McK Rioch, EA Weinstein (eds), Disorders of Communication (Proceedings of the Association for Research in Nervous and Mental Disease). Baltimore: Williams and Wilkins, 1964, pp 190–203.

Wernicke C. Das Aphasische Symptomenkomplex. Breslau, Germany: Cohn & Weigart, 1874.

Wernicke C. Lehrbuch der Gehirnkrankheiten. Berlin: Theodor Fischer, 1881.

Wernicke C. The symptom complex of aphasia. In ED Church (ed), Modern Clinical Medicine: Diseases of the Nervous System. New York: Appleton-Century-Crofts, 1908, pp 265–324.

Wertz RT. Review of word fluency measures (WF). In FL Darley (ed), Evaluation of Appraisal Techniques in Speech and Language Pathology. Reading, MA: Addison-Wesley, 1979, pp 121–149.

Wertz RT, Collins MJ, Weiss D, Kurtzke JF, Friden T, Brookshire RH, Pierce J, Holtzapple P, Hubbard DJ, Porch BE, West JA, Davis L, Matovich V, Morley GK, Resurreccion E. Veterans Administration Cooperative study of aphasia: A comparison of individual and group treatment. Journal of Speech and Hearing Disorders 24:580–594, 1981.

Wertz RT, LaPointe LL, Rosenbek JC. Apraxia of Speech in Adults: The Disorder and Its Management. New York: Grune and Stratton, 1984.

Wertz RT, Weiss DG, Aten JL, Brookshire RH, Garcia-Banuel L, Holland AL, Kurtzke JF, LaPointe LL, Milianti FJ, Brannegan R, Greenbaum H, Marshall RC, Vogel D, Carter J, Barnes NS, Goodman R. Comparison of clinic, home and deferred language treatment for aphasia. A Veterans Administration Cooperative study. Archives of Neurology 43:653–658, 1986.

Whitaker H. A case of the isolation of the language function. In H Whitaker, HA Whitaker (eds), Studies in Neurolinguistics, Vol 2. New York: Academic Press, 1976, pp 1–58.

Whitty CWM. Cortical dysarthria and dysprosody of speech. Journal of Neurology, Neurosurgery, and Psychiatry 27:507–510, 1964.

Whitworth RH, Larson CM. Differential diagnosis and staging of Alzheimer's disease with an aphasia battery. Neuropsychiatry, Neuropsychology, and Behavioral Neurology 4:255–266, 1988.

Whurr R. An Aphasia Screening Test. London: Whurr, 1974.

Wigan AL. The Duality of the Mind. London: Langman, 1844.

Wildmore LJ, Wilder BJ, Mayersdorf A, Ramsay RE, Sypert GW. Identification of speech lateralization by intracarotid injection of methohexital. Annals of Neurology 4:86–88, 1978.

Wilkins R. A comparison of elective mutism and emotional disorders in children. British Journal of Psychiatry 146:198–203, 1985.

Willmes K. Statistical methods for a single-case study approach to aphasia therapy research. Aphasiology 4:415–436, 1990.

Willmes K, Poeck K, Weniger D, Huber W. Der Aachener Aphasie Test. Differentielle Validitat. Nervenarzt 51:553–560, 1980.

Wilson SAK. Disorders of motility and muscle tone with special reference to the corpus striatum. Lancet 2:1–10, 1925.

Wilson SAK. Aphasia. London: Kegan Paul, 1926.

Wittrock MC. Education and recent neuropsychological and cognitive research. In DF Benson, E Zaidel (eds), The Dual Brain: Hemispheric Specialization in Humans. New York: Guilford Press, 1985, pp 329–339.

Wolpert I. Über das Wesen der literalen Alexie. Monatsschrift für Psychiatrie und Neurologie 75:207–266, 1930.

Wong L, Atwood A. Syndromes of autism and atypical development. In DJ Cohen, AM Donnellan, R Paul (eds), Handbook of Autism and Pervasive Developmental Disorders. New York: Wiley, 1987, pp 3–19.

Woods BT. Developmental dysphasia. In JAM Frederiks (ed), Handbook of Clinical Neurology, Vol 46: Neurobehavioral Disorders. Amsterdam: Elsevier, 1985a, pp 139–146.

Woods BT. Acquired aphasia in children. In JAM Frederiks (ed), Handbook of Clinical Neurology, Vol 46: Neurobehavioral Disorders. Amsterdam: Elsevier, 1985b, pp 147–158.

Woods BT, Teuber HL. Changing patterns of childhood aphasia. Annals of Neurology 3:273–280, 1978.

Woods RP, Mazziotta JC, Cherry SR. MRI-PET registration with automated algorithms. Journal of Computer Assisted Tomography 17:536–546, 1993.

Wyler AR, Ray RW, Aphasia for Morse code. Brain and Language 27:195–198, 1986.

Wylie J. The Disorders of Speech. Edinburgh: Oliver and Boyd, 1894.

Yamadori A. Ideogram reading in alexia. Brain 98:231–238, 1975.

Yamadori A. Right unilateral dyscopia of letters in alexia without agraphia. Neurology 30:991–994, 1980.

Yarbus AL. The Role of the Eye Movements in the Perception of Pictures. Moscow: Nauka, 1965.

Yarnell P, Monroe MA, Sobel L. Aphasia outcome in stroke: A clinical and neurological correlation. Stroke 7:516–522, 1976.

Yasuda Y, Akiguchi I, Ino M, Nabatabe H, Kameyama M. Paramedical thalamic and midbrain infarcts associated with palilalia. Journal of Neurology, Neurosurgery, and Psychiatry 63:797–799, 1990.

Young AW, Newcombe F, Ellis AW. Different impairments contribute to neglect dyslexia. Cognitive Neuropsychology 8:177–193, 1991.

Young RM. Mind, Brain and Adaptation in the Nineteenth Century. New York: Oxford University Press, 1970/1990.

Yu-Huan H, Ying-Guan Q, Gui-Qing Z. Crossed aphasia in Chinese: A clinical survey. Brain and Language 39:247–256, 1990.

Yudofsky SC, Hales RE (eds). The American Psychiatric Press Textbook of Neuropsychiatry, 2d Ed. Washington, DC: American Psychiatric Press, 1992.

Zaidel E. Lexical organization in the right hemisphere. In PA Buser, A Rougeul-Buser (eds), Cerebral Correlates of Conscious Experience. Amsterdam: Elsevier, 1978, pp 177–197.

Zaidel E. Language in the right hemisphere. In DF Benson, E Zaidel (eds), The Dual Brain: Hemispheric Specialization in Humans. New York: Guilford Press, 1985, pp 205–231.

Zangwill OL. Cerebral Dominance and Its Relation to Psychological Function. Springfield, IL: Charles C. Thomas, 1960.

Zangwill OL. Intellectual status in aphasia. In PJ Vinken, GW Bruyn (eds), Handbook of Clinical Neurology, Vol 4: Disorders of Speech, Perception, and Symbolic Behavior. Amsterdam: North-Holland, 1969, pp 105–111.

Zangwill OL. The concept of developmental dysphasia. In MA Wyke (ed), Developmental Dysphasia. New York: Academic Press, 1978, pp 1–11.

Zangwill OL. Two cases of crossed aphasia in dextrals. Neuropsychologia 17:167–172, 1979.

Zatorre RJ. On the representation of multiple languages in the brain: Old problems and new directions. Brain and Language 36:127–147, 1989.

Zurif EB, Caramazza A, Myerson R. Grammatical judgments of agrammatic aphasics. Neuropsychologia 10:405–417, 1972.

Index